Nordic health care systems

Recent reforms and current policy challenges

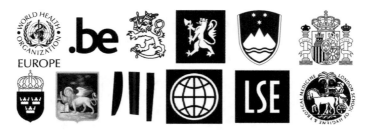

EUROPE

The European Observatory on Health Systems and Policies is a partnership between the World Health Organization Regional Office for Europe, the Governments of Belgium, Finland, Norway, Slovenia, Spain and Sweden, the Veneto Region, the European Investment Bank, the World Bank, the London School of Economics and Political Science, and the London School of Hygiene & Tropical Medicine.

Nordic health care systems

Recent reforms and current policy challenges

Edited by

Jon Magnussen
Karsten Vrangbæk
and
Richard B. Saltman

Open University Press

Open University Press
McGraw-Hill Education
McGraw-Hill House
Shoppenhangers Road
Maidenhead
Berkshire
England
SL6 2QL
email: enquiries@openup.co.uk
world wide web: www.openup.co.uk
and Two Penn Plaza, New York, NY 10121–2289, USA

First published 2009

A catalogue record of this book is available from the British Library
ISBN-13: 978-0-33-523813-2
ISBN-10: 0335238130

Library of Congress Cataloging-in-Publication Data
CIP data applied for

Typeset by RefineCatch Limited, Bungay, Suffolk
Printed in the UK by Bell and Bain Ltd, Glasgow

Fictitious names of companies, products, people, characters and/or data that may be used herein (in case studies or in examples) are not intended to represent any real individual, company, product or event.

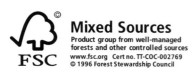

Mixed Sources
Product group from well-managed forests and other controlled sources
www.fsc.org Cert no. TT-COC-002769
© 1996 Forest Stewardship Council

FSC

The McGraw·Hill Companies

European Observatory on Health Systems and Policies Series

The European Observatory on Health Systems and Policies is a unique project that builds on the commitment of all its partners to improving health care systems:

- World Health Organization Regional Office for Europe
- Government of Belgium
- Government of Finland
- Government of Norway
- Government of Slovenia
- Government of Spain
- Government of Sweden
- Veneto Region
- European Investment Bank
- World Bank
- London School of Economics and Political Science
- London School of Hygiene & Tropical Medicine

The series

The volumes in this series focus on key issues for health policy-making in Europe. Each study explores the conceptual background, outcomes and lessons learned about the development of more equitable, more efficient and more effective health systems in Europe. With this focus, the series seeks to contribute to the evolution of a more evidence-based approach to policy formulation in the health sector.

These studies will be important to all those involved in formulating or evaluating national health care policies and, in particular, will be of use to health policy-makers and advisers, who are under increasing pressure to rationalize the structure and funding of their health system. Academics and students in the field of health policy will also find this series valuable in seeking to understand better the complex choices that confront the health systems of Europe.

The Observatory supports and promotes evidence-based health policy-making through comprehensive and rigorous analysis of the dynamics of health care systems in Europe.

Series Editors

Josep Figueras is Head of the Secretariat and Director of the European Observatory on Health Systems and Policies, and Head of the European Centre for Health Policy, World Health Organization Regional Office for Europe.

Martin McKee is Head of Research Policy of the European Observatory on Health Systems and Policies and Professor of European Public Health at the London School of Hygiene and Tropical Medicine as well as a co-director of the School's European Centre on Health of Societies in Transition.

Elias Mossialos is Co-Director of the European Observatory on Health Systems and Policies, and Brian Abel-Smith Reader in Health Policy, Department of Social Policy, London School of Economics and Political Science and co-director of LSE Health and Social Care.

Richard B. Saltman is Associate Head of Research Policy of the European Observatory on Health Systems and Policies, and Professor of Health Policy and Management at the Rollins School of Public Health, Emory University in Atlanta, Georgia.

European Observatory on Health Systems and Policies Series

Series Editors: Josep Figueras, Martin McKee, Elias Mossialos and Richard B. Saltman

Published titles

Primary care in the driver's seat
Richard B. Saltman, Ana Rico and Wienke Boerma (eds)

Human resources for health in Europe
Carl-Ardy Dubois, Martin McKee and Ellen Nolte (eds)

Health policy and European Union enlargement
Martin McKee, Laura MacLehose and Ellen Nolte (eds)

Regulating entrepreneurial behaviour in European health care systems
Richard B. Saltman, Reinhard Busse and Elias Mossialos (eds)

Social health insurance systems in western Europe
Richard B. Saltman, Reinhard Busse and Josep Figueras (eds)

Health care in central Asia
Martin McKee, Judith Healy and Jane Falkingham (eds)

Hospitals in a changing Europe
Martin McKee and Judith Healy (eds)

Funding health care: options for Europe
Elias Mossialos, Anna Dixon, Josep Figueras and Joe Kutzin (eds)

Regulating pharmaceuticals in Europe: striving for efficiency, equity and quality
Elias Mossialos, Monique Mrazek and Tom Walley (eds)

Purchasing to improve health systems performance
Joseph Figueras, Ray Robinson and Elke Jakubowski (eds)

Decentralization in health care
Richard B. Saltman, Vaida Bankauskaite and Karsten Vrangbæk (eds)

Health systems and the challenge of communicable diseases
Richard Coker, Rifat Atun and Martin McKee (eds)

Contents

Preface   ix
List of figures   xi
List of tables   xii
List of contributors   xiii
Acknowledgements   xv

Part I **Nordic health care systems: balancing stability
and change**   1

one   **Introduction: the Nordic model of health care**   3
           *Jon Magnussen, Karsten Vrangbæk, Richard B. Saltman and
           Pål E. Martinussen*

two   **Health care reform: the Nordic experience**   21
           Pål E. Martinussen and Jon Magnussen

three   **The political process of restructuring Nordic
           health systems**   53
           Karsten Vrangbæk

four   **Looking forward: future policy issues**   78
           Richard B. Saltman and Karsten Vrangbæk

Part II   Nordic health systems: key issues   105

five   **The changing political governance structures
               of Nordic health care systems**   107
               Terje P. Hagen and Karsten Vrangbæk

six   **Meeting rising public expectations: the
               changing roles of patients and citizens**   126
               Ulrika Winblad and Ånen Ringard

seven   **The changing autonomy of the Nordic medical
               professions**   151
               Peter K. Jespersen and Sirpa Wrede

eight   **Maintaining fiscal sustainability in the
               Nordic countries**   180
               Clas Rehnberg, Jon Magnussen and Kalevi Luoma

nine   **Harnessing diversity of provision**   198
               Unto Häkkinen and Pia M. Jonsson

ten   **Changing perceptions of equity and fairness**   214
               Johan Calltorp and Meri Larivaara

eleven   **Reforming primary health care**   233
               Allan Krasnik and Bård Paulsen

twelve   **Addressing the dual goals of improving
               health and reducing health inequalities**   255
               Signild Vallgårda and Juhani Lehto

thirteen   **Changing demands for institutional
               management**   274
               Lars Erik Kjekshus

fourteen   **The European Union: single market pressures**   294
               Dorte S. Martinsen and Paula Blomqvist

fifteen   **The Icelandic health care system**   316
               Tinna L. Ásgeirsdóttir

               Index   331

Preface

There has long been a standard assumption among European health policymakers that there was a 'Nordic Model' for health care systems. This model was understood to reflect a consistent set of parameters across all the Nordic countries: tax-based funding, publicly owned and operated hospitals, universal access based on residency, and comprehensive coverage. Moreover, this model was understood as a fixed, permanent component of the larger Nordic welfare state. This standard assumption was accepted as valid by most academics and policy-makers, both within and beyond the Nordic region.

The new study by a European Observatory on Health Systems and Policies team that is presented in this volume suggests that, while there certainly are important commonalities among the Nordic health systems, the reality is considerably more complex. In practice, while these systems share a number of core common aspirations, there is considerable variation at the structural level in the way that institutions are designed and at the policy level in the way strategies are conceived and implemented. As discussed in the chapters of Part I, it is this mix of consistency and divergence among the Nordic systems that characterizes the current health-policy environment, and that will undoubtedly colour the future direction that health systems development will take across the region.

This new comparative Nordic volume will be a welcome addition for health sector policy-makers and for students of health policy, not just in the Nordic countries but across Europe more generally. It draws on a comparative health services perspective that is well developed in the Nordic region. Starting in 1978, the Nordic Health Services Research Group has stimulated a wide variety of cross-Nordic studies, and a number of the chapter authors in the comparative chapters in Part II previously participated in the Group's research activities, as did the study's editors. This continuity reflects the emphasis that has been placed on comparative research in the Nordic region and its usefulness for making more evidence-based health policy.

May 2009, Copenhagen, Denmark

Finn-Kamper-Jørgensen
Former Chairman
Nordic Health Services Research Group

Director
National Institute of Public Health,
University of Southern Denmark
Denmark

List of figures

8.1 Share of central versus local financing of health care in
    2006.   185
8.2 Change in share of gross domestic product (GDP) spent on
    health 1985–2005.   188
8.3 Overall growth in purchasing power parity (PPP, in US$)
    adjusted spending per capita 1985–2005.   189
8.4 Per cent change in health care's share of public financing
    1985–2005.   190
13.1 An analytical model of the relationship between new
     governance structures, organizational structures and hospital
     performance.   278
13.2 Internal organizational developments in Norwegian somatic
     hospitals 1999–2007.   285
13.3 Merged hospitals organized in medical divisions with one
     medical director for each specialty.   288

List of tables

1.1 Country populations 2008   3
1.2 A framework for modelling Nordic health systems   8
3.1 Developments in health expenditures in the four countries   58
3.2 Key issues and problem areas behind Nordic government
     reform proposals   61
3.3 Country processes for launching and implementing
     structural reforms   66
6.1 Organization of the discussion of institutional factors   128
7.1 Three kinds of medical professional autonomy   156
8.1 Fiscal autonomy in the Nordic countries around 2004   184
8.2 Financing and provision of services   186
8.3 Health care expenditures as a share of gross domestic
     product, 1980–2005   187
8.4 Total expenditure on health per capita, 1985–2005   189
8.5 Public expenditures as a share of total health expenditures for the
     Nordic countries and mean values for European Union tax-based
     systems and social insurance systems, 1970–2004   190
11.1 Important features of the current organization of primary
     health care in Nordic countries   248
12.1 Comparisons of life expectancies: development in mean life
     expectancy in the Nordic countries 1970–2000   262
12.2 Comparisons of health inequalities: deaths in men aged 30–59
     years by socioeconomic group 1990–1994   263
13.1 Summarized responses regarding internal organizational
     development among Nordic physical care hospitals 2000–2008   282

List of contributors

Tinna L. Ásgeirsdóttir	University of Iceland
Paula Blomquist	University of Uppsala, Sweden
Johan Calltorp	Nordic School of Public Health, Sweden
Terje P. Hagen	University of Oslo, Norway
Unto Häkkinen	National Institute for Health and Welfare, Finland
Peter K. Jespersen	University of Aalborg, Denmark
Pia M. Jonsson	Karolinska Institutet, Sweden
Lars Erik Kjekshus	University of Oslo, Norway
Allan Krasnik	University of Copenhagen, Denmark
Meri Larivaara	National Institute for Health and Welfare, Finland
Juhani Lehto	University of Tampere, Finland
Kalevi Luoma	Government Institute for Economic Research, Finland
Jon Magnussen	Norwegian University of Science and Technology, Norway

Dorte S. Martinsen	University of Copenhagen, Denmark
Pål E. Martinussen	SINTEF Health Research, Norway
Bård Paulsen	Norwegian University of Science and Technology, Norway
Clas Rehnberg	Karolinska Institutet, Sweden
Ånen Ringard	Norwegian Knowledge Center for Health Services, Norway
Richard B. Saltman	Emory University, USA
Signild Vallgårda	University of Copenhagen, Denmark
Karsten Vrangbæk	University of Copenhagen, Denmark
Ulrika Winblad	University of Uppsala, Sweden
Sirpa Wrede	University of Helsinki, Finland

Acknowledgements

This study has benefited from generous contributions from a number of individuals and organizations. The editors are indebted to our chapter authors for their effort as well as patience. Pål Martinussen has been a research fellow on this study and has made substantial contributions to the chapters in Part I of the book as well as coordinated the efforts of the authors of chapters in Part II. We are also grateful to the external reviewers who provided comments on an earlier version of the manuscript: Terje P. Hagen, Anders Anell, Sven-Eric Bergman, Johan Calltorp, Terkel Christensen, Henrik Grossen Nielsen, Markku Pekurinen, Juha Teperi and Ilmo Keskimäki. The Norwegian Directorate of Health and the Health Organization Research programme at the University of Oslo both provided financial assistance, which made it possible to employ a research fellow on this project. The study also benefited from two workshops: the authors' workshop in Helsinki, hosted by Ilmo Keskimäki and STAKES, and the policy workshop in Stockholm, hosted by Henrik Lundstrøm and the Swedish Ministry of Health.

Finally this would still be a manuscript and not a book were it not for the efforts of Jonathan North and Jane Ward.

Part I

Nordic health care systems: balancing stability and change

chapter one

Introduction: the Nordic model of health care

Jon Magnussen, Karsten Vrangbæk, Richard B. Saltman and Pål E. Martinussen

1.1 The Nordic countries

The Nordic countries make up the Nordic region in northern Europe and consist of the five countries Finland, Sweden, Denmark, Norway and Iceland, along with their associated territories Greenland and the Faroe Islands (self-governing under Denmark) and Åland (self-governing under Finland). Total population was close to 25 million in 2008, of which the smallest country, Iceland, only made up 1 per cent (Table 1.1).[1] In English, the term Scandinavia is often used as a synonym for the Nordic countries, although within the Nordic countries the term Scandinavia is most often reserved for the three countries sharing the Scandinavian language: Norway, Sweden and Denmark.

The Nordic countries are commonly perceived as quite similar when viewed in a broader international perspective. This similarity relates to a historical background that for a long time had the countries united under one monarch in the

Table 1.1 Country populations 2008

Country	Population (× 1000)	Percentage of Nordic population
Finland	5 300	21
Sweden	9 183	37
Denmark	5 578	22
Norway	4 737	19
Iceland	313	1
Total	25 112	100

Kalmar union (1397–1523). Since then, the countries have been united in different constellations before they all gained their independence[2] in the twentieth century. A common history has led to the development of similar informal institutions; the Nordic countries share common customs, traditions and norms and have all adopted the Lutheran model of a state church. Language barriers are small between Norway, Sweden and Denmark (and those Finns who speak Swedish), and the countries have a similar climate. Finally (with the exception of Denmark), the Nordic countries have large areas that are sparsely populated.

1.2 Background: the Nordic welfare state model

The common history has been offered (Lundberg et al. 2008) as the main explanation for the countries' similar approach to social welfare, and in particular the dominant role of the state in the formation of welfare policies and a corresponding extensive public sector for the implementation of such policies. Many observers refer to a Scandinavian, or a Nordic, model of the welfare state (Esping-Andersen 1990). At the core of this welfare model lies the principle of universalism and broad public participation in various areas of economic and social life, which is intended to promote an equality of the highest standards rather than an equality of minimal needs. Although there are different specific attributes in each individual country, the list of characteristics commonly emphasized are a broad scope of social policies, universal social benefits, services free or subsidized at the point of delivery, a high proportion of gross national product spent on health and social services and emphasis on full employment, equal income distribution and gender equality.

Nordic health care systems are intrinsically related to the development of the welfare state, building on the same principles of universalism and equity. Central features have traditionally been an egalitarian ideology, promoting equal access to health services, low levels of cost sharing and high levels of tax-based financing to realize this ideology, public ownership of hospitals and decentralized responsibility for managing the services (Kristiansen and Pedersen 2000).

However, the health care systems in the Nordic countries have undergone a process of gradual change since the early 1990s. These reflect shifts in the economic environment as well as cultural and political developments. A common understanding has emerged about the need for prudent reforms, and as a result Nordic health care systems have also been subjected to a series of public reforms, commonly termed 'new public management' (NPM). The reform elements have been designed differently in the four countries, although with many similarities and with changing roles of patients and fiscal efficiency as key focus areas.

Universal social rights have been at the core of the Nordic welfare state model. When the state has the responsibility and individuals are given rights, however, the welfare state model runs the danger of turning individuals into passive recipients rather than active consumers or co-producers of services. This has been particularly evident within the health care sector because of the large informational asymmetries that exist between service providers and service recipients. With rapid developments in information technology, however, individuals are now better informed about both their own illnesses and the possibilities for treatment resulting from, for example, pharmaceutical and technological developments. Consequently, since the early 1990s patients have pushed to take on a more active role rather than merely being passive recipients of health care services. The Nordic countries have responded by expanding patient choice (see Chapter 6). Notably, this is still limited to choice of hospital for specialist health care – choice of physician within the hospital is not high on either the public or the political agenda. In contrast, choice of primary care physician is now an option in all countries, the recent 'vårdval' reform in Sweden being the latest example of a trend towards a health care model characterized by choice (and provider competition). However, the response goes beyond consumerism. Expansion of patient rights and facilitation of patient involvement have been at the centre of recent developments in the Nordic countries. Patients and patient-centred networks now play important roles in prevention, treatment, monitoring and developing services. Patient organizations, municipal social services and changing primary care physician practice all are part of this emphasis on integrated and patient-centred care.

The changing role of patients is one of several factors that affect the demand for health care services. Other factors are an ageing population and changes in the composition of population health. A growing share of old people not only implies that that demand for health care services increase, it also affects the types of service that are demanded. Similarly, lifestyle changes introduce new health care challenges, as is evident by obesity now being one of the main emerging challenges in the Nordic countries as elsewhere.

There have also been significant changes affecting operational efficiency on the supply side of health systems. Rapid pharmaceutical and technological developments have led to changes both in the possibilities for providing treatment and in the way patients are actually treated. While these developments have led to increased efficiency in the form of shorter length of stays and a rapid growth in the use of day care and day surgery, there has also been increased pressure on costs. Technological and pharmaceutical developments often imply both the use of more expensive equipment and/or medications and expanding 'the market for treatment' by offering treatment to patients that were previously excluded.

Moreover, these efficiency concerns along with technological advances have led to hospital restructuring. Increased specialization, a shift towards high-cost technological equipment and the necessity of having a sufficient patient volume in order to maintain quality for specialized services have resulted in decisions to reconfigure the hospital sector into fewer and larger administrative units. Yet Nordic countries still have substantial areas with a low population density. This creates a challenge to maintain geographical equity while at the same time exploiting both medical and economic scale efficiencies.

In the Nordic countries, as in much of the developed world, the overall fiscal sustainability of the system is under pressure. Within the framework of the welfare state, this has traditionally been handled by some combination of reducing benefits, increasing taxes and/or increasing efficiency. The content of the benefit package is of particular importance for health care, as pharmaceutical and technological developments have introduced clinical possibilities that are sought after but often increase overall costs. Within the Nordic model, this has led either to a slow implementation of new technologies or to certain types of rationing. Excluding certain services from the benefit package has been tried,[3] but with limited political success. Allowing people to purchase certain services outside of the public health care sector, creating a two-tier system, has generally not been regarded as a desirable policy for health care, although there are examples within dental care, physiotherapy and chiropractics. User charges have been implemented in some areas, but typically with extensive exemption schemes to secure equity in utilization. As a consequence, many of the health - care changes introduced since the early 1990s have led to an increased focus on the utilization of resources and on principles for prioritization. While still grounded in the core principles of the welfare state, Nordic health care systems are gradually putting more weight on economic incentives on the provider side, looking for more diversity in the provision of services, while at the same time seeking models of governance to handle the challenge of a more dynamic and market-oriented system.

1.3 A Nordic model of health care?

1.3.1 *The concept of a health care model*

The concept of the Nordic welfare state model is well defined and internation-ally recognized. While the health care sector is recognized as an integral part of the welfare state model in all Nordic countries, the concept of a 'Nordic model of health care' is less recognized and also less well defined. A health care system – or model – can be described by its structures and formal institutions.[4] How these structures and institutions arise and develop into their present form is the subject of a large, often conflicting, literature (Williamson 2000; Oliver and Mossialos 2005; Streeck and Thelen 2005). While some see institutions as rational solutions to the problems of coordinated action, other commentators contend that institutions have a more culturally embedded nature and that they persist more out of habit than as a rational solution to a specific problem. We follow a current definition of formal legal-political institutions as 'socially sanc-tioned', that is, collectively enforced expectations with respect to the behaviour of certain categories of actors or to the performance of certain activities. They typically involve mutually related rights and obligations for actors, distinguish-ing between "appropriate" and "inappropriate", "right" and "wrong", "pos-sible" and "impossible" actions and thereby organizing behaviour into predict-able and reliable patterns (Streeck and Thelen 2005, p. 9). Formal institutions in health care thus describe formalized rules that may be enforced by calling upon a third party. Examples include rules for referral, choice, payments, informa-tion, division of labour or use of technology. We assume that such institutional structures rest upon values and more or less explicit goals that are embedded in a society. As Williamson (2000) notes, at this 'social embeddedness level' one finds 'norms, customs, mores etc.', and at this level institutions change very slowly. This suggests that the pursuit of a Nordic model of health care should begin by examining values and goals that form the basis for structural and institutional arrangements. A second step concerns the specific structures and institutions that characterize health systems in the Nordic countries. Two central questions here are the degree to which these structures and institutions are changeable, and whether change can come gradually or needs to be the result of an exogenous shock. In either case, the structural and institutional setting (i.e. what we term *the health care model*) remains relatively stable over a reasonably long period of time.

At the same time, however, health care systems are also subject to more frequent changes in specific health policy measures and mechanisms. Moreover, within similar structural and institutional settings, there will be room for differences between countries in their design and implementation of health policy.

Therefore, a health care system can be understood and discussed on three different levels. Level 1 is where the goals and aspirations of a society are formulated. On this level, change is slow and rare. The institutional and structural design forms level 2. Again change does not occur often, but when it does it redefines the 'rules of the game' in a fundamental way. Finally, level 3 is the level of policy application within the structural dimensions. This is where systemic and institutional features are operationalized into specific delivery programmes and organizational designs. Pertinent questions at this level would include the degree of choice for patients, the mix of curative and preventative practices, the specific incentive structures and the assignment of responsibilities within particular programmes. At this level change tends to occur more frequently but these changes need not imply alterations in the more fundamental structural and institutional setting.

In Table 1.2, we specify a range of possible systemic features of health systems within the three levels. The list is extensive but not complete, only serving to illustrate a range of possible features at the three levels. The extent of differences between the Nordic countries is well described in the chapters in Part II of this book, but there are also many similarities as discussed in the following section.

Turning first to core values, two basic goals that characterize Nordic health systems are *equity* and *participation*. Equity is a term that can be subjected to different interpretations depending on whether one is most concerned about equal opportunities or equal results. Equal opportunities imply equal access or equity at the point of use. This is typically related to geography, social status, gender, ethnicity and so on, such that neither place of residence nor income will determine access to services. Interpreted as equal access for equal need, this implies a health care sector where the marginal benefit of health care services is equal for all individuals: that is, the health care sector will effectively maximize the total output of health. A different interpretation of the principle of equity, however, is in terms of equal result. Here the goal is not necessarily equal access for equal need, but equal health for all individuals. There is a fundamental difference between these two interpretations of equity that could potentially lead to differences in the structure of the health care system. Equity interpreted as equal access implies a system with universal access, e.g. a system with universal rather than targeted policies. Equity interpreted as equal result, by comparison, suggests policies that are targeted at groups with lower levels of health. Lundberg

Table 1.2 A framework for modelling Nordic health systems

Level	Possible systemic features
I: Goals and aspirations	
Equity	Geographical
	Social and economic
	Gender
	Between diagnostic groups
Public participation	Elected bodies
	Interest groups: formal and corporatist
	Advisory groups
	Informal interest groups
II: Structural issues	
Raising funds	Taxation (general or earmarked)
	Social health insurance
	Private health insurance
	Out-of-pocket payment
General governance structure	Centralized public
	Decentralized public
	Multilevel public
	Private
Political governance structure	Central
	Regional
	County
	Municipal
Delivery structure	Private for profit
	Private not for profit
	Public independently managed
	Public directly managed
III: Policy application (operationalization within the structural parameters)	
State versus market	Purchaser–provider split
	Privatization
Decentralization	To what level
	Content: types of decision
	Citizen participation
Patient choice	Content: hospital, primary care physician, specialist
	Degree of gatekeeping; by law or voluntary
Public health	Content: laws, regulations, campaigns
	Through institutional actions
	Through individual actions
Financing	Mix of incentives/subsidies/payments

et al. (2008) sum up the Nordic welfare state in three fundamental features: it is comprehensive, institutionalized and universal. This suggests that even if Nordic health care systems express a goal of equity in terms of results (i.e. as pursued by reducing social inequalities in health) this does not come at the expense of the principle of universalism.

The second goal highlighted in Table 1.2 is that of public participation. Such participation may take the form of voicing views, an example being the tradition for sending most policy documents out to a broad 'hearing' ('remiss') prior to adoption by either legislative or executive branch. Participation, however, also comes through formal and informal interest groups, through the use of ombudsmen and through regulatory and legal mechanisms (i.e. the right to see one's medical record). Even though governance and stewardship through elected bodies implies that decision-making in principle is based on public interest, direct participation is viewed as important in the Nordic world, and its existence reflects a key underlying value within these societies.

At the second, structural, level, four issues together describe the institutional setup of health systems: *funding, governance, political governance* and *delivery structure*. Funding decisions seek to control the magnitude of resources that a country wishes to devote to health care, but also how to distribute the financial burden between different groups within the population. There are four main forms of raising funds: through (general or earmarked) taxes, through social (public) insurance, through private insurance or through consumer payment (Saltman 1994; Evans 2001). Generally, European health systems tend to be described as tax or social insurance based: the traditional Beveridge/Bismarck distinction. In both cases, however, there also may be a mixture of funds generated from public(ly regulated) sources and private commercial insurance. Also, most systems have some type of cost-sharing mechanisms through which consumers pay a part of the total costs directly out of pocket.

Evans (2001) argues that, while there are substantial similarities between funding based on mandatory insurance and taxes, there are still two fundamental differences. First, a tax-based system will tend to be more progressive (e.g. high-income groups will tend to pay a relatively higher share than low-income groups). Second, a system where health care funds are taken out of the general tax revenue may be more prone to soft budgeting than a system based on fixed insurance premiums. Health care providers draw their resources from a common tax pool, which will seem more flexible than the upper limit given by insurance premiums. Therefore, the scope for political bargaining may be larger in tax-based than insurance-based systems. We note, however, that when taxes are earmarked, tax-based systems will also have a theoretical upper spending limit.

Table 1.2 lists 'governance' and 'political governance' as separate issues. This is a distinction between deconcentration – the transfer of responsibility to a lower administrative level – and devolution – the transfer of responsibility to a lower political level (Saltman et al. 2007). Also relevant is the extent of multi-level governance structures. While models may be devolved (i.e. in the form of elected local political bodies being responsible for financing and running of services), some decisions can still be centralized. This creates an environment where not only the administrative running but also the political governance of the health care sector needs to be coordinated across different levels; this is sometimes called 'multilevel democracy' in Nordic commentaries.

The final structural issue, delivery structure, has three dimensions: private versus public, for-profit versus non-profit in the case of private providers, and independently or directly managed in the case of public ownership.

The third level deals with policy application within the structural dimensions. The list of themes provided in Table 1.2 should be viewed as one of several possible lists; nevertheless, it captures essential elements of policy-making as it has been observed within both a Nordic and a European setting in the past few decades. Five themes are highlighted. The role of the state versus the market deals with issues as separate as purchaser–provider splits and the increased tendency towards privatization of the delivery of services. Second, decentralization, as will become clear throughout this volume, is a central characteristic of the Nordic health care systems, but a term that nevertheless can contain different practical solutions to important policy questions. Patient choice is a third issue, important both because the market for health care services is becoming increasingly globalized and because of the potential conflict between the state as the provider of welfare and health care and the individual as a recipient/ consumer of these services. Public health is included as a separate policy issue since the Nordic countries have traditionally placed strong focus on the role of governments in designing and implementing public health measures. Finally we include financing of services as an issue that play an increasingly important role in having health care providers face the right incentives. We shall discuss these five issues in more detail in Chapter 2.

1.3.2 Assessing common goals and institutions

A more detailed discussion of similarities and differences at these three systemic levels can help determine to what extent it is reasonable to talk about a distinct Nordic model of health care. Turning first to core health policy, the similarities of the four Nordic countries in history, culture, economy and social structure, as well as their close geographical proximity, suggest that it is not surprising that these countries also share a number of core *goals* and *aspirations*. Expressed in the political culture of the Nordic countries, these goals and aspirations have produced a set of fundamental health policy ideas. Health care systems, like other social sectors, have been built on the principle of universality: all inhabitants have the same access to public health services regardless of social status or geographic location. Thus the goal of equity has in the Nordic countries been closely related to equal access regardless of gender, age, place of residence and social status. The two last points have recently been in particular focus: geographical equity is an understandable concern given the number of low-density rural areas in these countries, while social equity reflects a long history of social democratic thinking.

This strong emphasis on equity has been combined with a tradition of decentralization to regional democratic control, by way of county institutions in Denmark, Norway and Sweden, and of the municipalities in Finland. Municipalities play an important role in all four countries, as they are responsible for providing all or part of primary health services as well as various prevention, rehabilitation and health promotion activities (plus specialized health services in Finland) for their inhabitants. Another distinguishing feature of Nordic health care systems, however, has been a tendency to oppose private expansion. The common understanding has been that health care should be under the ultimate control of democratically elected bodies, and not left to commercial market forces. This is partly because there is little tradition of voluntary or not-for-profit health care in the Nordic countries (after the Second World War), and 'private' is, therefore, usually equated with 'for profit' (Øvretveit 2003). Yet, this is also one of the areas where changes are currently taking place with a growth in voluntary health insurance and private delivery facilities.

A second core aspiration, public participation, has been and still is considered important in the Nordic countries. A key aspect of participation is the institutionalization of arenas for democratic decision-making at local, regional and national levels. This has been seen as an important way to ensure transparency and public participation in decision-making, and as a way to promote efficiency as decisions would fit the local and regional preferences and needs. Taken together, this is believed to improve the legitimacy of the public delivery systems. Another traditional argument has been that local and regional democratic government was an effective way to promote local innovation of organizational and management models. The decentralized structure would thus in essence serve as a series of local laboratories for developing solutions that might subsequently spread throughout the system (Baldersheim and Rose 2000; Vrangbaek 2007). With this focus on local governance, locally elected politicians have traditionally played an important role in the design, implementation and monitoring of health policy. This has been further accentuated by the role of organized local interest organizations such as the federation of county councils and/or the federation of municipalities in all four countries.

These two common goals – equity and public participation – have led the Nordic countries to develop health care systems that share several structural and institutional similarities. The Nordic countries belong to the family of public integrated single-payer health care systems. Similar to other Beveridge countries, Nordic health care systems are predominantly tax-funded health systems with only minor supplementary premium-based or out-of-pocket financing. In the Nordic case, private health insurance has often been marketed as a way to improve timeliness of access, rather than reduce the public costs of care. Denmark is the country with the largest share of supplementary insurance, in part a legacy from its recent history (up until 1972) of social insurance.

The governance structure of the Nordic countries has been (and is) decentralized, with the responsibility for service provision resting on a regional, county or municipal level – although often within a framework of centralized supervision, regulation or coordination. There are, however, considerable differences between the countries, both in terms of degree of decentralization and the interaction between the different levels. Norway has different degrees of decentralization for primary and secondary care: the first being the responsibility of the municipalities, the second of four regional health enterprises. Also, while tax funded, actual funding is a combination of locally raised (and regulated) taxes and matching central grants. This mixture of locally generated taxes and central funds can also be found in Finland, which is the most decentralized country, with responsibility for all service delivery held at the municipal level (hospital services are provided through hospital districts; however, each district is a federation of municipalities). Denmark, which in 2007 moved responsibility for its health services from counties to regions, has introduced separate national taxes to pay for health care, with health care budgets set annually in negotiation between the regions and the state. Finally, Sweden, with a mixture of regular (smaller) and merged (larger) counties, is the country with the least direct supervision of day-to-day service activity, also because counties finance roughly 75 per cent of health care expenses through their own local taxes.

What distinguishes the Nordic countries from other tax-based and/or decentralized systems, however, is its focus on political governance through locally elected political bodies. Thus the Nordic model has been one of devolution – transfer of power to a local political level – combined with the ability of these local units to raise taxes. Although tax financing is a common feature, there are substantial variations in how funds are actually raised and distributed. In Sweden[5] and Denmark there is a pattern of local discretion in setting tax rates, at least formally. In reality, the discretion has been reduced from the 1990s by tax stops and negotiated budget agreements between the state and the regions/municipalities. Norway, in contrast, has a system where tax rates and, therefore, available funds are a matter for the central government. Finland has a complex mixture of national funds (distributed through a social block grant) and municipally raised funds. To the extent that tax rates are centrally set or regulated, this effectively reduces the scope for both local decisions and financial accountability, and also implies that the costs of decisions made on a local level need not be internalized through higher local tax rates but can become a matter for negotiations between the different governmental levels. Therefore, in the context of rapid cost increases, centrally set tax rates combined with local decision-making may well put more pressure on overall public budgets than local tax discretion (Evans 2001).

Finland would seem to be the most decentralized of the Nordic countries. In reality, most municipalities are required by law to act together in hospital districts (called federations), thus to some extent 'recentralizing' to a regional level part of the actual responsibility for specialized health care. The Norwegian system also places the responsibility for primary care on municipalities, while secondary specialized care has been the responsibility of counties and, since 2002, regions. The Swedish system is based on counties. The Swedish system relies, however, to a larger degree on funds raised through local taxation: a key reason why it is run more independently from the central government. Norway also stands out with its peculiar distinction between primary care responsibility at the municipal level and hospital care at regional (previously county) level.

The specific form of multilevel public governance varies substantially between the countries, and these differences have increased after the recent Norwegian and Danish reforms. However, all four countries still share a tradition of centrally supervised local governance. This combination of elected political bodies and the possibility to raise local taxes is what has traditionally distinguished the Nordic countries from the more centralized tax-based National Health Service

(NHS) in the United Kingdom, a system that also belongs to the family of public integrated systems. The Norwegian hospital reform in 2002 implied both a recentralization of ownership and at the same time a change from devolution to elected county councils to 'deconcentration' to semi-autonomous regional health enterprises. This is in contrast to the Danish recentralization in 2007, where the new regions are still run by political elected regional governments. Even though appointed (not elected) politicians have since been reinstated on the boards of the Norwegian health enterprises, the 2002 reform marks a breach with one of the fundamental political governance structures that had characterized the Nordic health care model.

On the last issue in Table 1.2, delivery structure, the Nordic countries emerge as similar when it comes to specialized health care, with hospitals predominantly under public ownership. Private specialized health care exists, both in the form of private practitioners and some small private hospitals, but mainly as a supplement to the public hospitals. An increase in private suppliers is a political issue mainly in that it is a means of introducing contestability in the market for hospital services. The delivery structure for primary health care is, however, less similar within the four countries. In primary care, though, the question of private versus public does not seem to generate the same type of political debate as does the use of private providers in specialized health care.

Although differences exist between the Nordic countries with respect to the structural and institutional layout, the similarities are of a magnitude that still make it possible to talk about a distinct Nordic model of health care. Thus we can summarize *the Nordic model of health care* as characterized by:

- funding predominantly by taxes
- decentralized public governance structure (except Norway from 2002)
- elected local governments that can tax[6]
- public ownership (or control) of delivery structure
- equity driven, with focus on geographical and social equity
- public participation.

If we look beneath those broad similarities in goals, as well as basic commonalities in structures and institutions, however, we find that at the third level, policy design, there are more substantial differences. In essence, to the extent that it is possible to speak about a Nordic model for health care, it must be tempered with the recognition that the Nordic countries have in practice developed different combinations of service delivery policies and programmes.

1.3.3 A Nordic health policy?

Part II of this book provides in-depth descriptions and assessments on how the Nordic countries approach a variety of health care policy issues. In this introductory chapter, we briefly point to some key differences in the structural features as well as some elements of differences in design, attitude and timing of health policy initiatives. Of the five policy applications listed in Table 1.2, we focus on three: state versus market, decentralization and financial incentives.

State versus market

Within a predominantly public delivery and governance structure, the dominant question of state versus market is really not a question of private versus public ownership. Rather 'market' has mainly come to be synonymous with a variety of financial management mechanisms and tools that operate within the public sector and fall within the new public management framework (Saltman and von Otter 1992). On the supply side, these include regulated competition, the use of incentive-based contracts, the introduction of private providers to create contestability in a publicly dominated sector and independent management models. On the demand side, the introduction of choice and a strengthening of patient rights lead patients to behave more like consumers in 'ordinary' markets. As is discussed in more detail in Chapter 2, there are substantial differences between the Nordic countries in their approach to these issues. Sweden was the sole Nordic country to follow the Thatcher-inspired United Kingdom reforms and initiate a purchaser–provider split for hospital services in the early 1990s. It has, however, mostly returned to a less arms-length relationship between purchasers and providers, based more on cooperation than competition. Norway and Denmark have included patient choice as part of legally based patient rights, while Finland and Sweden have chosen not to. The overall picture that is painted both in the review of reform in Chapter 2, and in the chapters that form Part II of this book, is that NPM type policy changes have taken different forms, been introduced with different intensity and at different times, and also had different effects in the Nordic countries.

Decentralization

Decentralization has come to be a major policy strategy in many health care systems. The idea of decentralization as expressed by Saltman and co-workers (2007) is simply 'that smaller organizations, [if] properly structured and steered are inherently more agile and accountable than are larger'. As discussed above, the Nordic countries can all be characterized as decentralized with a strong role played by elected local governments. Within this broad heading of decentralization, there are, however, major differences between the countries. As noted earlier, Finland places formal responsibility for all services at the municipal level. Each municipality, however, is required to be a member of a hospital district, which then is given the responsibility for hospital services. Thus the degree of decentralization is different for primary care and hospital care. This is also the situation in Norway, which relies on the municipal level for primary care and on regional health enterprises for specialized care. In contrast, both Sweden and Denmark place the responsibility for all health care at the same level; Sweden on the county level and Denmark (since 2007) on the regions. Given the similarities in geography and population size, these differences in choice of governance level cannot be seen as insignificant. Rather, the differences reflect variations in the attitude towards decentralization and to what extent local authorities are viewed as best suited to provide public services for their population. In this context, it is noteworthy that the Norwegian hospital reform implies not only a centralization of powers from counties to regional health enterprises but also the removal of locally elected politicians from the regional boards.[7] Denmark, in contrast, when reforming in 2007 chose to retain local political control through regional boards with elected politicians. In Sweden, the health care sector is governed primarily by locally elected county councils, while elected municipal councils officially perform the same task in Finland.

Financial incentives

In all four Nordic countries, the public sector fills the role of both purchaser and provider. Traditionally, providers have been financed by global budgets, with little or no specification of expected volume or quality. The need to introduce incentives for providers to manage scarce resources as efficiently as possible has gradually emerged as a policy issue since the early 1990s. The generally successful efforts at maintaining macrolevel expenditure control had masked the importance of introducing more effective microlevel management mechanisms. This masking had faded by the 1990s, with the rapid growth in expensive medical technologies as well as concerns about the future costs associated with increased numbers of elderly.

There are, however, substantial differences between the countries in how such incentives have been introduced. Norway, in particular, has been eager to follow the rhetoric behind the introduction of the prospective payment system (PPS) in the United States in 1983. The introduction of an activity-based financing based on the diagnosis-related group (DRG) system in 1997 was built on the notion that activity-based financing would increase activity as well as efficiency. By that time, however, Sweden, which was the pioneer in introducing internal markets, had gradually reversed course back toward a more cooperatively based model. Denmark quite deliberately did not jump on the DRG bandwagon for incentive-based management and for many years held to the belief that global budgets were sufficient, although limited intraregional use of economic incentives has taken place as part of the negotiated soft contracts between counties and hospital managers in the 1990s, and national use of DRG rates for free-choice patients has been in place since 2000 (Street et al. 2007). In recent years and in particular after the 2007 reform, Denmark has, however, introduced DRG-based financing to a larger extent. Lastly, Finland uses DRGs but mainly as a system of distributing incurred hospital costs between the responsible municipalities.

1.3.4 Approaches to and timing of reform

The above points serve as examples of health policy differences between the Nordic countries. What is evident from the discussion of reforms in Chapter 2, and from the chapters in Part II of this book, however, is that at this third level of policy action, the Nordic countries not only differ on specific policy issues but they also take different approaches to reform and the timing of reform.

In Norway, major policy changes and recent reforms have been implemented through central initiatives and cover the whole country. In some cases, if there is doubt as to whether changes will work as expected, there may be 'local trials'. Such pilot projects were implemented before introducing activity-based financing in 1997 and before introducing the family doctor model for primary care in 2001. A similar general approach is taken in Denmark. Both the financial reform in 1999 (or rather, marginal change) and the structural reform in 2007 were centrally initiated and nationwide, yet many other policy initiatives have been taken at the regional levels or in collaboration between state and regions (Vrangbæk and Christiansen 2005). In contrast to this, both Sweden and Finland rely more on local initiatives and experiments. Both the internal market reform in Sweden starting in 1988 and subsequent follow-up initiatives, were characterized by different counties choosing different paths and to some extent different solutions. Alternatively, when nationally generated reforms are introduced, such as the 1985 Dagmar reform that channelled national social insurance payments for primary care directly to county councils, or the 1992 ADEL reform that transferred responsibility, facilities and funding for elderly residential care from county to municipal level, these reforms were designed to allow considerable discretion to local governments in how they were implemented. Yet, there are signs that the central level is taking a stronger steering role also in Sweden. An example is the strengthening of the National Board of Health in regards to planning of highly specialized services. Another example is the development of national monitoring systems for quality of service delivery. Finland is also characterized by an approach to reform and change that encourages local solutions and local initiatives. This approach reflects both the deep-seated historical role of municipalities prior to Finnish independence in 1917 and the shift in 1992 from national planning to a block-grant system in the health and social sector. While the national government in Finland also has begun to seek a greater steering role, to date the initiatives have been rather low profile, concentrating on instituting staffing and visit standards for certain municipally run services.

What this pattern indicates is that that the governance structures within the four countries have somewhat different configurations. Central state initiatives play an increasing role in Norway and Denmark, leaving local governments to enforce and manage centrally initiated policy reforms. This is not as dominant in Sweden and particularly in Finland, which by comparison, tend to be characterized by considerably more power at the decentralized levels when it comes to design and implementation of policy action.

As a final difference, we raise the issue of differences in timing and detailed design of health policy reforms and health policy initiatives between the Nordic countries. While there are many examples of cross-Nordic policy inspiration, it is also the case that on some significant policy areas there have been remarkable differences. A few examples follow. When Sweden introduced the internal market for hospital services in the early 1990s, no other Nordic country followed. When Norway introduced a prospective activity-based financing system in 1997, no other country followed. Ten years after, Denmark is now introducing stronger activity-based financing components in terms of the share of income that is directly related to activity, while at the same time the debate in Norway is whether one should revert to a system more based on global budgets. Norway centralized hospital ownership in 2002. Sweden and Finland have only voluntary plans to consolidate regional responsibilities in the health sector. Denmark, however, recentralized fiscal responsibility from regional to national level in 2007, as well as consolidating hospital ownership to larger regions.

The Nordic countries are not alone in grappling with multiple issues around how to maximize outputs from scarce health care resources. In this context, the differences in timing and policy solutions may be seen as an indication of a globalization of health care policy. The Swedish internal market experiments were influenced by the Thatcher reforms of the NHS in the United Kingdom, and the introduction of the Norwegian PPS meant adapting not only the principles of United States Medicare financing, but also the United States version of the diagnosis-related group system. As this process of cross-pollination suggests, the Nordic countries do look outside their own borders for solutions to challenges that are not specifically Nordic. Yet, it is also noteworthy that the international trends tend to be translated and adapted within national negotiation processes involving both state and regions as well as professional and patient interests. These consensus-oriented processes mean that international impulses are adapted to fit the national institutional structures. This can explain the lack of similarity in the timing of policy changes in spite of the many structural similarities and the subjection to similar reform ideas. It also means that the Nordic model should perhaps also be understood as a process model rather than an assembly of exactly similar structural and policy dimensions at any given point in time. We use the term 'public-negotiated health model' to capture these process-related dimensions of the Nordic health systems. Indeed, the Nordic countries may at the same time appear to be losing some of their specifically Nordic identity on some structural parameters while retaining a specific Nordic tradition for policy development in consensual and multidimensional democratic processes, albeit with some change in the balance of power between the different levels (as illustrated in Chapter 3 and in the chapters in Part II).

1.4 Why this book

The purpose of this book is *not* to compare the relative statistical performance of the Nordic countries, nor to compare the performance of the Nordic countries with that of other European countries. Other organizations such as the OECD in Paris and WHO Regional Office for Europe in Copenhagen already have sophisticated quantitative data series, and the reader who is primarily looking for numbers and advanced statistical analysis should look to those sources. In this volume, we base our analyses on various descriptive statistics as well as expert assessments and published primary and secondary material from the four countries.[8] What this book seeks to do is to provide a differentiated picture of Nordic health care systems for use in policy-making discussions both within the Nordic region as well as elsewhere in Europe and beyond.

While it is still possible to speak of a Nordic health care model in the very general terms used above, the term loses much of its usefulness when comparing the more detailed health sector policy designs of each country in the wake of the reforms since the early 1990s. In this sense, this study reinforces a recurring theme in Nordic health care research over recent years. Are we seeing the end of the Nordic tradition based on publicly administered hospitals and decentralized health care provision (e.g. Alban and Kristiansen 1995; Kristiansen and Pedersen 2000; Kuhnle 2000)? While all four countries are still broadly characterized by systems that are universally accessed, tax financed, publicly driven, decentralized and equity oriented, the many major recent changes have put the countries on different paths in terms of more specific aspects such as hospital funding, financing schemes and the role of the state. Moreover, the countries also differ when it comes to the timing and approach to reform, at least in recent years: the centrally initiated 'big-bang' hospital reforms of Norway and Denmark, which were implemented almost overnight, stand in contrast to the incremental and more voluntary changes in Sweden and Finland (Chapter 3). Given that recent reform processes create greater variability in the concept of a Nordic model, the question becomes that formulated by Lundberg (2006): how much national variation and internal flexibility the concept can capture without losing its contour. Indeed, some authors argue that there already exists a tendency for developed country health reforms to replicate themselves across countries and systems (Freeman 1998; Blank and Burau 2006), which would suggest that reformed Nordic health care systems are in the process of losing the unique characteristics that would justify referring to a Nordic model.

In addition, the performance of the Nordic model has become the subject of increasing debate. While the social welfare state approach is highly valued in the Nordic countries, observers outside the region sometimes find the Nordic approach to be too state orientated in character, with a strong governmental role that deprives the citizenry of important individual freedoms. Yet, traditional ideas of how to deliver welfare services in the Nordic countries have been challenged in the past three decades and pragmatic inclusions of market elements and private delivery forms have taken place. This gradual shift acknowledges that state monopoly of welfare provision may not be optimal, that maximum state-organized welfare is not necessarily an expression of the most progressive welfare policy, that voluntary organizations offer other qualities in welfare provision, that market competition can sometimes stimulate both better and more efficient health service delivery and that the tradition of government-run welfare can undermine individual initiative and threaten economic prosperity (Kuhnle 2000). However, given that the development of the Nordic model is so closely linked to the labour movement and social democracy, a key challenge becomes how to understand the distinguishing features of the Nordic model if they no longer can be explained by referring to the dominant position of the social democratic parties (Lundberg 2006).

Increasing internationalization also poses dilemmas for the Nordic model. With the European Union (EU) and the European Economic Area (EEA), the market for health is no longer limited to the territory of the nation state. This may well reduce the scope for public monopoly of health provision in the Nordic region (Kuhnle 2000). As noted in Chapter 14, the extension of the European market could lead to a rapid expansion of transnational insurance and the offering to firms, professional groups and individuals of a range of new 'packages' of private health schemes. Such developments towards more privatization of health care funding and services could result in organizational fragmentation, social segmentation and increased complexity in health systems, on the one hand, which may not be easily corrected even if a political majority should wish to change course. On the other hand, this would also allow patients and consumers more choice in a bigger policy space.

The remainder of Part I will consider these and other important analytical issues. Chapter 2 presents a thorough review of recent policy changes and reforms in the four countries. Chapter 3 discusses the political dimensions of the Nordic health reform process. Chapter 4 then draws on that political discussion to consider key factors and possible new paths as Nordic systems continue to evolve over the medium-term future.

Part II consists of 10 commissioned chapters dealing with broad themes. The changing role of the major participants; *politicians, patients and professions* are discussed in Chapters 5–7. In Chapters 8–10, themes related to *financing, production* and *distribution* are discussed. The final four chapters (11–14) each touch upon issues of particular relevance to the present policy debate. In Chapter 11, the role of *the primary care sector* and in particular the role of *integrated care* is discussed. Chapter 12 focuses on the (different) role of *public health* in the four countries, Chapter 13 on *internal management* while Chapter 14 deals with the challenges that are already present in an increasingly integrated EU market. Chapter 15 then discusses the situation in Iceland.

Notes

1. For most of this book, the descriptions and discussions will only cover Finland, Sweden, Denmark and Norway. A separate chapter (15) describes and discusses Iceland. For practical reasons, we choose not to dwell on the three autonomous regions.
2. Norway from Sweden in 1905, Finland from Russia in 1917 and Iceland from Denmark in 1944.
3. In vitro fertilization in Norway being one example.
4. While also acknowledging that informal institutions will be important for the day-to-day working of a system.
5. Except during the run-up to Sweden's entry into the EU of 1995, when the national government placed a 'tax-stop' on county and municipal rates in order to keep public expenditures within EU fiscal criteria.
6. In Denmark, municipalities can tax and regions cannot; since 2001, a regulation has prohibited any tax increase ('skattestop').
7. This represents a departure from the basic Nordic model as we have described it above. Although local politicians were subsequently allowed back on the regional boards, they were appointed, not elected.
8. Good sources are the Nordic Medico-Statistics Committee; http://nomesco-eng.nom-nos.dk/ as well as OECD health data.

References

Alban, A. and Christiansen, T. (eds) (1995) *The Nordic Lights: New Initiatives in Health Care Systems*. Odense: Odense University Press.

Baldersheim, H. and Rose, L.E. (2000) *Det kommunale laboratorium. Teoretiske perspektiver på lokal politikk og organisering.* [*The Municipal Laboratory. Theoretical Perspectives on Local Politics and Organization.*] Oslo: Fakbokforlaget.

Blank, R.H. and Burau, V. (2006) Comparing health policy: an assessment of typologies of health systems, *Journal of Comparative Analysis: Research and Practice* 8: 63–76.

Esping-Andersen, G. (1990) *The Three Worlds of Welfare Capitalism.* Cambridge: Polity Press.

Evans R.G. (2001) Financing health care: taxation and the alternatives, in Mossialos, E., Dixon, A., Figueras, J. and Kutzin, J. (eds) *Funding Health Care: Options for Europe.* Buckingham: Open University Press.

Freeman, R. (1998) Competition in context: the politics of health care reform in Europe, *International Journal for Quality in Health Care* 10: 395–401.

Kristiansen, I.S. and Pedersen, K.M. (2000) Helsevesenet i de nordiske land: er likheten større enn ulikheten? *Journal of the Norwegian Medical Association* 120: 2023–9.

Kunhle, S. (2000) The Nordic welfare state in a European context: dealing with new economic and ideological challenges in the 1990s, *European Review* 8: 379–98.

Lundberg, U. (2006) The *Nordic Model: Past Glory or the Way of the Future?* Stockholm: Institute for Future Studies.

Lundberg, O., Yngwe, M.Å., Stjärne, M.K., Björk, L. and Fritzell, J. (2008) *Health Equity Studies*, No 12. *The Nordic Experience: Welfare State and Public Health (NEWS).* Stockholm: Centre for Health Equity Studies (CHESS), Stockholm University/ Karolinska Institute.

Oliver, A. and Mossialos, E. (2005) European health systems reforms: looking backward to see forward, *Journal of Health Politics, Policy and Law*, 30: 7–28.

Øvretveit, J. (2003) Nordic privatization and private healthcare, *International Journal of Health Planning and Management* 18: 233–46.

Saltman, R.B. (1994) A conceptual overview of recent health care reforms, *European Journal of Public Health* 4: 287–93.

Saltman, R.B. and von Otter, C. (1992) *Planned Markets and Public Competition: Strategic Reform in Northern European Health Systems.* Buckingham: Open University Press.

Saltman, R.B., Bankauskaite, V. and Vrangbæk, K. (2007) *Decentralization in Health Care.* Maidenhead: McGraw-Hill.

Streeck, W. and Thelen, K. (eds) (2005) *Beyond Continuity: Institutonal Change in Advanced Political Economies.* Oxford: Oxford University Press.

Street, A., Vitikainen, K. Bjorvatn, A. and Hvenegaard, A. (2007) *CHE Research Paper 30. Introducing Activity-based Financing: A Review of Experience in Australia, Denmark, Norway and Sweden.* York: Centre for Health Economics.

Vrangbæk, K. (2007) Towards a typology for decentralization in health care, in Saltman, R.B., Bankauskaite, V. and Vrangbæk, K. (eds) *Decentralization in Health Care.* Maidenhead: McGraw-Hill, pp. 44–62.

Vrengbæk, K. and Christensen, T. (2005) Health policy in Denmark: leaving the decentralized welfare path? *Journal of Health Politics, Policy and Law* 30: 29–52.

Williamson, O. (2000) The new institutional economics. taking stock, looking ahead, *Journal of Economic Literature*, XXXVIII: 595–613.

chapter two

Health care reform: the Nordic experience

Pål E. Martinussen and Jon Magnussen

2.1 Introduction

Since the end of the 1980s, Norway, Denmark, Sweden and Finland have all implemented major changes in their health systems. This development has been paralleled by the market-oriented reform wave known as 'new public management' (NPM), which emphasizes the need to rethink how the public sector organizes and manages itself. In the Nordic countries particularly, the challenges related to cost increases and insufficient ability of hospitals to absorb patient inflows have led to the introduction of quasi-market mechanisms, such as waiting list guarantees, patient rights to free choice of hospitals and activity-based funding (ABF) schemes. These elements have been supplemented with other NPM-inspired reforms, as well as increased focus on patient pathways, integrated care, prevention and health promotion in coordination between different public authorities.

The main purpose of this chapter is twofold: first, to offer a systematic presentation of the major changes of the Nordic health care systems in the period from around 1990 until the present, and, second, to provide a discussion of the similarities and differences between the four countries. The chapter is organized as follows. The next section discusses the challenges of studying health care reform and outlines a framework within which to compare the health reforms of the Nordic countries. In order to describe the Nordic health systems, it is separated between *structure and institutions* (financing, government/steering, delivery structure) on the one hand and *goals and aspirations* (equity, democratic participation) on the other. Five different health reform themes are then explored within this general framework. Section 2.3 deals with the role of state and market, with the emphasis on purchaser–provider models and private health care services. Section 2.4 explores the de- and recentralization of stewardship and delivery organizations. The third reform theme, patient rights and empowerment, is addressed in Section 2.5, while Section 2.6 pursues the role of public health. A final central health reform theme is explored in Section 2.7, financing and payment. Section 2.8 contains the concluding remarks.

2.2 Health systems change: reform or gradual change

When embarking on a discussion of Nordic health care reforms, it is necessary first to decide upon a relevant framework within which to structure the study. First of all, there is the question of how to define reform. Saltman and Figueras (1997, p. 3) define reform as 'a process that involves sustained and profound institutional and structural change, led by government and seeking to attain a series of explicit policy objectives'. Hence, the key elements of health care reform are said to involve two dimensions: process and content. The key elements in the process dimension are that there is structural rather than incremental or evolutionary change, change in policy objectives followed by institutional change rather than redefinition of objectives alone, purposive rather than haphazard change, sustained and long-term change rather than one-off change, and a political top-down process led by national regional or local governments. The other dimension, the content dimension, is said to be characterized by diversity in the measures adopted and determination by country-specific characteristics of health systems. Second, in addition to the difficulties of defining health reform in general, there is also the challenge of identifying the actual change areas to study. Figueras (2003) warns against the simplicity of treating health care reform as an all encompassing and homogeneous social phenomenon without taking into accounts the large differences between countries. Arguing that the term 'health care reform' is increasingly unhelpful because it is interpreted in so many different ways, he suggests that the term 'reform' should be abandoned altogether in favour of more specific approaches that better reflect the nature of health care changes.

The question guiding this chapter is how the recent health care reforms have affected the key dimensions of Nordic health policy. We shall deliberately use the term reform more loosely than suggested by Saltman and Figueras (1997), thus discussing also changes that affect both the structural and institutional issues described in Chapter 1 as well as some of the changes that are more naturally labelled policy changes. In doing so, we believe the discussion will be more in line with public perception of what has constituted health care reforms in the Nordic countries since the early 1990s. Drawing on the publications of Saltman and Figueras (1998) and Hsiao (2003), we focus on five themes: the role of state and market, decentralization, patient rights, the role of public health, and financing and payment. These five themes can generally be said to capture the common challenges for health policy-makers, thus influencing the organization and behaviour of nearly all western European health care systems.

The greatest pressure for change has been in the *relative role of the private sector* in the operation and, in some countries, the funding of health care services. While the debate has a tendency to evolve around 'state versus market', market-style mechanisms may include solutions such as consumer sovereignty (patient choice), negotiated contracts and open bidding introduced on the funding, allocation or production subsectors of the system.

The second broad theme in European health care reform is that of *decentralization* (see also Saltman et al. 2007). This may involve both the decentralization of administrative (deconcentration) and policy (devolution) authority to lower levels in public and private sector. Decentralization is seen as a response to poor efficiency, slow innovation and lack of responsiveness to patients' demands, which may be some of the drawbacks of large, centralized public institutions.

Third, the *empowerment of patients* has emerged as a central theme in most European countries since the end of the 1990s. This trend reflects a demand for increased patient rights regarding both logistical and clinical matters: that is, in choosing physician and hospital as well as in participating more actively in elective medical decisions.

The fourth theme concerns the attempts to strengthen the *role of public health* in European health policy. Recognizing that many important determinants of health lie outside the health sector, there has been an increased focus on the role of intersectoral initiatives in health reforms.

Fifth, methods for *financing and payment* of service providers have been the subject of considerable interest in the past decades. The introduction of more accurate information systems (e.g. through diagnosis-related grouping (DRG)) together with the NPM-inspired ideas of separating purchaser and providers have resulted in an increased awareness that the use of economic contracts may be a vital policy instrument.

2.3 The roles of state and market

Since the early 1990s, there has been a gradual softening of the once-clear distinction between private and public in Nordic health care. In the following, we shall focus on two types of change areas that are of particular relevance in the Nordic context: purchaser–provider models and private health care.

2.3.1 Purchaser–provider models

Sweden

In the early 1990s, the purchaser–provider model became a popular management model for the Swedish hospitals. The experiments included resource allocation according to the needs of the residents, per-case payment schemes, total cost liability for departments and interdependent transfer pricing systems. The main idea was to redefine the role of politicians and professionals: the politicians would take on the role as purchasers of health services for their population while those responsible of delivering the health services would be reimbursed for their services after accomplishing their assigned tasks. Thus, the intention was that politicians would focus on the interests of the citizens rather than on the interests of the health service producers. These new arrangements were assumed to create competition between hospitals in terms of accessibility and quality of services, as well as to increase efficiency. By 1994, more than half of the 26 Swedish county councils at the time had introduced some form of purchaser–provider model. The type of purchasing organizations varied between – as well as within – county councils: from one large central county council purchasing organization to purchasing organizations at district or even local level (Harrison and Calltorp 2000)

At first, the competitive reforms were supported by a broad coalition of actors. Initially, the reforms also appeared quite successful, since waiting lists for elective surgery declined dramatically and hospital productivity and efficiency seemed to improve, without the quality of health services appearing to be affected adversely by the reforms (Hanning 1996; Bergman 1997).

However, research has later indicated that the purchaser–provider model was quite difficult to realize in practice (Siverbo 2004). It has furthermore been argued that the incentives for providers were limited by the weak split between purchasers and providers (Culyer et al. 1995; Anell 2005). According to Anell (2005), the contracts between purchasers and providers can best be described as 'letters of intent', meaning that the escape route back to traditional planning and management was always open for the county councils or for the providers when it became too difficult to perform as agreed. Adding to this is the fact that the same organization, the county councils, employed the personnel of both the purchasers and providers, and that the losses and gains across purchasers and providers in principle were the responsibility of the county councils. In practice, therefore, according to Harrison and Calltorp (2000), the new purchasing arrangements exposed the hospitals to intense pressure for productivity and cost reduction without generating much direct competition between hospitals. Both county council purchasers and patients generally retained strong loyalties to the hospitals that had traditionally provided services to each catchment area. With growing concerns that the market-based mechanisms would damage social equity and impact negatively on quality, the reforms, therefore, gradually aroused the opposition of a wide range of policy actors.

After the period of strong enthusiasm for market-inspired management models, these kinds of model were gradually viewed with scepticism within the health care sector (Brorström and Rombach 1996). Harrison and Calltorp (2000) argue that while the need for efficiency gains and cost control was still acknowledged, there was an increasing focus on problems that did not seem amenable to market solutions and could even be aggravated by too much stress on competitive incentives. The terms of discourse about health care finance and policy shifted from market terminology towards emphasis on reciprocity and integration among players. Cooperation both between and within county councils increased in order to improve the distribution of workload between hospitals, as well as to extend the administration of some hospitals over several nearby hospitals to increase efficiency. Today, purchasing organizations negotiate with health care providers to establish financial and activity contracts, which are often based on fixed prospective per-case payments (based on DRG), and complemented with price or volume ceilings and quality components (Glenngård et al. 2005).

Norway

In Norway, a purchaser–provider separation was first introduced for nursing and care services in the early 1990s. The models were variations of the purchaser–provider organization tried out in Sweden, and their implementation must be seen in relation to the introduction of competition and market-based solutions in the public sector in general. In addition, the purchaser–provider model was also perceived as particularly suitable for helping to clarify the responsibilities of local governments as both administrators and service providers (Norwegian Association of Local and Regional Authorities 2004). By 2004, almost 30 per cent of the 431 municipalities had implemented some form of purchaser–provider model within the nurse and care services. The main argument was a strengthening of the legal protection of the service clients, and to ensure equality in terms of service provision. The experiences with the model were mainly positive, with increased legal protection and better casework as a result (RO 2004). Furthermore, studies of the effects of the model suggest increased productivity and less-expensive services (NOU 2005). The municipalities have tended to use so-called 'soft contracts', which allow for much flexibility between the municipality and the provider (Johnsen 2006). Public health policy documents have emphasized two important premises for municipal purchaser responsibilities for health services: first, that it requires larger units than today's municipalities and, second, that it requires professional competencies which are difficult to develop in many units (NOU 2003).

Another distinct aspect of the market-based changes in Norway is the reorganization of hospitals into health enterprises, which took place within the 2002 hospital reform. The reform contained two main elements; the central takeover of hospital responsibility and the organization of hospitals as enterprises (Ministry of Health and Social Affairs 2000–2001). With the hospital reform, a purchaser–provider model was also, in theory, introduced for the specialized health services. Regional health enterprises can purchase health services from a variety of providers including local health enterprises and private providers. Since a complete division of roles between the regional health authority and its health enterprises would necessitate extensive use of auctions and competition tools, both the purchaser role and elements of the provider role rests with the former. Yet, in 2005, central government took measures to differentiate better between the regional health authorities and their health enterprises, by barring individuals from serving simultaneously on the boards of a regional health authority and a subordinate health enterprise, and by requiring the regional health authorities to establish in their organization a clear distinction between the role as owner of the health enterprise and their responsibility to care for health services (Johnsen 2006). Still, the regional health enterprises do not practice a purchaser–provider split but run their hospitals choosing a model of vertical integration.

Finland

With its decentralized hospital system, Finland should, at least in theory, be well suited to the introduction of purchaser–provider models. The natural split between the municipalities as purchasers and the 20 hospital districts as providers have, at least theoretically, a potential of allowing for realistic market competition. Certainly, the relationship between hospital districts and their owner municipalities has some elements of purchaser–provider splits in it, but in the end it is the municipalities that cover possible deficits or return possible savings to their accounts (Vuorenkoski et al. 2008). In the early 1990s, the municipalities were allowed more freedom in terms of purchasing services from public, non-profit and for-profit providers, and to contract out existing public services. This followed from a dismantling of various legal and administrative procedures that governed the municipalities' and health care providers' administration, personnel and user charges (Häkkinen and Lehto 2005). In the wake of these new relationships, there were continuous change and developments in terms of contractual or negotiation mechanisms, with a general move towards contracts on volumes and costs between municipalities or groups of municipalities and their hospital districts (Vuorenkoski et al. 2008). Yet, the attempts to create purchaser–provider splits with local purchasing authorities have created extremely small purchasing authorities that seem incapable of developing competitive health care markets. Therefore, it could be argued that the dominance of strong providers may even grow as a result of quasi-market reforms in Finland (Häkkinen and Lehto 2005). Even if the subject is under continuous debate, there is no classical purchaser–provider split in Finnish health care, as the municipalities still both fund and own the service provision organizations. The country's proponents of purchaser–provider separation, which includes private health care providers and the right-wing parties, build on the well-known arguments for such models: that true purchaser–provider splits will enhance management and make the municipal administration more transparent, and that it will better allow for the outsourcing of services to private actors who promise more efficient service provision (Vuorenkoski et al. 2008).

Denmark

No major efforts have been made to introduce purchaser–provider models in Denmark. Yet, as a response to the attempts in the United Kingdom to create internal markets, the use of explicit contracts between the county councils as purchasers and the county-owned hospitals as providers was introduced in the 1990s and is now in wide use. The contracts usually stipulate production and quality targets, research and teaching goals and areas which are to be developed, and provide funds to obtain these goals, but are neither legally binding nor developed in a competitive environment (Pedersen 2002, 2005). In its 2003 report on the organization of the Danish health care sector, the Ministry of the Interior and Health concluded that the experience from distinctive purchaser–provider models in other countries suggests restraint about introducing similar models in Denmark. It is pointed out that the difficulties of creating competition together with management-related aspects serve to restrict the purchaser's possibilities of acting as genuine purchasers within most treatment areas (Ministry of the Interior and Health 2003).

2.3.2 Private health care

Privatization strategies may take a variety of different forms; from the sale of public sector assets to private for-profit or non-profit providers, via the contracting-out of services to private providers, to more active market liberalization or deregulation to promote private health care through various incentive mechanisms. In the Nordic countries, the question of private health care is mainly a case of private versus public production within a system of public control and financing, as well as the question of supplementary private insurance.

Sweden

The universal access to health care in the Nordic countries implies that private health insurance will only have a supplementary function. Private health insurance was introduced in Sweden during the mid-1980s when insurance companies started selling it to key employees in the largest private companies as well as to private persons, offering the customers admission to some of the very few private providers of health care at this time (Norén 2007). The number of people purchasing supplementary private insurance is rapidly increasing, from 2.3 per cent of the population in 2004 (Swedish Insurance Federation 2004) to approximately 4.6 per cent in 2008 (Trygg-Hansa 2008). The voluntary health insurance mainly gives quick access to a specialist and allows for jumping the waiting queue for elective surgery (Glenngård et al. 2005). The Swedish Government policy regarding private health insurance has traditionally been restrictive, and in contrast to many other European countries there are no tax deductions tied to it.

While for-profit hospitals now exist in all four Nordic countries, they are generally of modest size and mainly specialize in particular niches of elective surgery. However, as for the purchaser–provider model, an exception is again to be found in Sweden. When the St Göran Hospital was sold to a private corporation in 2000, having been a public corporation up to then, with the county of Stockholm holding all shares, it became by far the largest privately owned and operated hospital in the Nordic region. The sale created much debate and led the social democratic government to introduce a law temporarily preventing the counties from selling (or managing) public acute hospitals to private for-profit actors (Pedersen 2005). The present conservative government has, however, reversed this law.

During the 1990s, Sweden also underwent important changes in its fundamentals for primary health care providers. The Family Doctor Act and the Act on Freedom to Establish Private Practice in 1994 enabled GPs to become independent entrepreneurs instead of public employees. Even though these two laws were withdrawn before they were fully implemented when a social democratic government replaced the non-socialist coalition the same year, several counties had already made reforms in their delivery of primary health care. Through the Family Doctor Act, all residents in a county were allowed to choose their own GP, even among private GPs who did not have contracts with the county councils. The Act on Freedom to Establish Private Practice revoked the county councils' regulation of the number and reimbursement of private practitioners.

Moreover, changes in the payment system also gave the family doctors financial incentives to attract patients. This has resulted in an increased privatization of primary care in many counties (Glenngård et al. 2005). In 2008, a public committee (SOU 2008) recommended that free choice of provider become mandatory in all counties. This should be coupled with a free right to establish practice and a payment system where the money follows the patients. No discrimination will be made between private and public practices.

Norway

Private health insurance plays a more marginal role in Norway than in Sweden. The estimated share of the population with such arrangements in 2003 amounted to only 0.6 per cent (NOMESCO 2006), but by 2008 the estimated share had increased to 1.8–2.3 per cent (Seim et al. 2007; Grasdal 2008). One explanation may be the introduction of a tax subsidy on this type of insurance in 2003. As in Sweden, this arrangement allows the clients to jump waiting lists by obtaining treatment from private providers paid by the insurance. Also, a number of private health care centres are being established in urban areas whose services are limited to members only (Johnsen 2006).

The first private commercial hospital in Norway was established in 1985. Yet, it was not until after the hospital reform of 2002 that this type of hospital ownership gained momentum. The parliamentary proposition for the reform (Ministry of Health and Social Affairs 2000–2001) outlined the use of private providers as a possible solution for solving the inherent capacity problems of the health care sector, causing the number of private hospitals to increase dramatically, from 6 in 2001 to 28 in 2004. From 1999 to 2004, the share of elective surgery performed at private commercial hospitals increased from 1 to 11 per cent. It is, however, only on the dimension related to production that the private hospitals are fully private. The state exercises control through its sanction authority over the number of beds and the technical and professional standards in the private hospitals (Midttun 2007).

Another important branch of the private health care sector is the private contract specialists. They have traditionally been an important link in the chain of tasks attended to by the specialized care sector. Following a law in 1998 stating that private specialists were to enter specific contracts with a county (then the owners of the hospitals) to be qualified for reimbursement from the National Insurance Scheme, there was a sharp increase in the number of private specialists with contracts. From 2005, however, there has been a decrease in the private activity, which mainly reflects political signals: when the new left-centre coalition took over government after the 2005 elections, it clearly stated in its letters of instruction to the regional health authorities that the use of private providers should be limited.

In 2001, Norway also liberalized its pharmacy system. Whereas pharmacies previously had to be owned and operated by a licensed pharmacist, the new regime opened the way for non-pharmacist investors. The main challenges with the old system were perceived to be inadequacy of the retail network, lack of competition and the associated high retail margins. The Pharmacy Act of 2001 allowed greater freedom in the establishment of pharmacies and in their ownership, and in 2003 Norway also followed Denmark in allowing the sale of selected non-prescription over-the-counter drugs in retail outlets. As a result of the liberalization of the pharmacy market, the number of pharmacies increased by 30 per cent from 2001 to 2003, while the many independent pharmacies previously in operation were replaced by three major integrated chains, controlling almost 90 per cent of the market (Johnsen 2006).

Encompassing changes also took place within the primary health care sector, where the introduction of a list patient system meant that the GPs were essentially privatized during the beginning of the 2000s. Inspired by the Danish organization of GPs, the new system was based on a registration system for choosing a GP. Aspects such as remuneration, size and composition of patient lists are regulated through national standards. The new model can be said to be in line with the NPM philosophy, since it implies a partial privatization of enterprises that previously were publicly owned and run. Today, approximately 90 per cent of the GPs have chosen to become self-employed contractors instead of public employees, and 98 per cent of the population have a regular GP (Johnsen 2006).

Finland

Private health insurance plays a modest role in Finland. The statistics on private voluntary health insurance is scarce, but the general impression is that this is mainly purchased as cover for child health care, and most usually in the urban areas where there is access to many private physicians (Vuorenkoski et al. 2008). In addition, there is also statutory Motor Accident Insurance and Occupational Accident Insurance, which are provided by private insurance companies. They also constitute a quite small proportion of the funding of services.

Unlike Sweden and Norway, Finland has had no changes in the employment status of GPs, and most are, therefore, still public, working in health centres or in occupational health. Yet, since the end of the 1990s, a new trend has emerged where private firms lease physicians to public primary health care (Vuorenkoski et al. 2007). These firms are most commonly owned by the physicians themselves, and since they offer better salaries and more flexible working conditions than municipalities, they are an attractive alternative for physicians. The municipalities basically use the services of these firms when they have difficulties of recruiting physicians, especially for out-of-hours duties. In 2004, approximately 5 per cent were employed by such firms (Vuorenkoski et al. 2008). The idea of a list system was also introduced in Finland during the early 1990s, and today approximately 50 per cent of the population is assigned to a personal doctor. Overall, approximately 8 per cent of the physicians have full-time private employment, while approximately one-third of those employed publicly have part-time private practice (Pedersen 2005).

Denmark

In Denmark, a large portion of health care has historically been financed through private health insurance, but these schemes were taken over by the county councils in 1973. The market for private health insurance is dominated by the non-profit mutual health insurance association 'Denmark', which grew out of the sickness fund that was abolished (Strandberg-Larsen et al. 2007). In 2004, Health Insurance Denmark covered approximately 29 per cent of the population and had a 99 per cent share of the private insurance market (Health Insurance Denmark 2007). Complementary health insurance provides full or partial coverage for services that are excluded or only partially covered by the statutory health care system, such as pharmaceuticals, dental care, physiotherapy and corrective lens co-payments. A major feature of this in Denmark is that it allows those insured to access a specialist without a GP referral. The purpose of supplementary schemes is to increase consumer choice and access to different health services, and traditionally it implies superior accommodation and amenities in hospital and allowing clients to jump waiting lists for elective surgery (Strandberg-Larsen et al. 2007). Private health insurance is becoming increasingly popular, because of increasing competition for employees and high levels of personal income tax (Mossialos and Thompson 2004). By making insurance premiums tax free for the insurance holder, the present right-wing government has signalled political support for a move towards more supplementary coverage (Pedersen 2005). It is estimated that nearly 15 per cent of the Danish population has supplementary private health insurance (outside of 'Denmark') in 2008 (Næss-Schmidt 2008).

The first private for-profit hospital in Denmark was established in 1989, and this was later followed by several other small private hospitals, mainly providing elective surgery. Even in Denmark, where private health insurance is far more widespread than in the other Nordic countries, this base is not big enough to provide a sustainable financial support for the existing private hospitals and clinics. While the common pattern has been that the counties contract with the private providers after a tendering process, this was replaced by a more automatic mechanism when a new national law that expanded free choice came into place in 2002. With this law, patients have the right to treatment at a private hospital or abroad after waiting two months for elective surgery at a public hospital. As in the other Nordic countries, the public–private relationship is regulated through national legislation: in 1993 the social democratic government took measures to prevent public hospitals from taking insurance or privately paid patients, and the counties were also prohibited from entering into commercial joint activities with private hospitals (Pedersen 2005).

The Danish pharmacy monopoly was changed in 2001, allowing a small, but gradually increasing, number of over-the-counter drugs to be sold by, for example, supermarkets (Pedersen 2005). No fundamental changes in the GP system similar to those in Sweden or Norway have taken place in Denmark. In principle, the GPs run private practices, but aspects such as income, the number of patients registered with each GP and the number of practising GPs per region are regulated through negotiations between the Organization of General Practitioners and the Danish regions (Strandberg-Larsen et al. 2007).

2.4 De-/recentralization of stewardship and delivery organizations

Since the late 1990s, decentralization has emerged as the preferred management strategy of many European health care systems (Saltman et al. 2007). The term decentralization refers to a wide variety of power-transfer arrangements and accountability systems, but generally it builds on the idea that smaller organizations are more responsive and accountable than larger organizations (Saltman et al. 2007).

All four Nordic countries have a history of decentralized management and political responsibility of health service delivery to either the county or municipality level. This phase of decentralization is now, in some countries, being replaced by a phase of recentralization.

Sweden

During the 1970s and 1980s, Sweden – like the other Nordic countries – had largely completed the aspect of decentralization that relates to delegating responsibility for and management of service delivery to lower-level governments. This development had already started in the nineteenth century, when the counties were made responsible for operating publicly financed hospitals (Saltman and Bankauskaite 2006). The second approach to administrative decentralization is associated with NPM strategies such as intra-public sector competition, purchaser–provider separation and performance measurement, and, as discussed in Section 2.3, Sweden was a forerunner in the Nordic region in that area too.

There are, however, several indications that the previous national policies of decentralization in Sweden are being reversed. This is perhaps most evident in the report from the Committee on Public Sector Responsibilities, which was delivered in 2007 (SOU 2007). The committee was commissioned to analyse whether changes were required in the division of responsibilities and structural arrangements in order to meet future public sector challenges. The main problem identified by the Committee was structural deficiencies arising from a confusing and fragmented regional level, with many actors and tasks that differ between sectors; this made coordination difficult. In order to create a new regional system with clearer roles and clearer division of responsibilities, it was, therefore, proposed that the 21 county councils[1] of today would be replaced by six to nine directly elected regional authorities with overall responsibility for regional development and health and medical care. While it was acknowledged that a decentralized health care system may stimulate both innovation and efficiency through different solutions and the spread of risks and development costs, the importance of units of a large enough size to meet the future challenges was emphasized. These changes are set to take place after the elections in 2014 at the latest.

As in the other Nordic countries, a large part of the funding of the Swedish health care system is through taxes. The degree of fiscal decentralization is quite high, with the bulk of the total health sector revenue for the county councils stemming from county-level taxes. The municipalities also generate a high share of their revenues through local taxes, with expenditure on care for the elderly and disabled constituting around a third of their total expenditure (Federation of Swedish County Councils 2004; Glenngård et al. 2005). Central government has implemented restrictions on local taxations rights, most recently in the period 1997–2000 when sanctions cut the state grants for county councils and municipalities that increased taxation (National Board of Health and Welfare 2002).

Norway

Norway makes for a particularly good example of the oscillation between political/administrative centralization and decentralization. With the Hospital Act of 1969, the responsibility for planning, building and managing the hospitals was formally given to the 19 counties. However, as described by Magnussen and co-workers (2007), the period up to the hospital reform in 2002 was characterized by this decentralized model being challenged and modified both in terms of regionalization and financial reforms. The small population of several counties combined with large geographical distances provided opportunities for economies of scale through centralization, and the country was, therefore, divided into five health regions in 1974. Recognizing that counties would not cooperate voluntarily, regional cooperation was deemed mandatory in 1999. When, in addition, the introduction of ABF in 1997 meant that more funds came directly from the state, and soft budgeting seemed to be the prevailing model, there was, in essence, little left of the original decentralized model upon entering the 2000s. The hospital reform of 2002 can, therefore, be said to represent the final and formal stage of an ongoing recentralization of the hospital sector.

The reform transferred the responsibility for all somatic and psychiatric hospitals and other parts of specialist care from the 19 counties to the state, with all specialized health care organized in five regional health enterprises under the Minister of Health. The main argument for state ownership, as stated in the Hospital Act (Ministry of Health and Social Affairs 2000–2001), was to provide the state with a position of total responsibility for the specialist health services by uniting sector responsibility, financial responsibility and ownership at the same administrative level.

The new organizational form implies that the hospitals are turned into separate legal entities. Hence, even though ownership is still public, the hospitals are no longer an integral part of the central government administration. Central regulations are primarily to take place through the enterprise meetings, which corresponds to the general meeting in ordinary companies. The introduction of enterprise organization signifies a distinct break with earlier administrative traditions, since it represents a new management philosophy: the enterprise structure implies an organizational division between the activity and the superior political body. In short, the argument for choosing enterprises instead of the common directorate model was to keep politicians at arm's length. The Hospital Act underlines that leadership should be allowed the control and responsibility of all input factors, the authority to choose an organizational structure that advances the purpose of the activity, and to have complete responsibility for the management, without interference from other administrative levels. The hospital reform can, therefore, be viewed just as much as a responsibility and leadership reform as an ownership reform. The central keywords are precisely the same as those associated with the NPM doctrine: distinct objectives, output demands and – not the least – professional and genuine leadership.

An interesting point to be made is the inherent duality in the reform. On the one hand, the reform implies a recentralization of the hospital sector: ownership was transferred back to the central state; the Minister of Health holds the overall responsibility, and the organizational unit for coordination and steering is the five regional health enterprises. On the other hand, the reorganization of health regions and hospitals into health enterprises represents decentralization. This signifies a change from devolution (to a lower political level) to deconcentration (to an independent lower administrative level) (Magnussen et al. 2007). At the time of the reform, there were 82 hospitals and clinics, but after a series of mergers this number reduced to approximately 25. Also, in 2007, the two largest regional health enterprises, East and South, were merged into one region covering 55 per cent of the Norwegian population.

In contrast to the other Nordic countries, there is little tradition for fiscal decentralization in the Norwegian system. A central characteristic of the former county model was vertical fiscal imbalance: demand decisions were decentralized while financing remained centralized. Counties were not able to fund their health services through taxes: the main financial sources were a fixed tax base, ABF of hospital services and a block grant from central government (Magnussen et al. 2007). This did not change with the hospital reform, as the state still maintains control over hospital financing.

Finland

A similar case of fluctuation between decentralization and centralization in health care can be found in Finland. In 1993, a reform decentralized all hospital financing to the municipalities, and it could be argued that the Finnish health care system thereby became more decentralized than any other country (Häkkinen 2005). The municipalities are small; more than 75 per cent have less than 10,000 inhabitants, and 20 per cent have less than 2000. As there is little detailed central regulation of the municipal health service provision, the municipalities enjoy relatively more autonomy in terms of deciding income tax rates, health care investments and organization of services (Vuorenkoski et al. 2008). Recently, however, there has been growing concern regarding the problems associated with the high degree of decentralization, such as continued waiting lists for elective procedures, diseconomies of scale, lack of expertise, geographical inequalities in access to services, increasing problems with sudden changes in expenditure, workforce shortages, poor regional and national cooperation and the potential impact of recent decisions on patient choice by the European Court of Justice (Mossialos and McKee 2002; Vohlonen et al. 2004; Vuorenkoski et al. 2008).

As a consequence of these developments, Finland has started the process of rebalancing national and local decision-making roles. Central government has begun deliberations about whether greater equity and efficiency could be achieved by more direct state control over the hospital sector (Saltman and Bankauskaite 2006). In discussing this development, Vuorenkoski et al. (2008) emphasize three reforms that are indicative of the reversion process of the decentralized tradition of health care decision-making. First, in 2005, the Ministry of Social Affairs and Health enacted a nationwide maximum waiting time and guidelines for access to treatment in elective specialized care. Second, in 2006, national supervision was reinforced by expanding the functions of the National Authority for Medico-Legal Affairs (NAMLA)[2] from supervising individual professionals to supervision of health care organizations, health centres, hospitals and other health service providers. Third, a project to restructure municipalities and services started in 2005 that aimed to decrease the number of municipalities and increase cooperation between municipalities. A Parliamentary Act that followed in 2007 states that primary health care and social services associated with health services is to be provided by organizations covering at least 20,000 inhabitants. In addition to these three reforms, Vuorenkoski and co-workers (2008) also point to the national four-year plan for social welfare and health care, which has been modified in order to increase its impact.

With regard to fiscal decentralization, national government played a relatively large role until the state subsidy reform of 1993, with health sector revenues split 50–50 between national and municipal sources (Saltman and Bankauskaite 2006). The most significant change in the financing of health care has been the shift from state to municipalities, with the municipalities in 2005 financing approximately 40 per cent and the state 21 per cent of total health care costs, while the rest was covered by the National Health Insurance (17 per cent) and private sources (22 per cent). The municipal income tax is the major source of tax revenue for the municipalities, constituting 87 per cent in 2005 (Vuorenkoski et al. 2008).

Denmark

With the administrative reform in 1970, local democratic governance was institutionalized as a dominant principle in Danish welfare policies, combined with an important change from specific and direct state subsidies to general block grants and county-level taxation. Since then, changes of both organizational and managerial kinds have been mainly within this general framework, with governance, ownership, financing and delivery of health services remaining predominantly public, and the decentralized nature of the system maintained (Vrangbæk 2005). The 25-year long period of incremental changes has led one commentator to argue that if the Danish health care system is unique, it is because of its lack of reforms (Green-Pedersen 2003). With the recent major structural reform, however, which erodes the counties' role as health care providers, Denmark has also chosen a strategy of recentralization. As Vrangbæk (2005) argues, the reform came as the result of gradual tensions that had been building up: in terms of governance between the use of hierarchical planning instruments and elements of market mechanisms; in terms of central versus decentralized management between the principle of county autonomy and increasing central regulations; and in terms of public versus private between pressures for new types of partnership and the need for new regulatory structures to handle such developments.

This structural reform was based on the findings of a public commission (Sundhedsvæsents organizering 2003) set up by the Danish Parliament in 2005 and was implemented in 2007. It reduced the number of regional authorities from 14 counties to 5 regions and the number of municipalities from 275 to 98. Both the regional and local levels are governed by directly elected politicians. The main responsibility of the regions is to provide health services, while the municipalities are responsible for prevention, health promotion and rehabilitation outside of hospitals. In order to ensure coordination between the two administrative levels, health coordination committees are established in which municipalities and regions are to enter into binding partnerships (Strandberg-Larsen et al. 2007). The reform is generally viewed as a response to uneven access to health services across the country, reflected in differences in waiting time, availability of medical technologies and rates of specific diagnostic and curative activities. The structure with the three political/administrative levels is said to have led to suboptimal decision-making and management, and the reform is the culmination of a series of interventions over the last decades attempting to strengthen coordination and centralize control. The main arguments in favour of the reform were broadly related to a reduction in bureaucratic costs and taxation levels and the need to create larger catchment areas (400,000 to 700,000 inhabitants) in order to support future specialization and to secure structural adjustments. In contrast to the common tradition with broad consensus between government and opposition when major structural reforms are introduced, the reform bill was passed by only a small majority in parliament.

Since 1970, Denmark has had a shared structure of health care funding between state and counties. The main financial sources have been general taxation at county and national levels, with redistributional mechanisms from central to county level and between counties based on demographic and economic criteria. With the structure reform, however, Denmark has reconfigured its health governance arrangements to resemble those of Norway, with fiscal decisions taken centrally and administrative responsibilities located within the five new regional units. The new financing scheme is a combination of central tax-based financing (80 per cent) through ABF payments and block grants, and municipal tax-based financing (20 per cent) through a combination of per capita and ABF. By removing the independent right to raise taxation at regional level, the system breaks with the tradition of having responsibility for management and financing at the same political level. Instead, health care activities are to be financed largely through a national earmarked health tax (8 per cent of income), which will be redistributed in terms of block grants to regions and municipalities. Earmarked health taxation is a novelty in Denmark and is thought to improve transparency in the sector and to reduce the potential of redistribution between health care and other service sectors. Furthermore, the idea behind the municipal co-financing is to create stronger incentives for municipalities to reduce hospitalization through, for example, investing in preventive activities (Vrangbæk 2005; Strandberg-Larsen et al. 2007).

2.5 Patient rights and empowerment

Strengthening the rights of patients generally refers to patients being allowed a greater say in logistical matters (selecting physicians and hospital) and in clinical matters (such as participating in elective medical decision-making), as well as participation in local policy-making (Saltman and Figueras 1997). The idea of free choice of provider has gained increasing support also in the Nordic countries, having been introduced in all four countries during the 1990s.

Sweden

Whereas Sweden was first among the Nordic countries to introduce patient rights, the legal position of patients has historically been rather weak. The right to choose a provider is not rooted in national legislation but has instead been adopted by the county councils on a voluntary basis. The process of implementing patient choice in Sweden has been thoroughly described by Winblad (2007), who relates this development to the general move towards increased freedom of choice within the public service sector during the 1990s.

The choice idea was manifested in practice through a string of reforms during the 1990s. In 1992, a National Guarantee of Treatment for patients was introduced, which allowed patients who did not receive care within three months the right to seek treatment at another hospital both within and outside the patient's own county. The choice of provider was further extended through the Family Doctor Act of 1994, which gave all residents within a county the right to choose a family doctor (GP). Perhaps most important, however, was the Federation of County Councils' adoption of the free choice recommendation in 1989. The recommendation was prepared centrally by the Federation of County Councils but was agreed upon by all county councils with little political dispute by 1991. The free choice recommendation entitled patients to seek care at hospitals or specialists throughout the whole country, except for highly specialized care. It was strongly emphasized that the freedom to choose applied to both public and private alternatives. The free choice recommendation was later revised in 2001, with the main difference being that patients were now also allowed to choose day treatment outside their own county. The revision was an effort to clarify and simplify the rules and applications, as the actual practice of patient choice varied significantly between the counties. The revised choice recommendation was, however, strongly opposed by the northern counties based on concerns that many patients seeking care in the southern parts of Sweden would be expensive; the northern counties did not accept the new recommendation until 2003 (Vrangbæk et al. 2007; Winblad 2007). Furthermore, a new treatment guarantee was introduced in 2005 based on the so-called '0-7-90-90' principle: instant contact with the health care system, GP appointment within 7 days, specialist consultation within 90 days and a maximum 90 days of waiting time between diagnosis and treatment (Glenngård et al. 2005).

In December 2008, the Government launched a proposition that the freedom of choice in primary care is to be regulated by law. The proposition recommends that the county councils should introduce systems for choice of providers that afford citizens the right to choose between different providers in primary health care. Every provider that meets the requirements stipulated by the county councils in the choice system has the right to establish practice in the primary care with public reimbursement. However, as of today (early 2009), many county councils (19 of 21) are critical of the proposition.

Norway

In Norway, the debate over patient rights began in the 1980s and early 1990s and was related to the problem of waiting lists for elective treatment. After an experiment with free choice of hospitals in two regions from 1994 to 1996, a first proposal for free choice was launched by the minority social democratic government. Reflecting the party's scepticism towards free choice, the proposal for choice was restricted to the patient's home county and the neighbouring counties, and only expenses above a ceiling of 1300 NOK would be reimbursed. Following negative reactions from the opposition parties, however, choice was extended to the whole country, and the co-payment ceiling for coverage of travelling expenses was lowered to 400 NOK. As was the case in Sweden, there was some concern that patients would prefer hospitals in the larger cities in the south, thus making it difficult to maintain a high-quality service within specialized medicine in the north (Vrangbæk and Østergren 2006).

The Patient Rights Act that was finally adopted in 1999 covered a broad package of rights that extended far beyond the free choice of hospitals. The Act was partly a simplification and consolidation of already existing legislation, and partly an implementation of new rights, and included the right to choose hospital; evaluation within 30 days; reevaluation; participation and information; access to medical records; and special rights relating to children, to complaints and to assistance from the Patients' Ombudsman (Vrangbæk et al. 2007). In 2003 and 2004, several amendments to the Patient Rights Act were made. First, child and youth psychiatric care was included in the scheme. Second, free choice of hospital was also extended to include the private hospitals that had entered into agreements with the regional health authorities. Third, a time limit should be determined in line with sound medical practice within which the necessary treatment must be provided. Fourth, the patient was given the right to be transferred to a private or foreign health care provider if the responsible regional health authority failed to provide treatment within the time limit, and the right to treatment abroad if adequate treatment could not be provided in Norway (Vrangbæk et al. 2007).

Finland

When Finland implemented the Act on the Status and Rights of Patients in 1993, it became the first patient law in Europe. The Act allows the patient the right to information, informed consent to treatment, to see any relevant medical documents, to complain and to autonomy. Also, a patient ombudsman is required in every organization providing medical treatment, to inform patients on their rights and, if needed, to help to make a complaint (Vuorenkoski et al. 2008). However, the degree of patient choice is more restricted than in the other three Nordic countries. Patients currently have very limited freedom to choose health - care provider unit or physicians in the municipal health care system. This is about to change with the proposed new Health Care Act, which will merge the Primary Health Care Act (from 1972) and the Act on Specialised Medical Care (from 1989) into a comprehensive Health Care Act. One of the most significant proposed changes is said to be increasing patient choice, by enabling patients freely to use the services of any health centre inside the same tertiary care region and by enabling patients – together with the referring physician – to choose any hospital within the same tertiary care region. While the bill was originally intended to be passed to the parliament in early 2009, the work with the Act has proven more complicated than estimated, and it is now said that it will be passed to parliament in early 2010 (Vuorenkoski 2008a).

Denmark

According to Vrangbæk and Østergren (2006, p. 377), the introduction of choice to the Danish political agenda can be seen as the result of 'a coalition between (some) patients demanding more flexibility and better service and national-level politicians seeking popularity and looking for ways to improve the legitimacy of the system'. While the choice issue was first and foremost carried forward by the liberal–conservative coalition government, it eventually gained support from all major parties. The counties initially opposed the scheme but still chose to enter into a voluntary agreement on extended choice before a parliamentary decision was made. This is seen as a defensive move in order to keep control over the design of the system.

The counties introduced freedom of choice in late 1992, and the scheme was formally implemented through law on 1 January 1993. The law allowed patients the right to choose between public hospitals at the lowest sufficient level of specialization. In outlining the specific details of the scheme, a cautious and pragmatic approach was chosen, with a number of restrictions and safeguards built into the policy in order to adjust to the institutional structures and policy objectives in the sector. In comparison with Norway, therefore, the Danish reform package was less comprehensive. Since 1992, the legislative and practical infrastructure has been adjusted several times, most importantly by improving the availability of waiting-time information and introducing DRG-based payments. Since the latter change has led to higher payment levels for most choice patients, the economic incentives to attract such patients have increased (Ankjær-Jensen 2002; Vrangbæk and Beck 2004). An 'extended free choice of hospitals' was introduced in 2002, when new legislation allowed patients to choose freely between a number of private hospitals and hospitals abroad if the home county cannot offer treatment in a public hospital within two months. This amendment of the choice scheme placed additional pressure on the counties to secure short waiting times (Vrangbæk and Østergren 2006).

2.6 The role of public health

Public health focuses on the population rather than the individual and involves mobilizing local, regional, national and international resources to ensure the conditions in which people can be healthy. The Nordic countries have been forerunners in this area during the last decades, with their adoption of comprehensive national strategies for public health.

Sweden

The Swedish National Institute for Public Health (SNIPH) was established in 1992, with three principal functions: to monitor and coordinate the implementation of a national public health policy with other central agencies, to be a national centre of knowledge on public health to the government and regional authorities and municipalities, and to exercise supervision in the fields of alcohol, tobacco and illicit drugs (Swedish National Institute for Public Health 2005a). Furthermore, the Centre for Epidemiology has the responsibility of monitoring and analysing the health and social status of the population. The majority of the public health work takes place at the local level and is undertaken by the county councils, the municipalities and nongovernmental organizations.

The stated overall aim of the national public health policy is 'to create social conditions that will ensure good health, on equal terms, for the entire population'.[3] It is also established that improving the public health of those groups most vulnerable to ill health is particularly important. In 2003, the Riksdag adopted a Public Health Bill that set out a new direction in this policy area. The new national public health strategy, which was outlined in the SNIPH report *Sweden's New Public Health Policy*, has a more distinct emphasis on health promotion than the former policy, focusing on health determinants rather than on diseases or health problems (Swedish National Institute for Public Health 2003).

The public health policy stipulates a number of objectives that are related to both structural and individual factors. Participation and influence in society is considered important, and among the fields assumed to be particularly relevant in obtaining this objective are labour market policy, media policy, gender equality, integration and disability policies. Second, the social security system is considered especially important in preventing economic hardship and combating mental health problems. Social services, the judicial system and criminal policy are further examples of areas of high relevance for socially deprived groups. A third public health objective is secure and favourable conditions during childhood and adolescence. A fourth objective deals with healthier working life, and the Public Health Bill stresses the considerable need for occupational medicine skills, and that the role of occupational health care needs to be strengthened; particular emphasis is placed on the importance of highlighting women's health. A fifth objective relates to creating healthy and safe environments and products. Finally, it is stressed that primary care is bound to play an important role in such a health promotion policy.

As emphasized in the national strategy for public health, however, the objectives are rather useless unless they are systematically monitored. After all, the objectives are estimated to involve 50 or so government agencies, and give the municipalities and county councils a major responsibility for public health activities on the regional and local level. Under the Public Health Bill, SNIPH is, therefore, responsible for monitoring the 11 objectives, and the intention is to draw up a public health policy report every fourth year presenting public health developments based on health determinants. In 2005, SNIPH delivered its first public health policy report to the Swedish Government, presenting the assignment received from the government and proposals for action (Swedish National Institute for Public Health 2005b). The report identifies 42 areas that are particularly important for improving public health work and for influencing current threats to favourable health development. These include areas such as rising alcohol consumption, obesity and lack of physical activity, work-related ill health, gender-related violence against women and impaired mental health.

Norway

There is a concern that improvements in health now seems to be slower in Norway than in countries that it naturally compares with, and that socio-economic disparities in health have grown since the 1970s (Ministry of Health and Social Affairs 2002–2003). The municipalities play a major role in the public health strategy, being responsible for health promotion, the prevention of illness and injuries, and the organization and management of school health services, health centres and child health care (Johnsen 2006). At the national level, several important structural steps have been taken through the reorganization of central social and health administration in order to strengthen the public health field. Several smaller agencies in the public health field have been incorporated in a Directorate for Health and Social Welfare, thus paving the way for better coordination and stronger implementation of public health policies (Ministry of Health and Social Affairs 2002–2003). Furthermore, the former National Institute of Public Health was merged in 2002 with the National Health Screening Service, the Medical Birth Registry and the Department of Drug Consumption Statistics and Methodology to create the Norwegian Institute of Public Health (NIPH). The main tasks of the NIPH are to monitor the development of the nation's state of health and employ new public health knowledge gathered worldwide, and to conduct research on why diseases emerge and on conditions that affect human health. Furthermore, the NIPH is also to follow up on public health activities by providing practical advice that promotes good health and prevents health hazards and disease – for the public health authorities, the public health service and the general public – and by cooperating closely with leading professional and technical actors in Norway and abroad in terms of research and initiatives.[4]

Norway followed Sweden in revitalizing its public health work at the beginning of this century (Ministry of Health and Social Affairs 2002–2003, p. 6). The new initiative is said to 'aim for a more systematic and comprehensive policy than hitherto', by drawing particular attention to the 'connection between the community's and the individual's responsibility for and possibility of influencing the health situation and to showing what the individual and the community have to gain from effective preventive health care'. The white paper gives particular emphasis to five general strategies: (1) to make it easier for people to take responsibility for their own health, (2) to build alliances to promote public health, (3) to encourage more prevention and less cure in the health service, (4) to build up new knowledge, and (5) to develop a strategy for women's health.

The first strategy aims to encourage individuals to assume responsibility for their own health and introduces four areas that are to receive particular attention: healthy lifestyle choices, reducing social inequalities in health, mental health and the surrounding environment.

The second strategy, aiming to build alliances to promote public health, stresses the need for a broad approach to public health. Such a strategy means mobilizing and coordinating a large number of players in society, and the white paper, therefore, calls for a national public health chain that is to provide the basis for more systematic cooperation with voluntary organizations, educational institutions and other bodies. Also, the new public health initiative promotes a municipal approach rather than a sector approach to public health work, clarifying local authorities' total and comprehensive political responsibility for public health work.

The third pillar of the public health strategy is to direct the focus away from medication as a first choice to concentrate on lifestyle action and effort on the part of the patient, and to strengthen preventive health services for children and young people. This strategy also calls for a stronger role for health care institutions in prevention. Fourth, in order to raise the level of knowledge, the following areas are considered particularly important: health surveillance, causal research, research on actions and intervention, systematic evaluation and cost–benefit analyses.

Finally, the new public health policy includes a strategy for women's health. The strategy seeks to strengthen research on gender differences in risk of disease, development of disease, diagnosis and optimum treatment and prevention, and to stimulate studies addressing gender differences in relation to the side-effects of medicines. There is also an increased focus on the health and living conditions of immigrant girls and women, and their use of the health and social welfare services, as well as on the prevention of violence and sexual abuse of women.

Finland

Following the focus in Finnish health care policy on health promotion and prevention of diseases since the late 1990s, public health has improved considerably. There remains, however, concern about increasing problems associated with obesity and the excessive consumption of alcohol, and the marked health differences between regions, socioeconomic groups and marital status groups. As in the other Nordic countries, public health and health promotion is carried out at both the national and local level. The Ministry of Social Affairs and Health is the main actor at the national level, being responsible for health protection, environmental health and chemical affairs, and tobacco and alcohol control. Closely linked to the Ministry of Social Affairs and Health is the Public Health Committee, which is appointed by the Finnish Government for a three-year term, representing various branches of government, the municipal sector, the health service system, nongovernmental organizations, professional organizations and health research. The tasks of the Public Health Committee include monitoring the development of public health and the implementation of health policy, as well as developing the national health policy and building up health-promoting cooperation with different sectors of administration and other bodies. On the local level, all professional public health activities except environmental health are located in the health centres, the most important being maternal and child health care and school health care. In addition, many nongovernmental organizations are working in the field of health promotion (Vuorenkoski et al. 2008).

The overall targets for Finland's public health policy are stipulated in the *Health 2015* public health programme, which was approved by the government in 2001 (Ministry of Social Affairs and Health 2001). Building on the Health for All policy of the World Health Organization (WHO), the programme presents eight targets for public health focusing on major problems requiring concerted action by a number of bodies: (1) to increase child well-being and health, (2) to reduce smoking and health problems associated with alcohol and drug use among young people, (3) to reduce accidental and violent death among young adult males by a third from the level of the late 1990s, (4) to improve working conditions and working and functional capacity among people of working age in order to increase retirement age by about three years compared with 2000, (5) to continue to improve average functional capacity among people over 75, (6) to enable Finns to remain healthy for an average of two years longer than in 2000, (7) to ensure that satisfaction with health service availability and functioning of health services will remain at the present level, and (8) to reduce inequality and increase the welfare and relative status of those population groups in the weakest position.

The concepts of 'settings' and 'course of life' play a key role in the *Health 2015* programme. The programme emphasizes that health is a process rather than a state of affairs and should, therefore, 'be studied throughout the course of life, striving to identify the important transition stages and critical periods and to help people to cope with them as well as possible' (Ministry of Social Affairs and Health 2001, p. 22). Background factors carry a different weight at different phases of life, thereby demanding different kinds of action. In addition to the eight public health targets, the programme also lists 36 statements concerning the lines of action stressed by the government within a number of defined areas: child health, young people's health, health during working life and health in old age. Furthermore, the 36 statements also stipulate lines of action related to the role of the municipalities, the health care system and health promotion, business and industry, nongovernmental organizations and civil action, research and training, international activities, and health impact assessments.

In addition, there are also some public health policy targets incorporated in the new national development programme. This scheme replaces the earlier 'four-year-plan', which was drawn up when a new government was appointed, stipulating the general aims of health care policy and the measures that will be taken in order to fulfil these aims. In the first National Development Programme for Social Welfare and Health Care adopted by the government in January 2008, the central theme is to strengthen the development activities of municipal services. The programme defines three main targets: to decrease marginalization of the people; to increase health and well-being and to diminish differences between population groups in this respect; and to increase quality, effectiveness and accessibility of services and diminish geographical differences in this respect. Several of the defined subtargets relate to central aspects of public health, such as alcohol consumption, obesity and smoking (Vuorenkoski 2008b).

Denmark

During the last decades, Denmark has seen the development of unfavourable trends in average life expectancy in comparison to other countries in the Organisation for Economic Co-operation and Development (OECD). Whereas, Danish men and women ranked fourth and fifth among the then 15 EU member states and Norway in 1970, they were number 15 and 16 on the same list of countries in 1996. Denmark was, consequently, the country that had the lowest increase in average life expectancy during the period 1970–1996 (Danish Ministry of Health 1999). In 2006, Danish men rank 18th among 20 OECD countries, while Danish women rank last (National Institute of Public Health 2007). This development mainly reflected the large number of smokers (especially heavy smokers) and the high level of alcohol consumption, exceeding even that found in certain countries in southern Europe. In addition, a high intake of calories and fatty foods combined with lack of physical activity adds further to this trend. As in the other Nordic countries, there is also increasing concern about the social differences in the population's health behaviour, morbidity, use of the health services and mortality (National Institute of Public Health 2007).

The public health services are partly integrated with curative services and partly organized as separate activities run by special institutions (Strandberg-Larsen et al. 2007). The National Board of Health is responsible for a number of tasks related to public health, which are undertaken by a number of divisions and centres dealing with related areas of expertise. This includes the National Centre for Health Promotion and Disease Prevention, which is responsible for the majority of the central initiatives in the field of prevention and health promotion. Its primary tasks involve monitoring, documentation, development of strategies and methodologies, dissemination, collaboration and planning, as well as advising the Ministry of the Interior and Health and other national bodies on issues regarding health promotion and prevention. Attached to the Board are also the medical public health officers, who are responsible for monitoring the health conditions in the respective counties.[5] The National Institute of Public Health conducts research on and monitors the health and morbidity of the population and the functioning of the health care system.

In response to the unfavourable development in life expectancy, *The Danish Government Programme on Public Health and Health Promotion 1999–2008* was launched in 1999 (Danish Ministry of Health 1999). The aim of the programme was to increase average life expectancy for men and women by at least two years, and to increase the number of disease-free life years through a reduction in chronic diseases. In order to obtain this, the programme built on three key elements: a multisectoral approach that involved large sectors of society, such as the health services, the social sector, traffic, working life, schools and the local community; a concrete and action-oriented approach that built on ambitious and realistic targets; and a 10-year perspective that made it possible to sustain the long-term efforts needed to improve public health in many areas.

In 2002, the health care programme *Healthy Throughout Life 2002–2010* was initiated by the new government (Ministry of the Interior and Health 2003). While keeping in line with the important goals and target groups from the 1998–2008 programme, the new programme – in contrast to the former – specifically focused on reducing the major preventable diseases and disorders. The new initiative emphasized that quality of life can be improved considerably through more systematic efforts in terms of counselling, support, rehabilitation and other measures in relation to patients; a key aspect is to provide individuals with the necessary knowledge and tools to promote their own health and care. The programme focused on eight major preventable diseases and disorders: non-insulin-dependent diabetes, preventable cancer, cardiovascular diseases, osteoporosis, musculoskeletal disorders, hypersensitivity disorders (asthma and allergy), mental disorders and chronic obstructive pulmonary disease. *Healthy Throughout Life* also contained an indicator programme, the purpose of which was to ensure the continued monitoring and documentation of trends based on available statistics and data.

2.7 Financing and payment

The funds raised to provide health care generally come from tax revenue, social insurance, private insurance or out-of-pocket payments. The choice of funding principle will determine the amount of funds available for health care, who controls the resources and who bears the financial burden. Also important are the institutional arrangements for contracting with and paying providers. In the Nordic context, competition between insurance providers is not an issue; therefore, in this section, the focus is on centralization versus decentralization of public financing and the methods of reimbursing service providers.

2.7.1 Provider financing

Sweden

Sweden was the first of the Nordic countries to introduce ABF for hospital services, when it was implemented in Helsingborgs Hospital (Skåne) and then in Stockholm. The so-called Stockholm model was based on using the DRG system as a basis for payment (Mikkola et al. 2001). In addition, DRG-based payments came into use for acute inpatient care in some county councils from 1991.

The use of ABF was introduced in Swedish health care in combination with other management reforms, such as purchaser–provider models and patient choice. The country's decentralized health care system implies that the county councils have much freedom in choosing models of hospital payment, and presently approximately half of the county councils have chosen to implement

ABF. Reviewing the experience with ABF in Sweden, Kastberg and Siverbo (2007) point out that the new financing system at first seemed to improve productivity and reduce waiting times. Yet, given that councils pay providers per received and diagnosed patient, ABF offers no incentives for the hospitals to keep production within any limits. Consequently, a side-effect was lack of cost control and difficulties in achieving cost cuts. Several county councils, therefore, moved to introduce limits on the type and number of activities for which providers would be fully reimbursed, as well as restrictions on the ability to produce more than the basic volume. Furthermore, several county councils implemented a policy of allowing no payment at all if production reached a predetermined volume, and regular adjustments of the payment levels were also commonly made, sometimes several times per year and in some cases retroactively. With regard to other problems commonly associated with ABF, Kastberg and Siverbo seem to conclude – even if results are somewhat mixed – that research so far suggests that DRG creep, DRG dumping, cream-skimming and DRG gaming have not occurred to any significant extent yet.

Norway

Norway implemented ABF for somatic hospital services based on the DRG system in 1997. The DRG weights are equal for all hospitals irrespective of cost structure, case mix and hospital type, and the price of a DRG-point – and thereby reimbursement – is equal throughout the country (Johnsen 2006). Since its introduction in 1997, the share between ABF and block funding has been changed frequently, varying between 30 and 60 per cent. The share of ABF was reduced from 60 to 40 per cent both in 2004 and 2006, and stayed at the latter level also through 2009. It is expected to decrease further from 2011.

Together with the waiting-time guarantee introduced in 1990 and increasing global budgets, the new hospital financing scheme was an attempt to handle the long waiting times for elective treatment that dominated in the late 1980s and during the 1990s. Yet, waiting times were still long at the end of 2001, despite the intended increase in treatment of patients realized by the introduction of ABF (Hagen and Kaarbøe 2006). Efficiency, however, increased (Biørn et al. 2003), though the increase was not substantial. As hospital activity has continued to increase in recent years, waiting times have finally been substantially reduced: from 2002 to 2006 there was a 24 per cent increase in hospital admissions, and a corresponding decrease in average waiting times of 30 per cent (Martinussen 2007). While the major challenges of Norwegian health care during the 1990s were related to lacking treatment capacity, and consequently long waiting lists for elective treatment, the situation after the hospital reform has rather been that the growth in activity has been larger than the signals given from central government. Hence, Hagen and Kaarbøe (2006) identify three dysfunctional effects related to the ABF system as it was implemented in Norway. First, they point out the increased financial dependence of the county councils on central government. Second, given that ABF only cover part of the marginal costs, increased production has resulted in larger deficits and further claims for supplementary funds. Hence, the same problems of productivity and total cost control encountered in Sweden soon also evolved in Norway. Third, the financing system is also said to have eroded the trust between central government and the county councils: because of the increased intervention from central authorities, there was developed a lack of transparency in the financing system and a blame game over responsibility for increasing deficits at county level.

Finland

In Finland, no national financing model has been introduced, and the system with the municipalities as purchasers and financiers of hospital services makes the conditions for using DRG quite different from those in the other Nordic countries. With the municipalities purchasing hospital services through their hospital districts, DRG first and foremost functions as a product description, enabling the hospitals to set the price of their services based on actual costs. Since the use of the DRG system is neither compulsory nor regulated, the hospital districts may choose between several types of price setting, such as average price per bed day, combinations of fee for service and average price per bed day, and case-based prices. The DRG system was first introduced to any great extent when case-based pricing systems based on DRG was implemented by three large hospitals in 1997 and 1998. Later there was a steady increase in the use of DRG, but mostly for other purposes than pricing, such as internal management of hospitals, benchmarking of hospital performance and health services research. By 2005, 9 of the 21 hospital districts base their service pricing on DRGs, while several others are now considering introducing it.

In their discussion of the use of DRG in Finnish hospital financing, Mikkola et al. (2001) point out that the introduction of similar DRG-based hospital financing models as the decentralized market-based model of Sweden or the centralized model of Norway would necessitate major reforms in the health care system. While the former type of model would call for a proper purchaser–provider split and freedom of consumer choice, a national implementation of a DRG-based hospital financing system would conflict with the decision-making autonomy delegated to the municipalities with the 1993 state subsidy reform. Given that the hospital districts operate as local monopolies with mandatory membership for the municipalities, and that municipalities rarely purchase services outside their own district, price competition seems like an unrealistic driving force. The patients themselves are unable to promote competition between hospitals, since – unlike in Sweden and Norway – their right to choose hospital is restricted. Furthermore, Mikkola et al. also emphasize the fact that the introduction of DRG-based financing in Sweden and Norway was seen as an effective incentive to reduce waiting lists and increase hospital productivity. In Finland, by comparison, the main concerns were cost containment and maintaining quality of care rather than increasing patient numbers.

Denmark

Denmark stands out from the other Nordic countries in several respects when it comes to the application of the DRG system. First, instead of following its neighbours in implementing some version of ABF during the 1990s, the country has until recently elected to stay with the traditional block financing of hospitals. Second, as prospective payment started to become increasingly more important in the financing of hospitals since the late 1990s, the country has chosen not to adopt the Nordic version of the DRG system (Nord-DRG).

The move closer to an ABF system in Denmark was mainly provoked by a combination of encouragement from central authorities and the development of the Danish case-mix system (Ankjær-Jensen et al. 2006). The problems encountered in the traditional bloc-grant system, particularly with waiting lists and budget deficits resulting from capacity shortages, also helped to stimulate a rising interest in new reimbursement systems (Larsen and Skjoldborg 2004). In addition, the realization that very few patients took benefit of the free hospital choice to seek treatment outside their own county also played an important role in this development (NOU 2003). In 1999, full DRG-based payment was consequently introduced for free-choice patients seeking treatment outside their home county, in order to stimulate increased patient flows and a more active use of the right to free hospital choice. In most cases, this has created incentives for counties to try to retain free-choice patients by reducing waiting lists (Strandberg-Larsen et al. 2007). This measure was combined with the introduction of a 10 per cent DRG-based distribution of the hospital budgets. Then, in 2004, an agreement was struck between central government and the counties that at least 20 per cent of hospital budgets should be activity based, with the intention of providing hospitals with an incentive to increase activity and efficiency. Even if it was solely up to the counties to decide how to implement the payment scheme, most chose to base it on the Danish case-mix system, while the actual percentage of the DRG tariff and the specific DRGs covered by the variable payment varied between the counties (Ankjær-Jensen et al. 2006). The active promotion of ABF from central government seems to have led to increases in activity levels, and it was, therefore, planned to gradually raise the level from 20 to 50 per cent in 2007 (Strandberg-Larsen et al. 2007).

As with the development of reimbursement principles, central government has also been the driving force behind the implementation and development of the Danish case-mix systems. Unlike the other Nordic countries, the health authorities have stimulated the development of a national version of Nord-DRG, and in 2002 the Danish case-mix system was introduced, consisting of the Danish DRG system (DkDRG) for inpatients and the Danish Ambulatory Grouping System (DAGS) for ambulatory patients. Since the medical specialists were strongly involved in the development of the system, it is widely accepted by Danish clinicians (Ankjær-Jensen et al. 2006).

2.8 Concluding remarks

The focus of this chapter has been on what could perhaps be termed 'the second wave' of Nordic health reforms. As we have seen, there are important differences in the detailed structures of the respective countries and consequently lessons to be learned by comparisons within the Nordic world. Far from being static, the Nordic model is constantly evolving through incremental and more radical change processes. The purpose of this chapter has been to provide the reader with a brief description of reforms and policy changes along five dimensions: state versus market, decentralization, patient choice, public health and financing. While the description confirms the assessment in Chapter 1 of Nordic health policy as uncoordinated, some general and important trends nevertheless emerge from this description.

First we seem to observe a trend towards increased formalization of regulation in health care. Examples of formalization policies included waiting-time guarantees, choice, patient rights legislation, quality regulation, complaints procedures, referral to treatment abroad and development of care packages for cancer and heart disease, with detailed specification of what to do when accompanied by monitoring and follow-up. The formalization is to some extent also a consequence of EU regulation (e.g. European Court of Justice rulings). The Nordic 'model' of informal, negotiated care delivery does not fit well with a more formalized and legalistic EU approach.

Second, the regulation is increasingly carried out by the central state, even in the two countries that have yet to recentralize: Sweden and Finland. Politicians at the national level are being increasingly blamed for health system irregularities, poor performance and so on. As an answer, they turn to more detailed regulation. This can be seen as an attempt to manage a quickly evolving, and to some extent 'unmanageable', field with many dilemmas and problems. The result is a thickening of the regulatory environment, where the regional political levels are being overruled or even dismantled. Yet the state is reluctant to take full responsibility for health care. This can be seen as a 'blame avoidance' strategy. It is nice to have regional scapegoats to blame, and to transfer the responsibility for difficult and unavoidable prioritizations.

Third, the strengthening of national policy-making goes hand in hand with an increased emphasis on evidence and documentation of performance. As the centre has limited direct insight, it needs more indirect measures. Also it needs tools to push the regional and organizational levels to self-regulation, and if this fails/succeeds to punish/reward. Productivity analysis, comparative analysis instruments, quality analysis and waiting-time statistics are all part of this.

Notes

1. Formally there are 18 counties, two regions (Vestra Gøtaland and Skåne) and one municipality (Gotland). For simplicity we use the term counties.
2. From 1 January 2009: National Supervisory Authority for Welfare and Health, Valvira.
3. As stated on the webpage of the Swedish National Institute of Public Health.
4. As stated on the homepage of the Norwegian Institute of Public Health: http://www.fhi.no/.
5. http://www.sst.dk/default.aspx?lang=en.

References

Anell, A. (2005) Swedish healthcare under pressure, *Health Economics* 14: 237–54.

Ankjær-Jensen, A. (2002) *DSI Rapport 2002: 04: DRG-afregning af frit valgs patienter.* [*DRG-Payment Choice for Patients.*] Copenhagen: DSI Institut for Sundhedsvæsen.

Ankjær-Jensen, A., Rosling, P. and Bilde, L. (2006) Variable prospective financing in the Danish hospital sector and the development of a Danish case-mix system, *Health Care Management Science* 9: 259–68.

Bergman, S.-E. (1997) Swedish models of health care reform: a review and assessment, *International Journal of Health Planning and Management* 13: 91–106.

Biørn, E., Hagen, T.P. Iversen, T. and Magnussen, J. (2003) The effect of activity-based financing on hospital efficiency: a panel data analysis of DEA efficiency scores 1992–2000, *Health Care Management Science* 6: 271–283.

Brorström, B. and Rombach, B. (1996) *Kommunal förändringsbenägenhet.* [*School of Public Administration Reports*, Report 1.] Gothenburg: University of Gothenburg.

Culyer, A.J., Graf van der Schulenburg, J.-M. and van de Ven, M.M.W.P. (1995) *SNS Occasional Paper No. 71: Swedish Health Care Revisited.* Stockholm: SNS.

Danish Ministry of Health (1999) *The Danish Government Programme on Public Health and Health Promotion 1999–2008: An Action Oriented Programme for Healthier Settings in Everyday Life.* Copenhagen: Danish Ministry of Health.

Federation of Swedish County Councils [Landstingsförbundet] (2004) *Sjukvårdsdata in Focus.* [*Health Care Data in Focus.*] Stockholm: Landstingsförbundet.

Figueras, J. (2003) Health system reforms and post-modernism: the end of big ideas, *European Journal of Public Health* 13: 79–82.

Glenngård, A.H., Hjalte, F. Svensson, M. Anell, A. and Bankauskaite, V. (2005) Sweden: Health System Review. *Health Systems in Transition*, 7(4): 1–28.

Grasdal, A. (2008) *Øker sosiale helseforskjeller.* http://www.forskning.no/artikler/2008/juni/183888.

Green-Pedersen, C. (2003) *Market-type Reforms of the Danish and Swedish Service Welfare States: Different Party Strategies and Different Outcomes.* Aarhus: Department of Political Science, University of Aarhus.

Hagen, T.P. and Kaarbøe, O. (2006) The Norwegian hospital reform of 2002: central government takes over ownership of public hospitals, *Health Policy* 76: 320–33.

Häkkinen, U. (2005) The impact of changes in Finland's health care system, *Health Economics* 14: 101–18.

Häkkinen, U. and Lehto, J. (2005) Reform, change, and continuity in Finnish health care, *Journal of Health Politics, Policy and Law* 30: 79–96.

Hanning, M. (1996) Maximum waiting time guarantee: an attempt to reduce waiting lists in Sweden, *Health Policy* 36: 17–35.

Harrison, M.I. and Calltorp, J. (2000) The reorientation of market-oriented reforms in Swedish health care, *Health Policy* 50: 219–40.

Health Insurance Denmark (2007) Sygehusforsikringen 'danmark' [What is 'danmark'?] www.sykehusforsikring.dk.

Hsiao, W. (2003) *What Is a Health Care System? Why Should We Care?* Cambridge, MA: Program in health care financing, Harvard School of Public Health [unpublished manuscript].

Johnsen, J.R. (2006) Norway: Health System Review. *Health Systems in Transition*, 8(1): 1–167.

Kastberg, G. and Siverbo, S. (2007) Activity-based financing of health care: experiences from Sweden, *International Journal of Health Planning and Management* 22: 25–44.

Larsen, J. and Skjoldborg, U.S. (2004) Comparing systems for costing hospital treatments: the case of stable angina pectoris, *Health Policy* 67: 293–307.

Magnussen, J., Hagen, T.P.and Kaarboe, O.M. (2007) Centralized or decentralized? A case study of Norwegian hospital reform, *Social Science and Medicine* 64: 2129–37.

Martinussen, P.E. (2007) Utviklingen i somatisk spesialisthelsetjeneste, 2002–2006.

[The development in somatic specialist health services, 2002–2006], in Petersen, S.Ø. (ed.) *SAMDATA Sektorrapport for somatisk spesialisthelsetjeneste 2006 3/07*. [*SAMDATA Sector Report for Somatic Specialist Health Services 2006 3/07*.] Trondheim: SINTEF Health Research.

Midttun, L. (2007) Private spesialisthelsetjenester [Private specialist health services], in Petersen, S.Ø. (ed.), *SAMDATA Sektorrapport for somatisk spesialisthelsetjeneste 2006 3/07*. [*SAMDATA Sector Report for Somatic Specialist Health Services 2006 3/07*.] Trondheim: SINTEF Health Research.

Mikkola, H., Keskimäki, I. and Häkkinen, U. (2001) DRG-related prices applied in a public health care system: can Finland learn from Norway and Sweden? *Health Policy* 59: 37–51.

Ministry of Health and Social Affairs (2000–2001) *Parliamentary Proposition No. 66: Om lov om helseforetak m.m.* [*On the Law of Health Enterprises, etc.*] Oslo: Ministry of Health and Social Affairs.

Ministry of Health and Social Affairs (2002–2003) *Parliamentary Report No. 16: Resept for et sunnere Norge. Folkehelsepolitikken.* [*Prescriptions for a Healthier Norway: A Broad Policy for Public Health.*] Oslo: Ministry of Health and Social Affairs.

Ministry of Social Affairs and Health (2001) *Government Resolution on the Health 2015.* [Public Health Programme. Ministry of Social Affairs and Health Publications 2001, No. 6.] Helsinki: Ministry of Social Affairs and Health.

Ministry of the Interior and Health (2003) *Healthy Throughout Life: The Targets and Strategies for Public Health Policy of the Government of Denmark, 2002–2010.* Copenhagen: Ministry of the Interior and Health.

Mossialos, E. and McKee, M. (2002) *The Impact of EU Law on Health Policy.* Brussels: PIE-Peter Lang.

Mossialos, E. and Thompson, S. (2004) *Voluntary Health Insurance in the European Union.* Copenhagen: World Health Organization on behalf of the European Observatory on Health Systems and Policies.

Næss-Schmidt, H.S. (2008) *Forskning og pension analyserapport 2008 No. 4: Sundhedsforsikringer: en løsning på fremtidens velfærd?* Copenhagen: Copenhagen Economics.

National Board of Health and Welfare [Socialstyrelsen] (2002) *Vård och omosrg ur ett samhällsperspektiv.* [*Health and Medical Services From a Societal Perspective.*] Stockholm: National Board of Health.

National Institute of Public Health (2007) *Public Health Report, Denmark 2007.* Copenhagen: National Institute of Public Health.

NOMESCO (2006) *Health Statistics in the Nordic Countries.* Copenhagen: National Board of Health.

Norén, L. (2007) The private health insurance and customers' demand for care. Paper presented at the Second Nordic Workshop for Health Management and Organization, 6–7 December, Gothenburg, Sweden.

Norwegian Association of Local and Regional Authorities (2004) *Bestiller- og utførerorganisering i pleie- og omsorgssektoren – en veileder. Agenda Utredning and Utvikling AS.* Oslo: Agenda.

NOU (2003) *NOU 2003: 1. Behovsfinansiert finansiering av spesialisthelsetjenesten.* Oslo: Ministry of Health and Care Services.

NOU (2005) *NOU 2005: 3. Fra stykkevis til helt. En sammenhengende helsetjeneste.* Oslo: Ministry of Health and Care Services.

Pedersen, K.M. (2002) *Working Paper 2002: 7; Reforming Decentralized Integrated Health Care Systems: Theory and the Case of the Norwegian Reform.* Oslo: Health Economics Research Programme, University of Oslo.

Pedersen, K.M. (2005) The public–private mix in Scandinavia, in Maynard, A. (ed.) *The Public–Private Mix for Health.* Oxford: Radcliffe, pp. 161–89.

RO (2004) *Bestiller–utførermodell i pleie- og omsorgstjenesten: en kartlegging av kommuner og bydeler.* [*Purchaser-Provider Models in Nurse and Care Services: A Mapping of Municipalities and Town Districts.*] Stjørdal: Ressurssenter for omstilling av kommunene.

Saltman, R.B. and Bankauskaite, V. (2006) Conceptualizing decentralisation in European health systems: a functional perspective, *Health Economics, Policy and Law* 1: 127–47.

Saltman, R.B. and Figueras, J. (eds) (1997) *European Health Care Reform: Analysis of Current Strategies.* Copenhagen: WHO Regional Office for Europe.

Saltman, R.B. and Figueras, J. (1998) Analyzing the evidence on European health care reforms, *Health Affairs* 17: 85–108.

Saltman, R.B., Bankauskaite, V. and Vrangbæk, K. (2007) *Decentralization in Health Care: Strategies and Outcomes.* Maidenhead: McGraw-Hill.

Seim, A., Løvaas, L. and Hagen, T.P. (2007) Hva kjennetegner virksomheter som kjøper private helseforsikringer? *Tidsskr Nor Lægeforen* 127: 2673–5.

Siverbo, S. (2004) The purchaser–provider split in principle and practice, *Financial Accountability and Management* 20: 401–20.

SOU (2007) *SOU 10. Hållbar samhällsorganisation med utvecklingskraft.* Stockholm: Ministry of Financial Affairs.

SOU (2008) *SOU 37. Vårdval i Sverige.* Stockholm: Ministry of Social Affairs.

Strandberg-Larsen, M., Nielsen, M.B. Vallgårda, S., Krasnik, A., Vrangbæk, K. and Mossialos, E. (2007) *Health Systems in Transition: Denmark.* Copenhagen: WHO Regional Office for Europe on behalf of the European Observatory on Health Systems and Policies.

Swedish Insurance Federation [Försäkringsförbundet] (2004) *Årsstatistikk från och med 1999* [Swedish Insurance Federation Statistics, 1999 and onwards]. Stockholm: Swedish Insurance Federation.

Swedish National Institute of Public Health (2003) *Sweden's New Public Health Policy: National Public Health Objectives for Sweden.* Stockholm: Swedish National Institute of Public Health.

Swedish National Institute of Public Health (2005a) *An Introduction to the Swedish National Institute of Public Health.* Stockholm: Swedish National Institute of Public Health.

Swedish National Institute of Public Health (2005b) *The 2005 Public Health Policy Report.* Stockholm: Swedish National Institute of Public Health.

Trygg-Hansa (2008) http://www.newsdesk.se/pressroom/trygg-hansa/pressrelease/view/kostnaderna-foer-privata-sjukvaardsfoersaekringar-oekar-251875.

Vohlonen, I., Ihalainen, R., Saltman, R.B., Karhunen, T. and Palmunen, J. (2004) Improving health security: a pilot study from Finland linking disability and health expenditures, *Health Policy* 67: 119–27.

Vrangbæk, K. (2005) Health policy in Denmark: leaving the decentralized welfare path? *Journal of Health Politics, Policy and Law* 30: 29–52.

Vrangbæk, K. and Beck, M. (2004) County level responses to the introduction of DRG rates for 'extended choice' hospital patients in Denmark, *Health Policy* 67: 25–37.

Vrangbæk, K. and Østergren, K. (2006) Patient empowerment and the introduction of hospital choice in Denmark and Norway, *Health Economics, Policy and Law* 1: 371–94.

Vrangbæk, K., Østergren, K., Birk, H.O. and Winblad, U. (2007) Patient reactions to hospital choice in Norway, Denmark, and Sweden, *Health Economics, Policy and Law* 2: 125–52.

Vuorenkoski, L. (2008a) The new health care act, *Health Policy Monitor,* October 2008; available at www.hpm.org./en/Downloads/Half-Yearly_Reports.html.

Vuorenkoski, L. (2008b) New national development programme, *Health Policy Monitor,* April 2008; available at www.hpm.org./en/Downloads/Half-Yearly_Reports.html.

Vuorenkoski, L., Bäckmand, H. and Korhonen, J. (2007) Menetetyt elinvuodet. PYLL-indeksi väestön hyvinvoinnin mittana [Potential years of life lost PYLL-rate in monitoring the wellbeing of a population], *Suomen Lääkärilehti* 62: 305–9.

Vuorenkoski, L., Mladovsky, P. and Mossialos, E. (2008) *Finland: Health System Review*. Copenhagen: WHO Regional Office for Europe on behalf of the European Observatory on Health Systems and Policies.

Winblad, U. (2007) Valfriheten: en misslyckad sjukvårdsreform? in Blomqvist, P. (ed.) *Vem styr vården? Organisation och politisk styrning innom svensk sjukvård*. Stockholm: SNS.

three

The political process of restructuring Nordic health systems

Karsten Vrangbæk

3.1 Introduction

Reform of the administrative structures for welfare services has been on the agenda in all four Nordic countries since the mid-1990s. Denmark and Norway have implemented major reforms affecting health care, while Finland and Sweden have chosen more voluntary approaches. Health care has been at the centre of the structural reform debates in all of the four countries.

Proponents of structural reforms in the Nordic health systems have argued that the changes represent prudent adjustments to meet future challenges. Opponents have argued that the reforms are costly and partly unnecessary undertakings that are primarily part of institutional power struggles. The aim of this chapter is not to investigate the merits of these two arguments but to analyse the differences and similarities in the policy processes and arguments leading to reform decisions in the four countries. This is particularly relevant for two reasons. First, the recentralization trends in the Nordic countries in this era represent a change compared with the dominating philosophy over the previous three decades. Second, traditional political logic points to vested interests, an abundance of veto points and likely resistance from voters as elements that make structural reforms unlikely (North 1990; Knight 1992; Christiansen and Klitgaard 2008). Why then have all four countries initiated structural reform processes and how can we explain the differences in outcomes of the policy process in the four countries? By analysing such questions, we can gain insight into health policy dynamics in the Nordic region in this period. The chapter provides descriptive analyses of the reform processes in the four Nordic countries. But the chapter will also point to some possible explanatory factors behind the reforms. It focuses on policy ideas related to the health sector, although this cannot be entirely separated from broader structural reform ideas. The reform debates are comprehensive in the sense that they entail changes in both the size of decentralized units and the distribution of tasks and functions between the units. The chapter does not aim to provide a detailed comparison of the contents of the reform decisions. They are described at various places elsewhere in this volume.

A typical political science perspective on structural changes (North 1990; Knight 1992) suggests that policy actors will pursue both substantive policy interests and institutional interests in terms of structures that can maximize their level of influence. Comprehensive structural reforms are prime examples of policies where both institutional and substantive issues are at stake. Such reforms are typically initiated at the central level and implemented in top-down processes. Key players in the process are governmental and parliamentary actors. Yet these actors must take the power of other stake holders into consideration. Of particular importance are the interests of regional and municipal authorities, but professional and industry organizations are also important. All of these actors can be expected to act strategically in order to maximise power and influence, and to promote their ideas about necessary changes and desired end states.

Based on this perspective, it can be suggested that decisions to embark on complex reforms can be understood by analysing a set of possible preconditions. The *first* issue to investigate is whether key actors were able to make convincing cases for general or specific challenges or problems indicating a need for reform. In the present case, we would be looking for clear arguments that the Nordic health systems were performing poorly, or troubled by specific problems. A *second* likely prerequisite for reform is the presence of strong governmental actors with a commitment to initiate change processes in spite of likely resistance. The commitment could be based on genuine concerns for underlying problems and/or expectations of rewards in terms of increasing share of votes, a stronger institutional position (e.g. more power, resources), a positive legacy and so on. A clear commitment means that the governmental actor stands unified in pushing a reform on to the political agenda and in seeking to gain support for the core elements of the reform despite opposition.

Equally important for understanding the success or failure of reforms is a *third* theme, namely the government's capacity to push the reform through the policy process. Two issues are particularly relevant in this regard. The first is the parliamentary situation, and, more specifically, whether the government commands a majority or must rely on ad hoc coalitions for its policies. The second is whether the government is facing a strong opposition to the reform. Opposing interests might be found in opposition parties, in factions within the government parties or in external organized interest groups such as unions, industry organizations, consumer organizations or federations of decentralized authorities. The worst case scenario for a reform-minded government is if such powerful interest groups form coherent coalitions that can veto or significantly alter the contents of the reform.

The ability to overcome or neutralize potential opposition and build support for the reform proposal is, therefore, a key requirement for the success of reformists. Skilful management of the reform policy process may help the governmental actor in pushing the reform forward. A *fourth* topic for investigation is, therefore, how the policy process is managed in the four cases outlined above. Important elements include decisions on when and how to provide information and to reveal policy options and preferences. Another important theme is the organization of arenas and access to arenas for potential opposition interests. A typical way to structure both information and access is to set up government committees to investigate the problems and possible solutions. By controlling the mandate, composition and timing of such committee work, governments might facilitate reform decisions. More generally, it has been suggested that a reform-minded government might benefit from clouding the reform process in a 'veil of vagueness' regarding policy options and preferences, as this will reduce or at least delay the strategic options for opposing interests (Christiansen and Klitgaard 2008). National norms and traditions for policy deliberation are likely to reduce the scope of such strategies. Governments that disregard the informal 'rules of the policy game' may incur 'costs' in terms of loss of voter support, legitimacy or trust in subsequent policy games. This is particularly relevant in a Nordic context with long-standing traditions for negotiation strategies and relatively consensus-oriented policy processes.

It is not possible to investigate all of these issues in detail in a short chapter. Yet an attempt will be made to provide some insight into the four main themes: (1) whether there was clear evidence for problems with the existing structure, including an assessment of general globalization-related pressures for the Nordic health systems and their translation into, and interaction with, specific performance problems; (2) whether there were governmental actors with a strong commitment to invest political capital in a reform process; (3) the strength of potential opposing interests; and (4) how the government managed the reform process in the face of national norms and traditions. The four themes are investigated for each of the four countries based on secondary data and existing analyses.

3.2 Evidence of performance problems in the Nordic countries

The first question was whether structural reform processes were initiated in response to clear evidence of major performance problems. The short answer is that all four countries appeared to have found a reasonable balance between policies addressing traditional aims of cost containment, equity, health outcomes and quality/service (Søgård 2004; Glenngård et al. 2005; Johnsen 2006; OECD 2007; Strandberg-Larsen et al. 2007; Danish Ministry for Health and Prevention 2008; Vuorenkoski 2008). Yet, in both the public debate and in various expert assessments throughout the 1990s and early 2000s, one can also find country-specific indications of shortcomings in performance in the four countries. In the Norwegian case, there had been a strong concern with the lack of economic steering capacity from the state level, and the recurrent budget overruns. This led to discussion of financing and state takeover during the 1990s, and the gradual implementation of an activity-based financing (ABF) system during the late 1990s. Unease about the national steering capabilities has also been a factor in Sweden, Finland and Denmark, leading to various gradual reforms in all three countries. Most of these reforms have been decided and implemented in dialogue between state and regional actors. Examples include the introduction of hospital choice for patients in Norway, Denmark and Sweden; experiments with purchaser–provider splits and internal contracting in Sweden and Denmark; and the introduction of diagnosis-related group (DRG) pricing and activity assessments in all four countries. Quality has been another important issue in the period since the early 1990s. This is particularly evident in Denmark, where relatively low life expectancies and a poor rating in *The World Health Report 2000* (World Health Organization 2000) sparked ongoing debates on quality and performance issues.

The longer and more detailed answer is thus that a number of tensions and national formulations of problems can be identified. At different points, this led to the formulation of structural reforms as potential answers to economic steering, coordination and quality issues. As a result, structural reforms became policy solutions to which a number of existing problems were attached. Waiting times, coordination, quality and the sustainability of current financing mechanisms have been important topics in all four countries.

In more theoretical terms, the answer is thus that the question cannot be answered in a simple manner. Performance issues in relatively well-functioning systems are always subject to political interpretation, as are the potential benefits and drawbacks of large-scale administrative reforms that affect many policy sectors and activities simultaneously, and where uncertainties of implementation are an inherent part. Causal linkages between institutional structures and performance (on multiple dimensions) are hard to establish and the politics of structural reform will, therefore, be a process of building plausible arguments based on the best available information and more or less clear ideas of the linkages between structure and performance. The problem is further complicated by the fact that health system objectives are multiple, and several competing objectives will emerge over time. Such uncertainties and interpretational contentions have led the Nordic countries to adapt gradual reform paths in the past, usually after negotiation processes between state, regions and various other stakeholders such as medical professions and patient organizations. This incremental policy style has worked relatively well, yet various performance issues have remained on the political agenda leading up to the structural reform processes in the four countries. Reform proponents have also applied an argumentation for reforms, based on a need to prepare for *future* challenges (e.g. the Danish Structural Commission). The assumptions about future challenges rest on the type of arguments we typically find in the general literature on the welfare state. These arguments are presented in more detail below. The short version is that a combination of globalization pressures with internal developments has created important changes in the functional conditions for the welfare states. Improving efficiency by creating larger and more specialized units has been seen as part of the answer to such challenges. Larger units are also seen as a necessity for improving quality and securing the best use of new medical technology developments. This is, in many ways, a specific Nordic issue because of small populations, sparsely populated areas (at least in Norway, Finland and Sweden) and a strong political tradition in favour of decentralization. Future problems are consequently a crucial part of the arguments for structural reforms in the Nordic area. Yet, they are combined with a number of nationally specific problems that have fuelled the policy process for structural reform. This will be discussed further below after a brief discussion of general challenges to the Nordic health systems by globalization and internal structural developments.

3.3 The combined challenges of globalization and domestic developments

Globalization trends affect the Nordic health systems in a number of ways, and the region is thus subject to many of the more general challenges and opportunities described in contemporary welfare state literature (Pierson 2001; Schwartz 2001). Advances in medical technology and the internationalization of knowledge and markets for health professionals, service concepts, drugs and equipment are particularly important factors. This changes the conditions for regional and national decision-making as local/national stakeholders become more aware of international trends, and the Nordic health systems have become more exposed to market forces for decision spheres that were previously sheltered and reserved for national/regional planning. This may entail benefits as local monopolies on labour supply and service delivery are challenged, but it also entails challenges for the national planning and prioritization ability.

The *internationalization of the knowledge base for medical practice* is therefore an important driver of changes. It specifically affects the Nordic health systems because of their tradition for regionalized decision-making. Regional variations in service delivery are increasingly contested by more general trends, and by stakeholders such as patients and professionals that refer to such international trends.

Professionals and patients have easier access to information on available practices in other countries. This creates a more informed basis for issuing political demands for access to the most recent treatments, and thus increases the pressure on the Nordic health systems, where political and professional decision-making used to be more uncontested.

The markets for pharmaceuticals and medical equipment are highly affected by globalization trends. This raises a number of regulatory concerns in order to secure the benefits of efficient international markets while at the same time safeguarding patient interest and securing research and development interest. European authorities have attempted to address such issues via regional regulation, such as the system for approving drugs in the EU. *Europeanization* is consequently a more general attempt to impose a common European regulatory framework in response to globalization and other developments. It impacts on the Nordic health systems in several ways, as described in Chapter 14.

The external factors of globalization and Europeanization are interacting with, and to some extent reinforced by, *internal factors* such as ageing of populations, changing epidemiological profiles, reductions in the revenue potential from taxation and increasing demands for individualized services. Ageing populations and changing epidemiological profiles (e.g. with higher prevalence of diabetes, heart diseases and cancer) are two major factors. The ageing populations also mean that the recruiting base for health personnel will change in

Table 3.1 Developments in health expenditures in the four countries

Country	Average annual growth in health expenditure per citizen (%)			
	1970–80	*1980–90*	*1990–2000*	*2000–06*
Finland	4.7	4.7	0.6	5.3
Sweden	4.4	3.1	4.1	4.3
Denmark	3.2	1.3	2.1	3.8
Norway	9	3.1	4.1	2.1

Source: OECD Health Database 2008.

the future. This is a major concern throughout the welfare sectors of the Nordic countries.

Cultural changes in the perception of citizen roles and the interaction between citizens and the public sector are also contributing to a general increase in demand for services, and for costly individualized high-technology services in particular. Rising education levels, changing family structures and urbanization trends contribute to such cultural changes affecting the demand structure.

The internal factors are interrelated and lead to upward pressure on the demand for health services, while at the same time posing challenges for financing and delivering health care. Ageing populations reduce the potential for raising revenue through income taxation in the future. These limitations in taxation potential are further reinforced by competitive pressures on local industry and the generally lower productivity growth in service sectors compared with the manufacturing sectors (Schwartz 2001).

An illustration of the political limitations of financing via taxation is the fact that both Denmark and Norway have had strong 'anti-taxation' views represented in their parliaments and that the current governments in Denmark and Sweden have maintained a 'tax stop' since they came into power. The political anti-taxation sentiments are paralleled by many, but not all voices in the economic advisory community.

Obviously the timing and importance of the globalization and structural changes have varied across the Nordic countries. This is partly because of differences in the linkages to the international economy. The Finnish economy suffered a serious economic crisis in the early 1990s after the downfall of the Soviet empire. The macroeconomic downturn in the open and financially integrated Danish economy in the 1980s led to austerity policies and a relatively high degree of willingness to accept expenditure controls. The Swedish state managed to postpone the impact of welfare state challenges until the 1990s, inter alia by pursuing more active labour market policies. The Norwegian and to some extend Danish economies have benefited from increasing revenues from oil and gas resources in the North Sea during the 1990s and 2000s. Table 3.1 illustrates developments in health expenditures in the four countries. It can be seen that particularly the Danish and the Finnish health sectors have experienced severe reductions in growth rates in the 1980s and 1990s, respectively.

3.4 National formulations of problems and policy options

The translation of general welfare state pressures into national formulations of problems and policy options has thus taken slightly different forms.

Lidström and Eklund (2007) mention the replacement of Keynesianism with monetarism and neo-liberalism, a gradual value shift from collectivism to individualism and a reemergence of nationalist/regionalist values and demands for territorial self-government as important ideational drivers for structural reform in Sweden. Although such trends can certainly also be observed in the other Nordic countries, they are less uniform than indicated. A better way to understand the developments may be as a series of ongoing tensions between several different value positions. Some of the most important value tensions include:

- neo-liberalism and markets versus collective welfare state solutions and democratic management
- choice and individualism versus equity
- decentralization versus geographical equity
- local democracy and participation versus centralization and control
- efficiency through local management versus efficiency through economies of scale
- quality through national standards and monitoring versus quality through locally adjusted solutions.

These tensions can be found in health policy formulations in all the Nordic countries, with different actors taking different positions. Each country thus displays a unique combination of emphasis at given points in time. In terms of specific national formulations, it appears that the Swedish reform proponents, in addition to ideas of enhancing efficiency through economies of scale and specialization, particularly emphasize two sets of ideas (Feltenius 2007). First, Sweden emphasized adjusting to Europeanization and particularly the notion of the 'Europe of Regions'. It was argued that larger regions with better coordination of business promotion and infrastructure were needed to get the full benefit of the EU membership. Second, renewed importance was given to the principle of equality of welfare provision. Apparently, the governmental actors found that the rather high degree of autonomy for Swedish counties/regions and municipalities had led to some differentiation in solutions and service levels in different parts of the country. The economic recession had exacerbated this problem as not all decentralized units were able to afford the same service level (Feltenius 2007). As in Denmark and Norway, this led to a reaction in terms of ideas that the state should guarantee a certain level of uniformity. Legislation on choice and waiting times were one set of state responses. Structural reform aiming at creating more uniform regional units and to strengthen the relative power of the state has been another part of the answer.

The Norwegian reform in 2002 appears to have been driven by an identification of several different problem areas. Unclear boundaries between counties and state, leading to ongoing 'blame games', budget overruns and reduced legitimacy for the county units are mentioned as particularly important (Stigen 2005, p. 18). Solution ideas were found in the concept of the 'new public management' (NPM) combined with experiences of autonomous organizational forms in the Norwegian public sector (e.g. Telenor and Statoil in the 1990s and 1970s) (Stigen 2005, p. 20). The dominant ideas in NPM were decentralization and the promotion of entrepreneurial management through separation from direct political management (Hagen and Kaarbøe 2006; Magnussen et al. 2007).

Danish reforms were based on perceptions at a national level of coordination problems across the public administration levels, and the idea that larger units would provide economies of scale in both administration and service delivery. This was supposed to lead to greater efficiency and better quality. There was also a concern that some municipalities and counties were unable to deliver services at an adequate level, or would be in the future. It appears that the previous trust in local democracy was eroding, at least at the national political level. Industry representatives argued that fewer administrative levels would imply less bureaucracy, and conservative politicians argued that the elimination of the middle taxation level would make it easier to control taxes.

The Finish reform process was based on rearticulation of two long-standing issues (Sandberg 2007, 2009). The first issue was that Finland, unlike the other three Nordic countries, had chosen to rely on intermunicipal cooperative structures rather than regional structures with direct elections. The second issue was the correct number and size of municipalities. Finland had maintained a very high number of municipalities throughout the period. A government proposal in 1965 suggested that the appropriate size would be approximately 8000 inhabitants, but many remained much smaller. There were some voluntary amalgamations (from 546 to 464) in the period from 1964 to 1977, partly in response to a reform decision in 1970, which introduced incentives for voluntary amalgamations. Municipalities of less than 8000 inhabitants that did not want to amalgamate were obliged to enter intermunicipal cooperation structures for secondary schools and health care. The reform process started in 2005. The government articulated a concern for the financial and quality-related sustainability of the municipalities and municipal cooperative structures. It also introduced a reorientation in reform strategy, as the voluntary and piecemeal approach was considered ineffective (Sandberg 2009).

Key issues and problem areas behind the governmental reform proposals in the four countries are summarized in Table 3.2.

Summing up, it appears that there was limited evidence for severe and acute crisis in the Nordic health systems that could trigger major structural reforms. Yet, a concern for future challenges and a number of country-specific performance issues can be identified. The severity of these challenges at the present time is subject to political interpretation but there is general agreement that the combination of ageing populations, increased technological possibilities and reduced financing potential in the public sector is problematic in the longer term. The challenges have been translated into different formulations of problems and policy ideas in the four countries based on the specific national conditions. We can therefore identify variations in the underlying arguments for reform, but we can also see a number of common traits.

To understand why radical reform decisions were implemented in two of the four countries (Denmark and Norway), while a more voluntary approach was chosen in Sweden and Finland, we need to look further at the actors, and their strategic options. The first part of the analysis looks at the strategic position of

Table 3.2 Key issues and problem areas behind Nordic government reform proposals

	Denmark	Norway	Sweden	Finland
Performance (efficiency and quality)	Concerns for the sustainability of small regions and municipalities particularly in terms of quality	Concerns for continued budget overruns and state–regional tensions	Concerns for differences in quality across regions: weak or differential implementation of some national initiatives	Concern for the sustainability of the many small municipalities and the intermunicipal cooperative structures in terms of financing and quality
	Issues of coordination problems and perverse incentives in 'grey zones' between different administrative and service delivery organizations	Specialization and 'economies of scale'	Specialization and 'economies of scale'	Specialization and 'economies of scale'
	Specialization and 'economies of scale'	NPM ideas of decentralization and entrepreneurship via creation of autonomous health regions run by boards rather than elected politicians		
	Incentives (municipal co-financing, ABF) and state control	Separation of purchaser and provider functions and extensive use of ABF; note, ABF started in 1997, 5 years prior to the reform: these are two very separate issues		
	Reducing emphasis on local democratic participation			
	Reducing the administrative costs by slimming the regional bureaucracy			

(Continued Overleaf)

Table 3.2 Continued

	Denmark	Norway	Sweden	Finland
Equity	Reduced acceptance of regional differences in service delivery	Reduced acceptance of regional differences in service delivery	Reduced acceptance of regional differences in service delivery	Reduced acceptance of geographical differences in delivery
State–region–municipality relations	Larger regions and stronger role for municipalities in health care intended to improve coordination across levels Strengthening the role of state in terms of financing, standard setting, monitoring and organizational issues	Separation of politics (at the state level) and management by autonomous regional health authorities Regional politics and preservation of equality between regions (east, south, middle, west, north) as an underlying condition	Strengthening the role of the state in health policy to overcome issues of implementation failure Long-term trend of urbanization (and migration from north to south) was undermining sustainability of some regions/municipalities	State level dissatisfaction with slow progress of the voluntary and piecemeal amalgamation process Long-term trend of urbanization and migration from north to south was gradually undermining the sustainability of some local administrations
National/regional competitiveness	Eliminating the regional tax level to improve possibilities for reducing overall taxation		Regional development and 'regions in Europe' perspective	Regional development

ABF, activity based financing, NPM, new public management.

the government, since major structural reforms are typically initiated top-down. The second part of the analysis looks at the opposing political forces in the four countries.

3.5 Government actors and their strategic position

Launching and implementing complex structural reforms is a particularly challenging policy task that involves a number of different actors and arenas (Scharpf 1997). An analytical discussion can be made between the parliamentary arena, the multilevel governance arena and the implementation arena.

3.5.1 *The parliamentary arena*

The parliamentary arena is the stage for formal political decision-making by nationally elected politicians. Party politics and ideology are important here. The government is a main actor but typically has to negotiate policies with opposition members of parliament. The rules of the negotiation game depend on the type of government and particularly whether the government is made up of a single party or a coalition, and whether it commands a stable majority in parliament or has to negotiate from issue to issue. An important aspect of the parliamentary game is consequently the ability to build supportive coalitions.

The relationship between national politicians and voters is another main dimension in the parliamentary arena. Politicians depend on popular support to maintain power and enact policies. Policies aimed to adjust or cut back welfare services are likely to be unpopular, and politicians proposing such policies normally have good reason to fear the reaction of voters at the next election. Framing of the structural reform initiatives is, therefore, of crucial importance if voters are to be convinced. Timing is another important dimension. Although governments are important in setting the policy agenda, they are not fully able to control how and when the issues enter the agenda.

3.5.2 *Multilevel governance arena*

The broader multilevel governance and interest organization arena is particularly important in the decentralized Nordic health systems. It is important for both agenda setting and developing support for policy decisions. The decentralized Nordic health systems have been dominated by relatively autonomous regions and municipalities with their own democratic decision bodies. Extensive responsibilities for organizing, delivering and financing health services have been decentralized to regions (Denmark, Norway and Sweden) and municipalities (Finland). This has naturally led to a strong position for the counties/regions and their interest organizations (kommunenes sentralforbund, amtsrådsforeningen, landstingsforbundet, Kuntaliitto) in health policy-making. Acceptance or rejection by regions/municipalities could traditionally facilitate or hinder policies, although obviously it has been a situation of give and take, where negotiation strategies, compromises and cooperation have been the dominant picture. This can best be understood by viewing the multilevel arena as a series of repeated games where the behaviour in previous games influences the negotiation climate for subsequent games. Both sides have an interest in maintaining a reasonable working climate in order to continue to have influence, and none of the participants can dominate the game all the time. Another important aspect of the game is that political parties are typically represented at both the national and decentralized levels. The implication is that parties may have split interests in structural changes. Local mayors might loose their position in case of amalgamation, and their power will be reduced if tasks are moved. Such internal divisions of interests particularly between rural and urban flanks have previously hindered reform, for example in Finland and Denmark.

A number of organized interest groups are active in health care. Health professionals (doctors and nurses) and their unions are important for policy development because of their specialized knowledge and central position in policy implementation. Policy-makers are dependent upon the skills and knowledge of professionals for designing and implementing policies and, therefore, have to provide a voice to these groups in the policy-making process. In spite of their importance in policy-making, it appears that the relative strength of different professional groups has changed over time. Medical doctors' associations used to be very dominant and represented a strong veto power in policy-making. This has gradually changed as more professional groups have entered the stage, and as the legitimacy of professional power in health governance matters has increasingly been questioned. The current picture is consequently more diverse, but still with a strong position for medical professionals. The mutual dependency and relative integration of professions and state in the Nordic countries has deep historical roots (Berg 1987; Jespersen 2005). It can be interpreted as a Nordic institutionalization of the basic contract, where the state guarantees a relative autonomy and a monopoly on employment while the profession, in return, provides crucial assistance in the practical prioritization and rationing of services (Blank and Burau 2004). The general picture with regards to the structural reform processes is that the professions have expressed limited direct concerns for what has essentially been seen as administrative matters. Yet, as the consequences in terms of hospital reorganizations have become more manifest in the implementation phase, there has been stronger input from health professions.

Broader interest organizations such as general industry and unions are not directly involved in financing and managing the health systems in the Nordic countries. This means that they have less direct influence than in countries like Germany with social health insurance. Yet, unions and employers typically play a more indirect role through political parties, or by attempts to influence the health policy agenda. Generally, both employers and unions have supported the universal health systems, although industry associations in recent years have also promoted the interests of the private health deliverers. In terms of structural reforms, it appears that industry interests, at least in Denmark, have been active in pushing reform on to the agenda, based on arguments of reducing the administrative burdens and facilitating tax cuts by streamlining the administrative structures (Christiansen and Klitgaard 2008).

3.5.3 The implementation arena

The implementation arena includes some of the same key actors but relates to the implementation phase of the policy process where policies are translated into behavioural practices by the actors in the field.

The decentralized authorities (regions and municipalities), hospital managers, health professionals and unions are all important in this translation process. All of these actors are linked to networks of other delivery organizations and civil society organizations such as patient interest groups. Any government wanting to implement unpopular decisions must first consider the potential for open or tacit resistance in the networks and organizations of key actors in the field.

One way to minimize the risk of implementation failure is to carefully consider the mix of regulatory instruments to get the most appropriate mix of 'sticks' (sanctions), 'carrots' (incentives/rewards) and 'sermons' (information/ persuasion) (Baldwin and Cave 1999; Vedung 2003). Although the Nordic countries are similar in many ways, there are also differences in what is considered to be the appropriate mix of regulatory measures.

The concepts of actors/arenas can be used to further analyse similarities and differences in the reform processes in the four countries. The analysis will point to key issues, while details of the parliamentary processes in all four countries cannot be presented in the limited space available.

3.6 Similarities and differences in the actor/arena constellations for reform

The specific country processes in the three arenas are discussed below and summarized in Table 3.3.

Norway

The parliamentary political process behind the Norwegian reform was rapid. It took one year from initial proposal in parliament to a decision. An important background was a shift of position within the Social Democratic Party. The party initially opposed the reform idea but changed its view to promote reform in spite of internal opposition. The reform decision was therefore made under the Social Democratic Stoltenberg Government in 2000. It was supported by the Conservative Party and the Progress Party, which had been in favour of removing the county level and creating a combination of state ownership and autonomous health enterprises for a number of years (Stigen 2005, p. 21).

The change within in the Social Democratic Party was fuelled by a frustration at the national level over the ongoing 'blame games' and budget overruns. There was a tendency for local problems to escalate to the national level in spite of the decentralized structure. One reason for this was the division of financing and delivery responsibilities. Centralized funding and decentralized decision-making can create accountability issues and 'blame games'. This can be addressed by aligning decentralized decisions with decentralized funding (i.e. benefit

Table 3.3 Country processes for launching and implementing structural reforms

	Denmark	Norway	Sweden	Finland
Parliamentary arena	Reform proposed by liberal/conservative government and supported by the Danish Peoples Party to create a relatively narrow majority for the reform decision; decision opposed by the Social Democrats Leadership of the liberal government party overruled the local level voices in the process	Reform proposed and decided by Social DemocraticParty in government; supported by the Conservative Party and the Progress Party Social Democratic leadership overruled the local level voices in the process	Reform process initiated by Social Democratic Party in government Committee on Public Sector Responsibilities recommended larger regions, but the conservative government settled for a process of voluntary mergers	Reform process initiated by coalition of Centre Party and Social Democrats; this was facilitated by a change in the internal power structure of the Centre Party (from rural to urban) A government commission presented a range of models for reform, and a broad compromise was struck between the government and opposition parties on a 'strong municipality' model without regions, and a voluntary reform process

Multilevel governance arena	Counties and Association of County Councils were opposed to reform but limited parliamentary support behind the counties

Municipalities were split, but largely supported the reform, as it became clear that they would gain importance in terms of tasks and responsibilities previously located at the county level

The state had gradually increased its role in health policy throughout the 1990s. Reforms initiated from this position of de facto change in relative power. | Opposing interests: counties and Association of County Councils; there was limited parliamentary support behind the counties

Stronger state position but 'blame games' and soft budget issues remain | Opposing interests: counties and Association of County Councils

Organization of the policy process enabled opposing interests to gather support and this led to a voluntary and bottom-up process | The interest organization of the municipalities was active in initiating the process, but supported a 'strong municipalities' solution with larger units, rather than a 'regionalization' or 'nationalization' model |
| Implementation phase | Relatively rapid implementation process

Top-down management of reform process, with some room for voluntary municipal mergers

Regions are currently in the process of adjusting the hospital systems | Relatively rapid implementation process

Top-down management

Political contention over the reform outcomes have led to adjustment and reinstatement of politically appointed management at the regional level | Voluntary merging (or non-merging) of counties into regions | Voluntary amalgamations in 2008–2013, supported by financial incentives

Forced participation in intermunicipal cooperation structures if not part of amalgamation

Government may intervene to force amalgamations after evaluation in 2009 |

taxation, or at least tax discretion). In the Norwegian system, this was not the case. Another reason was the relatively strong sentiments about regional and local service provision in Norway, based on geographical and historical conditions (Byrkjeflot and Neby 2005). The willingness to experiment with new organizational forms was also supported by the strong macroeconomic situation based on oil revenues. This probably made it difficult, on the one hand, to impose austerity programmes and control the counties, while on the other hand it made it less risky to experiment with new steering forms. The specific configuration of the multilevel governance arena in Norway and the macroeconomic situation has played a role in the pathway chosen.

In terms of implementation, it appears that the reform has not solved all the problems it was designed to address (Magnussen et al. 2007). Local issues continue to surface on national agenda. In addition, the creation of semi-independent health enterprises has not sheltered the political level (Opedal and Rommetvedt 2005; Nerland 2007). Structural adjustment (closing local hospitals) remains difficult, and geographical equity has remained a key policy issue. All regions have had economic problems, which has led to excessive soft budgeting from the state. Such issues have led to subsequent adjustments of the reform components.

Denmark

The process behind the Danish reform of 2007 was also relatively rapid. A government commission was established in the fall of 2002 by the Liberal/Conservative Government. It presented its main conclusion in January 2004. The commission concluded that structural change was needed and presented a number of different options for the politicians. Reading between the lines, it was clear that the commission, which had been dominated by ministry representatives, supported a reform comprising larger municipalities, fewer regions and more state power (Bundgård and Vrangbæk 2007). A final agreement was made by a relatively slim majority consisting of the government and the Danish People's Party in June 2004. The government had failed to get support from the Social Democrats and other opposition parties, thus breaching a long-standing tradition for broad support behind major structural reforms in Denmark.

The reform was fuelled by a combination of personal ambitions from strong government politicians and a frustration at national level over the inability to enforce policies on counties. The counties were perceived as 'foot-dragging' in regards to government reform ideas. This had led to a gradual increase in the level of state intervention via formal legislation and detailed budget agreements during the 1990s. Yet national politicians still perceived a need to demonstrate an ability to 'handle health care' to the voting population. The structural reform was, therefore, linked to tough rhetoric against the counties and to general rhetoric of 'economies of scale' through mergers and specialization (Bundgård and Vrangbæk 2007; Christiansen and Klitgaard 2008).

An internal shift in political power and attitudes in the major government party (Venstre) made the reform process possible. Powerful and ambitious actors at the state level managed to turn the party away from a decentralist, local democracy orientation, which was backed by the many Venstre mayors throughout the country. The party 'crown prince' (and current Prime Minister), Mr Løkke Rasmussen, was a very important player in this process. The parliamentary process was made easier by a weak and scattered opposition and limited political support for the counties. The smaller government coalition party (the Conservative Party) and the government support party (Danish People's Party) had been in favour of a state take-over of health care for a number of years.

The management of the policy process was probably also instrumental in getting the reform decision pushed through (Bundgaard and Vrangbæk 2007; Christiansen and Klitgaard 2008). It has been suggested that the structuring of the commission process, on the one hand, led the county opposition to assume that their voice would be heard, and on the other hand shrouded the process in a 'veil of vagueness' regarding the true preferences of the government until it was too late to mobilize other forces (Christiansen and Klitgaard 2008). The counties wrongly based their strategy on the assumption that the government would follow the general norm of seeking a broad majority across the centre for major structural reform. This norm had in previous instances led to blockage of reform attempts.

The implementation process was also fairly rapid. Municipalities were forced into 'voluntary' mergers (i.e. they could choose who to amalgamate with), while the institutional conditions for municipalities that refused to merge made this stance practically impossible. The previous counties were merged into five regions with responsibility for health care and regional development. The municipalities gained a larger role in health care and became coresponsible for financing via municipal contributions. The idea behind this was to create incentives for better coordination and stronger municipal public health efforts. The regions are currently in the process of making structural adjustments to their health systems. Hospital departments are merged and closed down and decisions are being made on new hospital infrastructure.

The regions are generally perceived to be under pressure to deliver on structural changes and providing services within budget. The Conservative Party and the Danish People's Party have already threatened to dismantle the regions if they fail. Ironically, the regions may also become irrelevant if they succeed in the difficult task of making structural adjustments. Consequently, many observers see the regions as a temporary solution en route to a more centralized system. In any case, their margin for failure seems very limited, and their scope for decision-making on economic issues (taxation) has been eliminated

Sweden

The Swedish reform process has been longer and less streamlined than in Denmark and Norway. A precursor for the reform was the establishment in 1997 of two experimental regions (Skåne and Västra Götaland) by the Social Democratic Government based on recommendations by 'the Regions Committee' in 1995. These experiments were evaluated in 2000 by the PARK Committee, which concluded that the experiment appeared to work well, although it was still too early for a full evaluation (Feltenius 2007, p. 462). This evaluation and a tendency for gradually stronger state intervention in municipal management led to a demand for a broader investigation of public sector responsibilities. The Social Democratic Government, therefore, set the mandate for the 'Committee on Public Sector Responsibilities' in January 2003. Unlike the Danish situation, the Swedish Government decided to include politicians and to have a fairly extensive process with an interim report as well as involvement of external experts along the way. This meant that the process was less controllable by the government than in the Danish process. The final report from the commission came in 2007. Its most important proposal was that the existing organization with county councils should be replaced by regional bodies covering a larger territory following the experiments in Skåne and Västra Götaland (Feltenius 2007, p. 469). The report did not specify an exact number of regions, but somewhere between six and nine was considered appropriate. The regions were to have responsibility for health care and regional development. They were supposed to be in place by 2010. The committee also suggested a formalization of the deliberations between state and the decentralized authorities to replace the existing informal meetings. This would bring the relations between the state and decentralized authorities more in line with the Danish situation.

A change of government took place in 2006, where the Conservative Party (Moderaterna) replaced the Social Democrats, who had been in power for the past decade. The new Prime Minister Fredrik Reinfeldt declared that he was 'sceptical' about the proposition to create larger regions (Feltenius 2007, p.470), and in 2007 it became clear that this view was shared by the other government parties. They did not support a reform dictated from above, only a reform derived from bottom-up initiatives. The creation of larger regions thus became voluntary.

The Swedish case can be interpreted as a reflection of political/administrative traditions for long and careful deliberation of reforms. It also reflects a situation with a comparatively stronger position of regions and the regional interest organization (landstingsforbundet) compared with other Nordic countries. This has led to more agreement-based policies in the Swedish case, with stronger veto options for regions. An illustration of this can be found in patient choice regulations, where voluntary agreements were chosen instead of legislation as is the case in Norway and Denmark. The result appears to have been a more hesitant implementation by the counties (Winblad 2003). It should also be noted that Sweden already had established six large medical care regions, within which the county councils cooperated to provide the population with highly specialized care. The need for a full-scale reorganization may therefore have been more limited, although the reliance on 'medical regions' can also be seen as a further illustration of the strength of the counties to avoid more comprehensive amalgamations.

In conclusion it appears that the relatively strong position for Swedish county councils combined with particular circumstances in the parliamentary arena in the period led to a structural reform based on voluntary implementation and acceptance of diversity in institutional forms.

Finland

The Finnish reform process was rooted in recurring discussions concerning administrative size since independence in 1917. Unlike the other Nordic countries, Finland did not implement a major amalgamation reform in the early 1970s to establish larger municipalities and a regional level. Instead, a process of voluntary amalgamations supported by national incentives, and forced introduction of intermunicipal cooperation for health care, was commenced. The relatively slow progress of this voluntary and piecemeal approach led governmental actors to initiate a new reform process in 2005. The new reform process was unusual in several regards (Sandberg 2009). First, the government coalition of the Centre Party and Social Democrats was seen as the least likely to introduce comprehensive reform. While the Social Democrats had traditionally supported centralization, the Centre Party with its strong presence in local democracies, and a very strong traditional rural flank, had been firmly opposed to any attempts to forced changes in the administrative structure. Second, the reform represented a more comprehensive and top-down approach to reform than previously seen. This surprising reform initiative can be explained by several political factors (Sandberg 2009). First, movement of political power had taken place from rural to urban areas and from north to south. This had led to a reorientation of the Centre Party, particularly from 2003 and onwards. The change was also fuelled by general demographic and urbanization developments and by reorientations after the financial crisis in the 1990s and the membership of the EU in 1995. Second, the local government interest representation had been amalgamated into one organization, as had been the case for some time in the other Nordic countries. Within the Association of Finnish Local Authorities (AFLA; now Association for Local and Regional Authorities (Kuntaliitto)), there had been a shift in power from smaller to larger municipalities, and the AFLA was a particularly important actor in setting the process in motion by its approach to the government in 2004 with an initiative for a parliamentary investigation of the local government structure. Inspired by the Danish reform, the government started the process, despite the fact that reform had not been on the governmental agenda presented in 2003. The amalgamation and new direction of the AFLA implied fewer possibilities for blocking alliances between national level parties and the different interest organizations and thus a more manageable reform process for the government. The third factor promoting the reform was the use of new reform strategies with more rapid processes and closer control of the preparatory work by the government. The emphasis on dialogue with the decentralized actors was maintained, but now with more willingness to steer the process by top-down management and the use of incentives. A compromise reform decision was reached between the government and the opposition in 2007. The main ingredients in the reform were that all municipalities were obliged to submit a detailed plan for the local implementation of the reform (i.e. amalgamation or not) by August 2007. Amalgamations were supported by financial incentives, and municipalities that chose not to amalgamate would have to transfer the responsibility for social services and primary health care to joint municipal bodies covering at least 20,000 inhabitants. Municipalities of 16 urban areas had to present plans for future development of transports, zoning and local government service. The implementation of the reform was to run from 2008 to 2013. The government signalled an intention to evaluate progress in 2009, and possibly introduce more top-down management if the voluntary process once again were to prove insufficient.

3.7 Management of the policy process

The management of the policy process was mentioned as an independent factor that might facilitate structural reforms. Governments need to persuade actors about the benefits of reform, and to neutralize possible opposition. That policy management is important in reform processes is intuitively obvious. Yet in empirical terms, it can be very difficult to trace the process decisions and their relationship to actor strategies. There are several reasons for this. First, strategies are not always openly formulated, as this would reveal preferences to possible opponents and weaken the negotiation position. Second, strategies might change over time, and in hindsight actors are likely to try to portray their own role in the most positive light. There are, therefore, obvious limitations to how detailed we can get in our presentation, and how sure we can be of the results. Nevertheless, a number of interesting differences in process dimensions appear when looking across the four countries. First, it appears that the relatively tightly controlled processes in Denmark and Norway provided benefits for these governments in being able to push the reforms through. Note that the Stoltenberg Government was overturned before the reform was implemented and it was a centre/conservative government implementing the reform. It appears that the Danish Government strategically controlled the timing and dissemination of information, and that it delayed the presentation of its preferences to the last possible moment in order to reduce the strategic options for the county interests (Christiansen and Klitgaard 2008). The Danish Government also surprised the potential opponents by not living up to traditional norms of seeking a broad parliamentary backing for this type of reform. The stable majority with the Danish Peoples Party made it possible to disregard this norm, and the relatively weak parliamentary opposition reduced the potential future costs of pursuing such a strategy.

The Finnish case also highlights the importance of process management. Compared with previous reform attempts, the 2005 reform process was organized with a more rapid preparation phase, which was closely controlled by the government. Similar to the Danish case, the Finnish Government organized the preparatory work without parliamentary appointed politicians. The government also used a more top-down approach than in previous periods, with a combination of 'sticks' and 'carrots' to induce municipalities into amalgamation. The 'sticks' included the overt threat of government intervention after 2009 if the voluntary process proved unsatisfactory.

The Swedish process, in contrast, implied lengthy commission work with both political and administrative actors, and with many opportunities for opponents to influence the process and provide information. This meant that it was easier for the counties and related interests to mobilize opposition to the reform. It also meant that the political landscape shifted during the process, and that the governmental actors that initiated the process were succeeded by other and less-committed actors while the commission was working. All in all, this led to a more open decision process, and finally to a less radical reform decision and more open implementation process.

3.8 Concluding remarks

Structural reforms have been on the agenda in all four countries, although the outcomes of the political processes have been different. Health care has been a crucial element in the discussions in all four countries and the reforms have been promoted as ways to secure the efficiency of the public health systems in the face of changing internal and external circumstances such as ageing populations, rapidly increasing technological possibilities and internationalization of markets for professionals, patients and service concepts. Denmark and Norway have implemented reforms following relatively fast and government-controlled processes. Sweden and Finland have had a longer period of consideration and both countries have ended up with a weaker reform decision based on voluntary mergers.

The answers to the questions raised in the introduction are, therefore, that a set of changes in internal and external circumstances have opened the discussion of how best to readjust the Nordic health systems. The reform processes have further been carried forward by a combination of functional arguments of economies of scale and specialization, and a number of political factors in the parliamentary and multilevel governance arenas. The combination of functional arguments and political circumstances created 'windows of opportunity' for change of formal structural regime since the late 1990s. As in the previous reform period in the early 1970s, there appears to have been a degree of cross-Nordic inspiration, which has contributed to the processes. The differences in national configurations of ideas, actors and arenas have led to somewhat different outcomes. In particular, it appears that the stronger traditions for bottom-up and piecemeal solutions in Finland and Sweden have been continued with the current reform decisions.

The coming years will show whether the chosen solutions are sustainable, or whether a phase of more volatility in structural parameters of the Nordic health systems will be entered. The Norwegian experience indicates that this could be the case. The differences in timing and content of the structural reforms potentially place the countries on different development paths for the future.

A number of specific points about health reform policies in the Nordic region can be drawn from the presentation. First, a concern for future sustainability in terms of financing, quality/service, skilled manpower and so on has been prominent in all four countries. Structural reform has been presented as one of the ways to respond to such challenges, although to some extent this has been based on hopes and aspirations rather than solid evidence. There is also an implicit hope that restructuring the administrative structures will help to facilitate adjustments of the delivery structure. This has been on the agenda in all four countries but it is a topic which has been notoriously hard to address. One of the reasons for the continued existence of a regional level is probably that state actors see it as expedient to have an intermediate political/administrative level to take the blame for tough readjustment decisions, closure of hospitals and other unpalatable decisions.

A second general observation is that coordination issues are at the forefront in all four countries. Coordination pertains to practical interaction across administrative and organizational levels in delivering health care. The aspiration of the structural reform is to facilitate such coordination by creating larger functional units under the same administrative leadership. The Danish reform further addresses the coordination issue by introducing incentives for cooperation between municipalities and regions. Yet it seems obvious that functional coordination issues cannot be removed entirely as the reforms also create new relationships and divisions of responsibilities. Problems may, therefore, simply move to new relational settings. Coordination issues also relate to the overall aims and means across the different government levels. This is an issue that has sparked considerable tensions in recent years. On the one hand, politicians at the state level have been frustrated by the lack of budget compliance (particularly in Norway) and with the occasionally slow and differential implementation of policy measures across regions/municipalities. Regional and local politicians, on the other hand, have been frustrated by the increase in both quantity and quality of steering ambitions from the national level and have complained that these were not always accompanied by sufficient funding. Structural reforms have been presented as ways to create a better balance in the steering relationship between state and decentralized authorities. Yet success or failure is likely to depend on the practices that develop based on the structures. The Norwegian case illustrates that it is not easy to escape tensions by structural design. The conditions for the game may change somewhat, but the underlying issues and tensions remain and will have to be managed within the revised setting. Regarding coordination, primary health care in Norway is a municipal responsibility whereas the regional health enterprises are responsible for specialized health care. This leads to problems of coordination, which would be expected to be higher than in the other countries. Also there is fear that the reform will shift the balance of power more in favour of the regional health enterprises.

The increased national steering ambitions are related to a third general trend in the Nordic health systems, namely a reduced acceptance of geographical differences in service delivery. To rely on decentralized democracy for health service delivery is also to accept that the solutions chosen in different areas can be somewhat different. Previously, the decentralized democratic management was seen as a positive feature in the Nordic context, as local/regional democracies could adapt to local circumstances, provide testing grounds for local experiments, facilitate political participation and be a training ground for political actors. Such ideas are still present, but it appears that the pendulum has swung in favour of more state steering and less acceptance of the possible consequences of relying on decentralized democracy. More focus is now on the aspirations of efficiency gains through benefits of scale than on the potential benefits of participation, small-scale systems and proximity in decision processes and service delivery.

A fourth general observation is that the circumstances must be right for large-scale structural reform to take place. The differences in timing and outcome, and the failed attempts in both recent and distant past in several countries (e.g. Denmark and Finland), point in that direction. The necessary circumstances include a relatively strong and committed government and a weakening of the potential opposition both within and outside parliament. It is also necessary to manage the reform process in order to build a case for the necessity of the reform. All four countries have used preparatory committees, but it is important to note that there seems to have been a shift away from traditional slow-working general committees with parliamentary appointed politicians and experts, and towards a much more tightly controlled process where the government administration has the dominant role. Only Sweden has maintained the more traditional committee approach, and it is Sweden that has had the lengthiest process, and the least radical reform decision.

A fifth general observation is that in each country there was the argument that administrative costs may be reduced by having fewer administrative/political entities. Although some such benefits are likely, it is unclear exactly how big the potential is. There might also be diseconomies of scale in both production and administration as the control span becomes larger and the distance between decision-making and 'production' increases. Larger control span and greater distance from decision-makers tend to increase the need for coordination and control mechanisms. This may, in turn, lead to increases in administrative costs. The growth in evaluation and quality assessment technologies can be seen in this light. Nevertheless, the centralization idea harnesses powerful symbolic rhetoric from the wave of private sector mergers. It clearly serves the purpose of communicating the ability to act in accordance with commonly accepted wisdom in the voting population.

From a broader comparative perspective, it should be noted that the general features of universal coverage, tax funding and decentralized management have largely been maintained in all countries, although with important developments and differences in the distribution of tasks and rights.

The structural reforms can consequently be interpreted as continuations of the attempts to adjust to a number of internal and external challenges for the Nordic welfare states.

In political terms, the reforms can be interpreted as ways to shift power in the health policy arenas by eliminating some of the previous veto points in the decision process. Politicians at the national level in all Nordic countries have from time to time been frustrated by the lack of direct power over implementation and service delivery. The strong position of decentralized authorities has previously created veto points and a fairly slow, negotiated and consensus-based policy process. Such a process has advantages in taking detailed and complex information from 'the ground' into consideration, and not least in getting everybody to concur in the decisions. However, it can be more problematic when seen from the perspective of a national politician under pressure from the voters.

An additional political institutional aspect is that recentralization not only weakens veto points in the policy process but also creates better opportunities for pursuing competition strategies. Larger regions imply larger and potentially more attractive markets for private suppliers, which no longer have to adapt their service concepts to many small administrative units. The larger regions are also better equipped with legal and economic expertise to do contracting and follow-up on contracts.

Finally, in light of the globalization trends, we can also interpret the structural adjustments as functional attempts to adjust the Nordic systems to the regional structure in the EU and to the potential for more competitive pressure in terms of contracting out and movement of patients across borders. Larger units present a better fit with EU regionalization concepts and programmes. They also have a potential to provide more administrative capacity to deal with contracting, applications, lobbying and other matters.

References

Baldwin, R. and Cave, M. (1999) *Understanding Regulation: Theory, Strategy, and Practice*. Oxford: Oxford University Press.

Berg, O. (1987) *Medisinens logikk: studier i medisinens sosiologi og politikk*. Oslo: Oslo University Press.

Blank, R.H. and Burau, V. (2004) *Comparative Health Policy*. Houndsmills: Palgrave Macmillan.

Bundgaard, U. and Vrangbæk, K. (2007) Reform by coincidence? Explaining the policy process of structural reform in Denmark, *Scandinavian Political Studies* 30: 491–520.

Byrkjeflot, H. and Neby, S. (2005) Norge i Norden: fra etternøler til pioner i reformeringen af sykehussektoren, in Opedal, S. and Stigen, I.M. (eds) *Helse–Norge i Støpeskjeen: Søkelys på Sykehusreformen*. Bergen: Fagbokforlaget, pp. 47–62.

Christiansen, P.M. and Klitgaard, M.B. (2008) *Den utænkelige reform. Strukturreformens tilblivelse 2002–2005*. Odense: Syddansk Universitetsforlag [University Press of Southern Denmark].

Danish Ministry for Health and Prevention (Ministeriet for Sundhed og Forebyggelse) (2008) Det Danske sundhedsvæsen i internationalt perspektiv. [Danish Ministry Benchmarking report] Copenhagen: Government of Denmark; http://www.sum.dk/ IMEVEREST/Publications/imdk%20x2D%20dansk/SSTAT/SIT/international%20Sit/ 20080929201306/CurrentVersion/Det%20danske%20sundhedsvæsen%20i%20 internationalt%20perspektiv.pdf.

Feltenius, D. (2007) Relations between central and local government in Sweden during the 1990s: mixed patterns of centralization and decentralization, *Regional and Federal Studies* 17: 457–74.

Glenngård, A.H., Hjalte, F. Svensson, M. Anell, A. and Bankauskaite, V. (2005) Sweden: Health System Review. *Health Systems in Transition*, 7(4): 1–128.

Hagen, T.P. and Kaarbøe, O. (2006) The Norwegian hospital reform of 2002: central government takes over ownership of public hospitals, *Health Policy* 76: 320–33.

Jespersen, P.K. (2005) *Mellem profession og management: ledelse i danske sygehuse*. Copenhagen: Handelshøjskolens.

Johnsen, J.R. (2006) *Health Systems in Transition: Norway*. Copenhagen: WHO Regional Office for Europe on behalf of the European Observatory on Health Systems and Policies.

Knight, J. (1992) *Institutions and Social Conflict*. Cambridge: Cambridge University Press.

Lidström, A. and Eklund, N. (2007) Decentralisering eller maktdelning på allvar: vad är sannolikt i Sverige? in Karlson, N. and Nergelius, J. (eds) *Federalism på Svenska*. Stockholm: Ratio, pp. 165–99.

Magnussen, J., Hagen, T. and Kaarbøe, O. (2007) Centralized or decentralized? A case study of Norwegian hospital reform, *Social Science and Medicine* 64: 2129–37.

Nerland, S.M. (2007) *Effekter af sygehusreformen. Fire essay om mål og virkemidler i styringen af specialisthelsetjenestene.* Oslo: Faculty of Medicine, University of Oslo.

North, D.C. (1990) *Institutions, Institutional Change and Economic Performance.* Cambridge: Cambridge University Press.

OECD (2007) *Health Data 2008.* Paris: Organization for Economic Co-operation and Development.

Opedal, S. and Rommetvedt, H. (2005) Foretaksfrihet eller stortingstyring? in *Helse-Norge i støpeskjeen. Søkelys på sykehusreformen.* Bergen: Fakbokforlaget, pp. 64–85.

Pierson, P. (ed.) (2001) *The New Politics of the Welfare State.* Oxford: Oxford University Press.

Sandberg, S. (2007) En fråga om politisk logic: om forsaken at förstärka och omorganisera den regionale nivån i Finland och i Sverige på 1990-talet, in Karlson, N. and Nergelius, J. (eds) *Federalism på Svenska.* Stockholm: Ratio, pp. 128–64.

Sandberg, S. (2009) The art of the possible: territorial choice in Finland, in Baldersheim H. and Rose, L.L. (eds) *Territorial Choice: The Politics of Boundaries and Borders.* London: Palgrave & McMillan.

Scharpf, F. (1997) *Games Real Actors Play: Actor-centered Institutionalism in Policy Research.* Boulder, CO: Westview Press.

Schwartz, H. (2001) Round up the usual suspects! Globalization, domestic politics, and welfare state change, in Pierson, P. (ed.) *The New Politics of the Welfare State.* Oxford: Oxford University Press, pp.17–44.

Søgård, J. (2004) Om sundhedsvæsenet, in Bakka, J.F. and Petersen, U.H. (eds) *Hvorhen Danmark? Perspektiver på Kommunalreformen.* Copenhagen: Samfundslitteratur, pp.195–220.

Stigen, I. (2005) Innledning, in Opedal, S. and Stigen, I.M. (eds) *Helse–Norge i Støpeskjeen: Søkelys på Sykehusreformen.* Bergen: Fagbokforlaget, pp.15–25.

Strandberg-Larsen, M., Nielsen, M.B. Vallgårda, S., Krasnik, A., Vrangbæk, K. and Mossialos, E. (2007) Denmark: Health System Review. *Health Systems in Transition*, 9(6): 1–164.

Vedung, E. (2003) Policy instruments: typologies and theories, in Bemelmans-Videc, M.-L., Rist, R.C. and Vedung, E. (eds) *Sticks and Sermons: Policy Instruments and Their Evaluation.* New Brunswick, NJ: Transaction.

Vuorenkoski, L. (2008) Finland: Health System Review. *Health Systems in Transition*, 10(4): 1–168.

Winblad, S.U. (2003) *Från beslut till verklighet. Läkarnas roll vid implementeringen av valfrihetsreformer i hälso- och sjukvården. Avhandling.* Uppsala: Acta Universitatis Upsaliensis.

World Health Organization (2000) *The World Health Report 2000.* Geneva: World Health Organization.

chapter *four*

Looking forward: future policy issues

Richard B. Saltman and Karsten Vrangbæk

4.1 Common Nordic challenges

Nordic health systems have demonstrated a notably complex mix of stability and change over the past 20 years of reform. Chapter 1 presented a three-part framework that can help to explain how this mix has evolved (see Table 1.1). At the first level of goals and aspirations, there has been near rock-solid stability in Norway, Denmark, Sweden and Finland. Key values-based issues such as equity (both socioeconomic and geographic) and extensive public participation in government and decision-making continue to be central health sector touch-stones, even with recognition that their specific interpretation within countries has typically evolved over time.

At the second analytic level of basic health system architecture, the picture becomes a little more mixed. On the one hand, there has been fundamental stability in the broad overarching structures of funding (overwhelmingly tax based), governance (multilevel, public sector) and service delivery (public versus private providers) across all four countries. Moreover, these structures continue to be organized and managed by democratically elected and accountable bodies, consistent with the goal of public participation at the first level. On the other hand, there have also been several major changes in system governance. One structural change – from county to region in both Norway and Denmark – has reconstructed (Denmark) or shifted (Norway) the meso- or intermediate level of government. More far reaching has been the transfer in governmental responsibility for funding in Denmark (from intermediate to central government) and for ownership and operation of hospitals in Norway (also from intermediate to central government). Similarly, the shift of Sweden's 1992 ADEL Reform from county to municipal responsibility for both care and financing of the elderly involved a major institutional change. However, taken overall, these can be observed as shifts inside the basic structure of multilevel democracy, and so the balance at the second level has leaned more towards overall stability than towards change.

At the third level in the analytic framework, that of policy application, all four Nordic countries have seen major change. Numerous policy questions, including the degree of patient choice, the configuration of financial payment systems, the content and focus of primary care and public health initiatives, and the mix of state command-and-control with market-style management mechanisms, have all evolved considerably since the late 1980s. Moreover, these and other policy questions, again as noted in Chapter 1, often have developed in the four Nordic health systems in quite different directions and/or at quite different speeds. Consequently, at the third level, one can observe at least as much change as stability in the overall direction of Nordic health systems.

Taken together, this three-part framework suggests a central difficulty in proclaiming the existence of a uniform Nordic health care model. The changing patterns over time at levels two and three, as well as divergent strategies on particular issues adopted on level three across the four countries, limit structural commonalities to the existence of common aspirations and, to a degree, core institutional components. In addition, one can point to a common process-oriented form of decision-making, what is termed in Chapter 1 as the 'public negotiation model', with its emphasis on multilevel democracy and pragmatic solutions and which can be found in various forms in all four countries. Overall, while there are commonalities in the structural building blocks (objectives, institutional components) and in decision-making processes, the actual health system outcomes vary noticeably across the four countries, leaving little sense that there is a consistent Nordic model of how to construct a health care system.

Within these changing patterns and divergent strategies, moreover, there appears to be an intriguing shift in the focus of policy innovation among the four countries. In the early 1970s, when the central thrust of Nordic health reform was focused on developing publicly operated primary health centres, intended to improve both socioeconomic and geographical equity as well as reducing dependence on expensive hospital outpatient care, the focus of Nordic policy innovation was in Finland (1972 Primary Care Act) and Sweden (1973 Primary Care Act). Both countries succeeded over the next decade in shifting nearly all (Sweden) or a large portion (Finland) of first-contact clinical care into these primary health facilities. During that period, neither Denmark nor Norway was particularly interested in this new structural configuration of primary health care. While Denmark developed a small number of primary care centres in Copenhagen, most primary care remained in the hands of private GPs. Similarly, Norway continued with private GPs who provided services on contract to municipal governments.

In the late 1980s and early 1990s, when various purchaser–provider arrangements were introduced in an effort to stimulate market-style competition and, it was hoped, greater efficiencies within the public sector, as well as widening patient choice, again Sweden was the main innovator. In the early 1990s, a number of county councils developed and introduced their own planned market 'model' (Saltman and von Otter 1995). These models faced considerable resistance both conceptually (fearing market-style arrangements would harm equity and/or quality) and institutionally (organizational inertia). Moreover, as these reforms were being introduced during an economic recession, there was concern that market-style mechanisms were merely disguised means to reduce staff and close facilities (Harrison and Calltorp 2000). In part for these reasons, this reform impetus largely faded as the 1990s unfolded. During that time, also, there was minimal interest in these market-influenced reforms in either Finland or Denmark, and little real experimentation with these ideas in Norway.

By the start of the twenty-first century, renewed concerns about social and geographic equity, as well as continued pressures to improve efficiency and choice, had pushed innovative health policy thinking toward the centralization of political and fiscal authority into larger intermediate/regional and especially national governmental bodies (Saltman 2008). It was with this policy shift towards recentralization that the mantle of reform innovation in the Nordic region shifted to Norway (2002) and Denmark (2006). Norway adopted a 'big bang' approach in 2002, and Denmark followed in 2007, with a more comprehensive reform covering both regions and municipalities and after a slightly longer decision process. Both countries succeeded in implementing a major recentralization of their health system lines of authority.

From a Swedish and/or Finnish perspective, however, these recentralization pressures have run directly contrary to the generation-long process of decentralization in their health sectors, and consequently have evoked a complicated policy response. On the one hand, national governments in both countries share the same concerns about growing social and geographic inequity, as well as regional variations in service quality. There also was similar concern in Sweden and Finland that local government units (counties in Sweden; municipalities in Finland) were too small to meet coming health sector challenges either financially or managerially. On the other hand, these two countries both had a higher threshold before the national government could intervene in the decisions of local government, and such interventions tend to be based on carefully negotiated compacts in which county councils (Sweden) or municipalities (Finland) agree to the proposed changes.

The solution to these contradictory policy pressures has been that both countries have adopted a stronger national steering role, but one that is notably less sweeping than the major structural changes introduced in Norway and Denmark. In Sweden, national funds given to counties to develop specific services (e.g. the access and care guarantees in 2005) are now linked to performance on a negotiated set of indicators. Moreover, since 2007, certain high specialization services now require (as they did before the 1982 Health Services Act) operating permits from the National Board of Health and Welfare, which has begun to concentrate those services into only a few locations in order to safeguard both quality and expenditures. Services regulated in this manner to date include organ transplantation, eye cancer, paediatric surgery and treatment of severe burns, with additional services likely to be added in the near future. In Finland, an initial step toward reasserting a national role in sensitive service delivery issues was the introduction in 2005 of nationwide access guidelines. National policy-makers are currently establishing standards for certain municipally operated services including healthy child centres (staffing ratios and frequency of child visits) and elderly nursing home and home care services (S. Kokko, personal communication, 23 April 2009). In addition, in an effort to increase the size of local health-providing units, both Swedes and Finns point to the voluntary (in Sweden) and negotiated (in Finland) process of ongoing local-level consolidation into larger operating units (Section 4.3.5 below).

The less-interventionist postures of these two national governments reflect multiple factors, including the historical legitimacy and constitutionally protected role (Finland) and political strength (both Sweden and Finland) of local government. Further, it can be argued that the importance of multilevel democracy, if not of decentralization itself (e.g. of what is still the core Swedish and Finnish strategy), has been underscored by recent reform decisions that continue to support some forms of local political control in Denmark and Norway even as they centralize other elements. Denmark has maintained directly elected politicians as the leaders of its five new regional governments, and increased municipal responsibilities for prevention in addition to a wide range of other welfare services, while Norway revised its strategy after the start of the reforms by appointing local politicians to sit on the controlling boards of its five (now four) state-operated 'regional health enterprises'. Indeed, overall, the efficiency and effectiveness of the new recentralization strategy in Norway and Denmark has yet to be fully assessed (Saltman 2008).

Viewed overall, the fundamental question in all four countries can be interpreted as one of the appropriate mix and balance of decentralized and recentralized activities, with the general conclusion being that Sweden and Finland are also seeking to recentralize some health system activities, only fewer and by following a considerably different (slower and less imperative) path than that adopted by Norwegian and Danish policy-makers. This shifting pattern of stability and change, both substantively in terms of specific health reform strategies and nationally between countries, suggests two general observations. First, the impetus for innovation in Nordic health systems has undergone substantial evolution since the late 1980s. While reform activity has been a part of the policy picture throughout this period, the content of these reforms has shifted noticeably over time. Second, different countries have responded more strongly to different policy initiatives. Decentralized, publicly operated primary health care strongly motivated Swedish and Finnish reform, while, more than two decades later, recentralized national responsibility and creation of larger decentralized regions to improve efficiency and quality influenced Norwegian and Danish reform. Both points serve to highlight the degree of difference that can be found within Nordic health systems, and, again, the difficulty in describing a Nordic health model that moves beyond the most general level of goals and aspirations.

4.2 Accommodating a shifting context

The range of pressures that are currently pushing Nordic health policy-making, and that influence the future mix of stability and change, have been richly documented in Part II of this volume. Whether one looks within health systems at the pressure for more effective governance (Chapter 5), for more effective institutional management (Chapter 13), for greater patient choice (Chapter 6), for more professional autonomy (Chapter 7) or for more effective primary care (Chapter 11) and public health (Chapter 12), or outside health systems for persistent demands for more effective fiscal management (Chapter 8), greater diversity of providers (Chapter 9), greater equity of access and provision (Chapter 10) or the increasing intrusion of EU regulations and courts (Chapter 14), Nordic policy-makers face important challenges as they go forward. How likely is it, then, that the current balance of stability and change will shift in the near or medium term? How likely that the four countries will respond to what are relatively similar pressures in a relatively similar manner? Are there crucial factors in the differences among existing health sector structures, or of national history and culture, that will lead different Nordic countries down quite different reform paths? In short, even as these systems remain faithful to the same goals and aspirations, what will be the likely degree of similarity and difference between these four health care systems if one looks down the policy road five or ten years from today?

4.2.1 The economic context

The degree of policy-making freedom in Nordic health systems, as in all countries, is closely intertwined with the economic and political contexts within which that decision-making necessarily operates.

Turning to the economic context first, the overall condition of the national economy, as discussed in Chapters 2 and 3, inevitably influences the scope and character of the decision process within the health sector. When national economies are struggling, as was the case in Denmark in the 1980s, in Sweden and (especially) in Finland in the early 1990s, or in all four countries in early 2009 as this book goes to press, the range of near-term policy options in the health sector becomes heavily constrained. Conversely, when an economy has dramatic surpluses, for example from large-scale oil production, as in Norway since the 1980s, decision-making in the health sector, while still financially constrained in the short term, inevitably encompasses an opportunity to consider and fund a wider set of potential options.

One important factor in this near-term consideration is the impact of international trade, as all four Nordic economies generate a high proportion of exports. Since the mid-1990s, the globalization of industrial activity and the rise of low-cost manufacturers in central and eastern Europe as well as in Asia have created fears about future employment levels in Sweden and Finland with their industrially based economies, and, to a lesser degree, also in Denmark. This is much the same as elsewhere in western Europe (Tremonti 2008) and the industrialized world (Kagan 2008; Shapiro 2008). As a result, despite recent efforts among health policy researchers to emphasize the investment dimensions of additional health sector spending (Figueras et al. 2008), budget makers in three of the four Nordic countries remain concerned about the rapidly changing international economic environment and near-term fiscal controls remain tight. Reflecting these concerns, recent Nordic health policy debate has focused on short-term issues including the current rate of economic growth as well as potential employment threats, which will limit taxation levels and, with them, public expenditure. This economic debate is likely to intensify in the aftermath of the recessionary conditions in late 2008 and in 2009. The lingering effects of substantial declines in housing prices coupled with extensive public transfers to the banking industry may well leave a major financial problem for the public sector as a whole.

The economic context for health policy-making, however, also incorporates a less-discussed but nonetheless influential dimension. This is the long-term growth in the overall wealth of these four countries since the end of the Second World War, and especially in Finland since the economic hardships of the early 1990s. Beyond the many social infrastructure programmes, which have also been influential in forming the self-image that Nordic citizens have of themselves and of their countries, there have been the direct physical manifestations of increased wealth creation, both in private lifestyles and in expensive purpose-built public sector infrastructure. Examples of the latter include the advanced high-speed trains on Swedish rails, the major new bridge that spans the Oresund linking Sweden and Denmark and the new Opera House in Oslo.

This visible private and public sector wealth serves to reinforce the perception of the general public that society overall is substantially better off economically than it was previously – a perception that can directly influence political debate about the appropriate level of health care access and quality. It can be difficult for health policy-makers at national or regional level to carry on conversations with their constituents about limited resources and the need to prioritize services (e.g. rationing access to necessary care) when the same constituents have such direct evidence about society's financial capacity.

Overall, the important dimension here for policy formulation lies in the sharp tension between the first, near-term economic discussion, focused on economic and employment worries and on budget and tax constraints, and the second quite different perception of substantial societal wealth. This tension inevitably spills over into the political context for the ongoing health policy debate in these countries. The health sector's political context itself, in turn, serves to influence the future direction of decision-making for the entire social sector: that is for the Nordic welfare state as a whole.

4.2.2 The political context

The political component of the policy-making context in the Nordic countries, like the economic context, reflects a number of different, sometimes contradictory, elements. These include the 'common aspirations' that make up the Nordic health sector objectives: the introduction of self-managed and/or privately managed approaches to provider institutions; the general weakening of mid-twentieth century political ideologies among the electorate; the rise of quality of care as a core patient-driven concern, including rapidly changing capabilities in medical technology and the dilemma of waiting lists and other forms of rationing care; the challenge of expanding chronic care services, especially for the elderly; and the stronger steering role of elected politicians. Each is considered briefly.

As noted above, the 'common aspirations' that underlie the Nordic welfare state (discussed in Chapter 1) continue to define the broad policy framework within which health sector decisions are made. Both by law and by cultural preference, such principles as equity of access, public responsibility, public financing and broadly decentralized operational management are important elements within all four Nordic health systems. These objectives form the basic values that politicians and citizens alike understand as the core of the Nordic approach to the health sector, and which set the framework from which policy debate begins.

A second dimension of the political context has been the recognition that provider institutions need better incentives to operate efficiently and effectively. Beginning in the early 1990s in Sweden, efforts have been underway to shift directly managed public hospitals and health centres into quasi-independently managed public firms or, in some cases, into various types of private not-for-profit and for-profit entities (Saltman and von Otter 1995). The restructuring of Norwegian hospitals in 2002 into 'state enterprises' pushed further into this 'new public management' (NPM) territory. This ongoing process of provider diversification both within and beyond the public sector has created new political constituencies and new demands within the Nordic countries' policy-making systems.

A parallel, third dimension reflects a general retreat of political ideologies, and an accompanying weakening of citizen ties to the political parties of both left and right (Chapter 3). As incomes have improved and more workers have entered the solid middle class, voters are increasingly drawn to traditionally pragmatic values tied to demonstrable results. Thus, the core public-delivery focus of prior welfare state models, which reflected these institutions' social-democratic origins, is now giving way to more diverse, public–private mixtures of providers and, in certain instances, regarding funding for less-intensive services. This shift in organizational arrangements reflects the additional impact of several related factors, including the rise to power of national centre-right governments, the growing external pressure from various EU bodies, especially the European Court of Justice and the European Commission's Single Market project (c.f. Chapter 14), and the more welcoming political climate towards private involvement in the health sector in other tax-funded countries (often for similar reasons) elsewhere in Europe, such as the United Kingdom.

A fourth dimension of the political context is increasing pressure from citizens for their public health systems to ensure the timely delivery of high-quality diagnosis and treatment. This pressure for quality has been a key force behind a substantial number of recent national health policy decisions, including the introduction of quality assessment schemes that post benchmark results on the internet, stimulating diversity of public and private sector providers (Chapter 9), and the rapid growth of patient choice and patient rights, including the opportunity to select a primary care physician as well as a provider institution (Chapter 6). The desire to improve quality has also been a major factor in recent decisions in Norway, Denmark and some regions in Sweden to recentralize operating authority into larger regional and/or national bodies.

As one Nordic Ministry of Health official noted regarding the main motivating factor for health reforms in 2008, 'today it's quality of treatment, not localness of care'.

This emphasis upon quality generates a major challenge for future Nordic health sector arrangements. This quality-focused approach will need to be pursued, moreover, within the economic environment already described: continued tight constraints on near-term health-related public expenditure occurring within societies that 'feel' wealthy overall.

Quality concerns, in turn, also incorporate two additional elements that play a role in the political context: new medical technologies, and waiting time and other rationing measures. The continuing rapid developments in clinical technologies, pharmacology and information systems (particularly electronic patient records) create difficult choices for Nordic health policy-makers at both national and local levels. The essence of the dilemma is that these technological developments are driven by international research, and set an ever-higher international standard for patient care and related services. To the extent that these new capabilities improve patient care and outcomes (not always a given), and that they will require higher levels of expenditure (again not always a given), budget holders find themselves trapped between patient demands for higher quality and fiscal pressures to restrain expenditure.

This dilemma, in turn, contributes to decisions by some budget holders that result in longer waiting times for some diagnostic and elective treatments. Recent policy changes that create maximum waiting periods (0:7:30:90 in Sweden; 30 days from referred to treatment for most conditions, shorter for serious conditions in Denmark; individual physician determined in Norway; procedure-specific maximums in Finland) have further reduced the policy latitude to delay elective treatment. In the case of some of the newer, very expensive pharmaceuticals (particularly for cancer care), however, some budget holders have refused to pay on the grounds that (1) these drugs often have low rates of long-term effectiveness, and (2) the available funds will produce more benefit if spent farther upstream on preventive individual or population-based public health programmes. These and similar policy decisions continue to be controversial in all four countries, and they can be expected to become more so as the clinical outcomes produced by these drugs improve.

A further element of the political context in Nordic health policy-making concerns the changing mix of epidemiology and demography within the Nordic population. The rapidly increasing rate of chronic disease linked to the overall ageing of the population has been a major worry for Nordic policy-makers for at least a decade (Lagergren et al. 1998). Recent reviews have demonstrated that dealing with large numbers of frail elderly need not be as expensive or as fiscally destabilizing as first feared; however, more acceptable economic and social outcomes will require a wide range of coordinated policy initiatives that are consistently pursued over an extended period of time (Saltman et al. 2006). An additional dilemma is the growing number of obese individuals, as well as continuing concerns over the consequences of related lifestyle issues, including alcohol and tobacco use.

Lastly, the political context for the health sector includes a stronger steering role taken by elected politicians at both national and local levels. The Nordic model of locally elected (county, municipal, or, now in Denmark, regional) councils has traditionally made politicians responsible for broad operational decisions in Nordic health systems. As noted above and in Chapter 1, this direct electoral accountability is one of the hallmarks of the Nordic approach to health care. Beginning with the development in Sweden of county-level purchaser–provider models, however, elected politicians began to inject themselves more directly into day-to-day management decision-making (Maino et al. 2007). This level of intervention went beyond the normal administrative role of the 'landstingsrad' or political executive and has raised concern from medical professionals that their clinical decision-making autonomy has been infringed (Chapter 7). Now, as issues of efficiency have been joined by concerns about equity and quality, and as national politicians feel that they are being blamed by the general public for increasingly visible inadequacies, pressure has grown to intervene more forcefully. This issue of how best to balance political versus professional responsibility for management decisions continues to be part of every tax-funded health system, both within and beyond the Nordic region.

4.2.3 The overall context

Viewed overall, the combined economic and political context in the coming years appears likely to focus on efforts to develop a more quality-driven yet still financially sustainable framework, with emphasis on treating the chronically ill and/or elderly. However, in all four Nordic countries, this more targeted service delivery framework will need to be built on a structural and organizational infrastructure first put in place to deal with a very different set of mid-twentieth century clinical and fiscal problems. This pressure to rethink industrial era institutions for roles in a new century is already underway and is not, of course, unique to these four countries or to tax-funded health care systems generally. How to achieve an appropriate institutional shift – and to do so without weakening the loyalties of the citizenry to an equitable, universal, health system – will be a key political challenge over the next period of years.

4.3 Key future factors

The complex, often contradictory, nature of both the economic and political contexts creates a difficult environment for future policy-making. One useful perspective may be to focus on key organizational and institutional factors that have recently influenced Nordic health care reform, and then consider what likely future changes these and other similar factors might generate. An initial listing of key factors would include the following: (1) diversity of providers, (2) choice of provider, (3) integrating care across institutional borders, (4) pursuing sustainable funding, (5) reconfiguring the role of local government, (6) the impact of the EU, and (7) a pragmatic approach. The first three of these factors focus on quality and effectiveness, reflecting the growing pressures from patients to improve timeliness, appropriateness and outcomes of care. The fourth factor concerns funding care, and the continuing need to balance restraints on public sources of revenue with expanding clinical capabilities. The last three factors focus on governance and strategies. Here, there is a dual emphasis on balancing expectations of local government with the requirements of the supranational EU, and of the role of national government in coordinating these two seemingly opposite pressures. The final factor in this group – a pragmatic approach – reflects a core Nordic value orientation that has strongly influenced health sector policy-making in the past and that now appeals politically to the growing number of independently minded voters.

4.3.1 Diversity of providers

Prior to the onset of this period of market-oriented reform, Nordic health systems were typically characterized by broad public ownership and operation of health sector institutions. There were occasional exceptions for a few – small – private not-for-profit hospitals in Sweden (Carlanderska; Sophiahemmet) and Finland (Mehiläinen, Eira), for specialized institutions that treated arthritis or tuberculosis on contract from the public sector (Denmark), as well as for religiously organized facilities, mostly nursing homes (Diakonysis in Denmark and Norway). The overwhelming proportion of hospitals and health centres, however, were part of the public sector: owned, operated and funded by elected political actors and staffed by publicly salaried physicians and other health professionals.

The great advantage of this uniform public sector was its ability to provide broad access for all inhabitants to acute, primary and custodial care, and – importantly – to be able to do so at a known, publicly budgeted cost. The great disadvantage to this structural arrangement, of course, was that it was, as health economists frequently noted (Rehnberg 1995; Anell 2005; Pedersen 2005), a public sector monopoly: bureaucratic, arguably slow to innovate, often with long waiting lists and sometimes with questionable service quality.

Beginning in Stockholm County in Sweden in January 1988, the monolithic character of public sector health services began to crumble (Saltman and von Otter 1992). In the first phase of the process, purchasing was separated from provision within the elected public sector bodies responsible for the provision of health services. A public sector purchasing function was created; provider institutions (particularly hospitals) were reconfigured as publicly owned corporations (offentliga ägda bolag), and funds were allocated on the basis of negotiated contracts. Importantly, nothing was privatized – all this policy change took place within the preexisting public sector institutional structure. Subsequent evaluations of the Stockholm County reforms found that overall productivity increased by 11 per cent in the period 1992–93 (Bruce and Jonsson 1996). Moreover, by the early 1990s, half of the 26 county councils in Sweden had their own, more-or-less similar reform 'model' in place.

While much of this intra-public-sector reform process faded away in Sweden's hospital sector over the course of the next 10 years (one exception was Stockholm County, which expanded its restructuring to most hospitals and, in South District, to primary health centres), more extensive diversification took hold in a neighbouring country. In 2002, as part of Norway's major structural reform in the hospital sector, all hospitals were transformed into 'state enterprises' (Chapter 2). Recently, Finland too has begun to look at restructuring its hospitals into some type of public firms (I. Vohlonen, personal communication, October 2007). In several counties in Sweden, interestingly, some health sector actors are considering a return to directly managed public hospitals, especially in terms of looking for a payment mechanism that can create better incentives for more efficient and more effective performance (J. Calltorp, personal communication, December 2007).

Beyond diversification in governance arrangements at the institutional level, there also has been a considerable broadening inside public sector institutions in the range and diversity of management styles and medical treatment options. Managerially, there have been numerous experiments with new organizational forms, for example, in Denmark, with matrix-like structures based on function-bearing units and also models that span across multiple institutions based on patient pathways. Clinically, there have been efforts in both Denmark and Sweden to create a more diverse public hospital structure, moving away from the traditional general hospital model to specialized surgical units, and also to set up different arrangements for ambulatory and day care services. These and similar developments have helped to create a picture of considerable dynamism within public sector institutions.

Beyond changes in the public health sector, there has been substantial growth in the roles of various types of private provider in all four Nordic countries. This has been particularly true in primary health care in Sweden and Finland (Norway and Denmark have private GPs), as well as in home-care services. In the South District in Stockholm County, for example, 16 primary health centres were put out to bid, resulting in a variety of private contractual arrangements (including small private companies composed of the health centre's previously public employees). In Finland, a number of municipalities, including Kotka, Lahti and Kouvola, have contracted out the operation of their health centres to private for-profit companies (Chapter 9). Also, short-term hiring of temporary primary health care personnel, supplied by a private agency, has grown considerably. In home-care services in Sweden, some municipalities have shifted service delivery from publicly managed employees to contracted private, sometimes for-profit, companies. Health sector employment figures in Sweden now show some 25 per cent of primary care employees as 'private', many reflecting this growth of contracted-out health centres as well as various municipal care services, especially for the elderly.

In the hospital sector in Denmark, private surgical procedures contracted out from the public sector grew by an average of 61 per cent in 2007 (Kjellberg et al. 2009), and the rapid growth of private supplemental insurance has fuelled a similar increase in privately paid procedures. In Norway, private hospitals emerged at the time of the 2002 reform, performing elective procedures either on contract from the public sector or with out-of-pocket patient payments, with an overall growth in number of treated patients of 350 per cent in the period 2002–2005. There are currently 28 private clinics and hospitals working in Norway, most small and engaged primarily in day surgery. However, the centre-left government, which came into power in 2005, has announced publicly that the use of private hospitals should be reduced, and there was a reduction of 15 per cent in the number of patients from 2005 to 2006.

To date, neither the start-up of private hospitals nor the contracting-out of publicly built hospitals to private management companies has played a substantial role in any of the four Nordic countries. Most publicly built hospitals remain publicly operated (although some as public companies) in the Nordic world, and a very high proportion of patients (well over 90 per cent) receives care in these facilities. In Sweden, for example, the core private hospital sector continues to consist of two small hospitals, Carlanderska in Goteberg and Sophiahemmet in Stockholm, both of which have traditionally had a considerable volume of their business in providing elective procedures on contract to the county councils, typically utilizing publicly employed physicians working extra hours. Only one publicly built hospital, Sct. Gorans in Stockholm County, is still operated on contract by a private management firm. Similar contracts in two Skane hospitals have now been discontinued, with the hospitals returned to direct public management. In Finland, there are four small long-standing private hospitals whose patients receive partial reimbursement – officially 20 per cent but in practice somewhat less – from the public Social Insurance Institution. In both Sweden and Finland, efforts to start new private hospitals have failed, often (as with the 20 bed 'heart hospital' in Kuopio) despite a business plan based on providing contract services to the public sector.

In sum, there have been three major developments regarding the growing diversity of providers in Nordic health systems. First, a substantial number of publicly operated institutions have been restructured as quasi-independently managed public firms. Second, a growing number of primary health centres and long-term care services are being contracted out to various types of company, both public and private. Third, public hospitals to date (with one current Swedish exception) have *not* been either contracted out to private management or (through sale) privatized; however, the role of the private sector in contract areas such as elective surgery is currently growing in Denmark and Norway as a result of waiting-time guarantees, voluntary choice options and Voluntary Health Insurance. Overall, diversification of hospitals in the Nordic health systems to date has been driven largely by change in the structure and operations of the public sector, rather than by privatizing or privatized ownership. A key future issue will be whether this pattern continues as before, and private institutions remain only a small segment of the hospital sector even as they grow more prominent in other, less-intensive parts of these health systems.

4.3.2 Choice of provider

The topic of patient choice of provider has a complicated history in the Nordic region. It incorporates two different if related aspects of patient influence over health care service delivery, which can be simplified as (1) where care is received and (2) who provides it. The first issue is the ability to choose a provider institution. At the secondary care level, this has meant giving patients the ability to choose which public hospital to go to for elective procedures (acute intake – emergencies – remains governed by proximity and capacity). At primary care level, in those countries with public primary health care centres (predominantly Sweden and Finland), it means patient choice of health centre. The second issue regarding patient choice concerns choice of physician. At the primary care level the question is one of allowing patients to choose their doctor inside primary health centres – since countries where primary care is delivered by private GPs (Denmark and Norway) have long had choice of doctor. At the secondary (hospital) level, however, patients in all four countries are typically assigned to a clinic, and the question of choice of physician has, so far, rarely been raised.

Since the late 1980s, the dominant question for provider choice has been regarding public hospitals (Chapter 6). Although change has taken time, and hospitals and physicians have frequently been reluctant to implement choice-related measures, choice of hospital has gradually emerged as an accepted norm in Sweden (1991), Denmark (1993) and Norway (2001). Finland, however, continues to have fixed catchments. The recent introduction across the region of waiting-time guarantees for elective procedures (as noted above) further reinforces choice in that, if the time limit cannot be met by a patient's local hospital, he/she is entitled to seek care at another public (in some instances, also private) hospital. Choice is also extended to treatment facilities in other European countries. Standing behind the latter changes, acting as a political spur, is a decade of decisions by the European Court of Justice, which has gradually expanded the right of patients who cannot get timely care in their home country to seek care in another country, with the home country's health system obligated to pay (Chapter 14).

With regard to choice of primary care centre, Sweden has seen two separate reform efforts. In the first reform wave in the late 1980s (Stockholm County) and the early 1990s, a number of counties allowed patients to select which health centre they preferred. This opportunity was seen as particularly valuable for individuals who worked at some distance from where they lived, making it possible to choose to receive regular care near their workplace (among other advantages, reducing job absenteeism). A second, more varied movement under the general label 'care choice' ('Vårdval') is currently underway and this can include choice of either health centre (Halland County) or of primary care doctor (Stockholm County) (Anell 2008).

In Finland, although individuals cannot choose which publicly operated health centre they prefer, if they have personal resources they can decide to receive primary care from private GPs (sometimes these are public GPs working after hours) with partial reimbursement from the Social Insurance Institution. Also, if they are employed, they can choose to receive care from the occupational health service at their workplace (also subsidized by the Social Insurance Institution). Recently, there has been considerable growth in employed individuals seeking primary care services from occupational health providers, a trend that raises equity issues regarding care for the non-working population, but which appears to reflect insufficient staffing levels and delays in obtaining appointments for visits in some primary health care centres.

Although there continues to be concern that individual choice of public provider upsets the planning-based logic of Nordic systems – and that it can interfere with the crafting and delivery of continuous and/or integrated services, especially for elderly chronic care patients (Chapter 11) – the demand from the citizen for more flexible, more responsive and more personal service continues to grow (Chapter 6). This is not surprising given the overall increase in affluence of the citizenry in the Nordic region. Indeed, it is this basic demand, combined with efficiency concerns, that also drives the shift toward provider diversification.

The second form of provider choice – choice of doctor – has to date been mostly a concern within the primary care sector. In primary care, it has been long recognized that continuity and quality of care are best served by seeing the same physician regularly. This recognition is reflected in the list system for primary care physicians in Denmark, the GP reform in Norway in 2001 effectively introducing family physicians, and in a series of efforts in both Sweden ('husläkare' programme in early 1990s and the 'vardval' initiative currently underway in 2008) and Finland (personal doctor programme (Vohlonen et al. 1989)).

In the hospital sector, however, patients are still largely seen as patients of a clinic rather than of specific physicians. This means that the physician who performs a procedure for a patient – up to and including difficult surgery – is assigned by the clinic, often on the day of the procedure. It is possible to select one's specialist only in Finland, by becoming a private pay patient utilizing the Social Insurance Institution, or in Sweden or (to some degree) Denmark by utilizing private health insurance. Inside public hospitals, it remains difficult to see how choice of physician might work. Hospital administrators argue that efficient management of staff requires flexibility in how they assign physicians. Hospital physicians themselves see patients as belonging to a clinic, and speak of 'our patients'. Moreover, the current labour contracts for hospital physicians do not deal with the salary or regulatory process for this type of patient choice. Lastly, older Nordic patients – like the politicians that run the Nordic systems – often say that 'all our physicians are qualified doctors, and I trust our doctors'.

Overall, the issue of patient choice of provider institution (and of primary care physician) continues to influence policy decision-making across at least three of the four Nordic health systems. Choice of hospital is increasingly seen as a standard option (except in Finland), and choice of primary care provider and/or health centre is also increasingly common. Both of these forms of choice can be expected to grow in the near future, and there will likely be increased pressure on policy-makers to find strategies to combine choice with an efficient and high quality public delivery system.

4.3.3 Integrating care across institutional borders

Delivering services across the parallel areas of acute, primary and social/home care has emerged as a pressing concern for Nordic systems as for countries with well-developed health systems in general. Among numerous care-coordination issues, the increasing proportion of the elderly in the population will likely result in the provision of chronic care and home care consuming a growing percentage of health sector resources. Moreover, there will be a growing emphasis on coordinating patient self-care with services delivered by professional providers (Coulter and Magee, 2003). However, knowledge about how best to integrate services across these separate sectors is not well developed (Chapter 11), and the traditional bureaucratic solution of 'coordination committees' has not always worked very well from a managerial perspective (Axelsson et al. 2007).

In 1993, Sweden followed the Danish county of North Jutland in harnessing the power of economic incentives across public budgets to improve coordination between inpatient hospital and nursing home/home care. With the ÄDEL Reform, municipalities had five working days to take back 'finished' patients who require long-term care. If a municipality did not receive a patient within those five days, it had to pay the full direct cost of continued inpatient services. The result was quite powerful: in the first year, Swedish municipalities, using additional resources reallocated from the counties, were able to take back 85 per cent of 'finished' patients and provide adequate care (Johansson 1997). A similar arrangement is considered to work quite well nationwide in Denmark and in Norway; however, in Finland this approach has been less effective because of municipal cross-ownership of hospitals.

There are continued difficulties in coordinating the complex mix of acute-care, primary care and home-care services for the chronically ill elderly. A variety of care programmes have been established, including 'individual plans' in Norway and in Denmark (Kaye 2007). Primary care reforms in Denmark and Norway have sought to make the GP the locus of coordination for patients requiring chronic care. In Denmark, in what is expected to be the first phase of a broader programme, GPs will receive an additional fee for each diabetes patient for preventive and counselling visits and also for coordination time spent with social welfare agencies (Chapter 11). There is, moreover, considerable work underway with various patient pathway and other pilot programmes. Again in Denmark, as a way to eliminate cross-border grey-zone problems, the 2006 reform requires explicit agreements between the new regions and the municipalities on coordination issues. These agreements must be approved by the National Board of Health, which, tellingly, rejected the first set of plans, sending them back for more specific details.

Despite this progress, however, inadequately resolved issues still remain, in particular coordination between public hospitals and private primary care and home-care services. As new treatments successfully transform acute conditions such as the acquired immunodeficiency syndrome from terminal into chronic conditions, and as the number with diabetes mellitus and other lifestyle-related conditions grows, all creating younger patients who will need long term, integrated provision of acute, primary and/or domiciliary services, issues of cross-institutional coordination will further increase in importance.

4.3.4 Pursing sustainable funding

Viewed at the macro level, Nordic health systems have been relatively cost-effective since the beginning of the 1990s. There is considerable variation between Finland at the lower end (8.2 per cent of gross domestic product in 2006) and Denmark (9.5 per cent), with Norway (8.7 per cent) and Sweden (9.2 per cent) between these. Differences grow when one looks at annual per capita expenditures (Finland at US$2668 while Norway is US$4520). If one considers the average for 2006 published by the Organisation for Economic Co-operation and Development (OECD 2008), which is 8.9 per cent, then the Nordic countries spend just above or below the median for their peer counterpart countries.

Despite past performance, however, the issue of sustainable funding requires looking into the future, and, not surprisingly, this is where some Nordic health policy-makers become nervous. In an era of economic globalization, the Nordic countries that rely on exports for a substantial share of their overall economy cannot continue to raise taxes and social security levies as they have in the past, for fear this will price their exports out of international markets. Similarly, EU maximums on budget deficits will continue to place restrictions on increasing public sector deficit spending without raising taxes. With fiscal policy more (Finland, a member of the EURO zone) or less (Norway, Sweden and Denmark retain their national currencies) constrained by European Commission deficit standards, Nordic health systems may well find themselves financially constrained if they continue to rely on predominantly public revenue. Yet if they seek to raise an increasing amount through private households, especially through higher co-payments, deductibles and co-insurance, the central principle of solidarity will suffer. Beyond the unlikely saviour of permanent strong economic growth in the overall economy, health policy-makers in the Nordic region will likely grapple with this core funding dilemma every time expensive new bioengineered pharmaceuticals or new diagnostic or treatment techniques join the 'international standard' of quality of care that their citizens expect from their public health care system. The problem will no doubt intensify in the near term (2009–2010) because of the ongoing global recession. As one senior national policy-maker bluntly put it, 'we still have large cost drivers we can't establish mechanisms to control. If we can't succeed in this, more reforms will be necessary'.

Beyond strictly economic notions of sustainable funding, the concept also incorporates elements of social acceptability, for example the levels of expenditure and sources of funding that a broad majority of the population can be expected to continue to support. At this level, sustainability refers to the exquisite calculus that a population makes between willingness to pay, on the one hand, and level and quality of services received, on the other hand. To date, in all four Nordic countries, that calculus has supported, and continues to support, the existing tax-funded arrangements; indeed, in Sweden, the general population has been willing to increase support. It remains to be seen, however, as lifestyle-related conditions such as obesity and diabetes generate an increasing percentage of costs, whether current funding arrangements will continue to be socially acceptable in the future.

4.3.5 Reconfiguring local government

Since the mid-1990s, there has been substantial restructuring of both regional and municipal government arrangements in the Nordic region. This pattern does, however, reflect the split noted above between Norway and Denmark – which have embraced restructuring – and Sweden and Finland, which have had some difficulty in pursuing major nationally led change. The first phase of restructuring was initiated in the 1990s by two voluntary regroupings of Swedish county councils, each of which decided to form a larger, area-wide county, one around Gothenburg (combining four county councils), the other around Malmö (combining three). With Stockholm County, which had earlier amalgamated Stockholm municipality and Stockholm County, Sweden now has three large counties as well as 18 'regular' county councils.

The main development of meso-level restructuring has occurred since 2000, in Norway (health responsibilities removed from 19 counties and given to five new health regions in 2002, reduced to four regions in 2007) and in Denmark (14 counties replaced by five health regions in 2007). As Chapters 3 and 5 highlight, both countries have engaged in a major transformation of their national–regional governance relationships, based in the expectation that political (and in Denmark fiscal) recentralization back to the national level, combined with regional consolidation of administrative responsibility into larger units with stronger national steering, will be more economically efficient and also – an important point – be able to guarantee more equitable access and better quality for geographical and demographically disadvantaged groups.

In Sweden, however, the national government now seems unlikely to adopt proposals from a 2007 State Commission report to consolidate its 18 'regular-size' counties into six to eight larger units (although local counties can still decide on their own to merge). Similarly, the Finnish Government also has scaled back earlier consolidation plans and is now expected to reduce the number of central hospital districts from 22 to only 21 (J. Tepari, personal communication November 2008).

Regarding consolidation at the municipal level, there is now a parallel pattern reflecting efforts to create larger governmental units that can better pay for and manage the needed health sector and social services. In 2007, Denmark reduced the number of local governments from 274 to 98. Finland initiated a national programme in 2007 to consolidate health sector management into health-specific and/or fully merged municipal units of at least 20,000 inhabitants; however, results have been achieved more slowly than expected. The number of municipal primary care units has been reduced so far by 69, leaving some 370 still in place (S. Kokko, personal communication, 24 April 2009). Further, individual municipalities, no matter how small, mostly continue to pay hospitals separately for secondary and tertiary clinical services provided to their inhabitants (Vuorenkoski et al. 2008). Sweden had an earlier municipal reform that by the early 1970s had reduced the number of municipalities from approximately 2500 (many being small parishes) to 289 units large enough to administer welfare state programmes (Olsson 1990).

Despite differing outcomes to date, all four governments continue to struggle with a common set of issues that produced this desire to shrink the number of units and increase the size of regional and municipal bodies (Saltman 2008). There is concern across all four national governments about inequity in access, and especially regarding health outcomes between regions. Further, there is worry that existing regional governments will not be able to pay for expensive new treatments and equipment. Positively, there is the enabling capacity of information technology, which has made it possible to supervise provider institutions more effectively from a distance. Lastly, but importantly, there is the 'blame factor': national politicians feel that they are held responsible by the voters when the health system underperforms, and, as a consequence, they increasingly feel that they should have adequate levers to correct the problems that generate the underperformance.

This restructuring of local government alters two important balances in the Nordic countries: the balance of power between state and sub-state governments, and the balance between local democracy and economic efficiency as a prime health sector objective. Regarding state versus sub-state bodies, recent restructuring in Norway and Denmark has reflected a complex set of power shifts that rearranged authority relationships among national, regional (including county councils) and municipal government bodies. The overall impact is to strengthen the hand of central government – fiscally and politically in Denmark, politically and administratively in Norway – while simultaneously strengthening, in Denmark, the power of local municipalities regarding chronic care and prevention, and, in Norway, creating the capability for hospitals to manage themselves as quasi-independent public firms. In effect, the recent reforms serve both to recentralize and to decentralize different components of decision-making power, with the meso-level being the obvious loser to both the state above them and to municipalities and/or individual provider units below them. This element of recentralization back to the central state is a new phenomenon in the Nordic region, running contrary to the established pattern since the Second World War of continuous decentralization in the health sector both in the Nordic region and across Europe generally (Saltman et al. 2007; Byrkeflot and Neby 2008).

Regarding local democracy versus efficiency objectives, the strong efficiency dimension of this recentralization movement suggests that the traditional democratic argument – that health care should be locally controlled in order to serve the needs of the local population better – continues to apply to administrative but less to political and fiscal forms of decentralization (Saltman and Bankauskaite 2006).

As Nordic policy-makers look to the future, there is likely to be a strong impetus toward increased recentralization on both political and fiscal dimensions. This will continue to be a political issue in both Sweden and Finland in the coming years, as national governments may feel compelled by the same litany of pressures to revisit the question of how to achieve major structural changes lower down in the delivery system. This will be particularly true in Sweden if voluntary efforts by regular-size counties to merge together falter, and in Finland if the current process to increase the minimum population size for public primary health care providers does not succeed. In both Denmark and Norway, there already is speculation that the state's role in the health sector, already considerably strengthened, may have to grow further over the coming years. As this process of consolidation of governance continues, additional decision points will likely emerge at which the balance between state and local power and between democracy and efficiency may need to be reconsidered.

4.3.6 *Impact of the European Union*

An increasingly influential element in the Nordic health policy mosaic is being woven outside the region, in Brussels (the European Commission) and, importantly, in Luxemburg (European Court of Justice). Although formally only three of the four Nordic countries are member states (Sweden, Denmark and Finland), Norway is bound economically to honour EU decisions through its European Economic Area agreement, is affected politically by the content and approach of EU decisions, and is subject judicially to decisions taken by the European Court of Justice. Consequently, in practice, all four countries must take under consideration the current direction of EU policy (Chapter 14).

Economically, there has been continued pressure within the EU since the early 1990s to include aspects of publicly operated health care systems within the purview of the European Single Market (Mossialos and McKee 2002). Pressures are particularly intense from commercial insurance companies, who want greater opportunity to compete for a portion of what they see as large revenue streams currently running through a protected tax-based structure, and from pharmaceutical corporations who want to override specific national pricing regimes to create a single pan-European market in which power in the market place – not government – could determine the prices paid. From the efforts of the Bangemann Commission in 1997 onward, these corporate concerns have received a sympathetic hearing in some quarters within the European Commission.

Politically, there is growing pressure to acknowledge and legitimize what is an implicit EU health policy framework. This implicit framework has been created piecemeal and often unintentionally, as a by-product of what are formally economic and/or other sectoral regulations (Mossialos and McKee 2002; Mossialos et al. 2009). Therefore, although the EU is authorized by the Maastricht Treaty only to have a public health function, in practice it has a considerable de facto health system impact as well. Further, beginning in 2001 with the establishment of a High Committee of Reflection, now followed by an EU health strategy from DG Sanco in 2008, there is considerable EU effort underway to define and develop what a proper EU health policy should look like. Simultaneously, there was a decision by the Competition Directorate, headed at the time by Fritz Bolkestein, to include the health sector within efforts to deregulate the EU's service sector. The initial directive on this issue did include the health sector, although it was subsequently removed from the directive before it was finalized. Thus politically, from a variety of different directions, there continues to be substantial pressure to construct an EU-wide health policy, and to fold that policy into existing deregulation strategies elsewhere in the EU economy.

Finally, judicially, health systems in the Nordic region, like their counterparts throughout the EU, have been subject to 10 years of increasingly interventionist decisions from the European Court of Justice. Beginning with Kohll/Dekker, these decisions have developed a widening set of precedents that enable citizens who do not receive services in a timely manner to seek care in another legal jurisdiction, without requiring permission from their home jurisdiction, and requiring the home jurisdiction to pay the full cost of that care. Invoking the European Declaration of the Rights of Man, decisions of the European Court of Justice have forced EU health systems to reexamine waiting times as well as service restrictions. In the Nordic region, concern that patients could decide to seek expensive care outside the country has been an element in the emergence of care guarantees in Sweden and Denmark.

Taken together, the economic, political and judicial impact of the EU on Nordic health systems can be expected to continue to grow in the future. As the range of areas influenced continues to expand, how EU institutions take decisions will increase as a factor that Nordic policy-makers need to consider and accommodate.

4.3.7 A pragmatic approach

A striking characteristic of Nordic policy-making in the health sector has been how pragmatic it has been. Pragmatism, defined as finding practical, consensus-based solutions that respond flexibly to the economic and political context, has been a core component of modern Nordic political life at least since the 1920s, when Rickard Sandler first proposed to the Swedish Social Democrats that they compromise ideology by supporting capitalism but then redistributing the wealth it produced (Tilton 1991). Writing in 1967, Adler-Karlsson described this approach to economic decision-making as 'functional socialism', a framework which Scott (1977, p. 546) contended, in his history of Sweden, 'illustrates the Swedish pragmatic approach and the rejection of the doctrinaire'. More broadly, pragmatism in the Nordic political arena reflects agreement among all parties on a core set of values and principles, including general assent to the broad objectives of what Esping-Andersen (1990) termed the social democratic welfare state, as well as common recognition of basic economic concerns for both individuals and the state.

This pragmatic perspective has been particularly apparent since the late 1980s in the structural and organizational reforms in the health sector (Saltman and Bergman 2005). The major organizational measures put in place in all four countries have typically been driven by practical necessity, as indicated by the fact that, with rare exceptions, they have not been reversed when the then-opposition parties have come to power. Some of this durability has reflected a political need for minority-led governments to pursue consensus-based solutions in order to secure support from opposition parties, as well as a series of political traditions that reinforce a broadly participatory and democratic decision-making process. However, policy outcomes in the Nordic health sector also have typically been more practical than ideological in nature. This under-lying pragmatism of both process and outcomes has led in the past, despite rather different political contexts, to an increasingly similar set of conceptual (although not necessarily structural) solutions across all four countries, along lines similar to if not exactly resembling those outlined in the previous six key factors noted above.

The observation that pragmatism rather than political ideology has largely driven the current health reform process may seem overstated to some politi-cians and also some professional staff within these health systems, who have witnessed various political parties taking different positions on key issues, some initially driven by explicit political beliefs. It also runs counter to commentaries by non-Nordic observers who argued that NPM reforms in the early 1990s must have been stimulated by British neo-liberals such as Mrs Thatcher. However, as already noted, the consensus agreement and long-term stability around many reforms within countries, as well as the above-noted convergence among the four countries around key organizational measures, suggest that deeper, more organic forces have been at work. This emphasis on pragmatic processes and outcomes remains valid despite recently emerging differences between Denmark and Norway, on the one hand, and Sweden and Finland, on the other, as to what the exact content of a pragmatic approach should involve.

How these systems respond to future challenges also will be shaped by practical aspects of day-to-day operational concerns. Although pragmatism, along with an accompanying deliberative policy approach, may not sound particularly exciting to political partisans, in practice it can serve as the policy-making glue to keep organizational reform on a broadly moderate, steady path.

4.3.8 Summarizing the key factors

How these seven key factors, which have characterized the ongoing process of health reform since the late 1980s, will influence future policy – along with the demographic and technological factors discussed in Chapter 1 (ageing, information systems, advances in medical technology) – is not predetermined. Other policy elements that are likely to affect policy outcomes include the shortage of trained medical professionals, particularly physicians, and ongoing efforts to improve public health outcomes by adjusting the balance of responsibility among state, regional and municipal governments. Moreover, which factors a particular cohort of policy-makers can choose to ignore, which factors they are able to steer and harness for their own policy purposes, and which factors they will have little choice but to accommodate also will shift with future circumstances. Overall, however, it would appear likely that these seven factors will continue to play a substantial role in how Nordic systems evolve. Indeed, it would be surprising if any of the seven does not contribute to the development of new reform policies in the future.

4.4 Concluding observations

The policy direction in which Nordic health systems will likely move over the near to medium term, and the degree to which all four systems will evolve in parallel rather than in divergent directions, is in considerable degree dependent on the specific character and mix in each system of the elements and factors detailed above. While the existence of a variety of common pressures suggests a similar development, one can point to equally central elements that appear to be pulling these systems in quite divergent directions. It is worth highlighting that divergent strategies currently exist not only at the overall system reform level but also within such signature policy areas as primary health care (Chapter 11) and public health (Chapter 12).

Relying on the three-level model of health system analysis presented in

Chapter 1, it would seem likely that the same historical, geographical and cultural similarities that generated 'common aspirations' for these four health care systems will continue to exert strong influence over their goals and objectives. The commitment to universality, equity and democratic public participation can be expected to remain as the normative touchstones of these systems. At the second and third levels of structural issues – funding, governance and delivery – and specific policy applications, however, existing patterns suggest that the four systems may continue to follow different speeds if not different paths. As detailed in Section 4.1, the four Nordic countries appear to have separated on to two tracks since the mid-1990s, each pathway premised on a differing mix of national, intermediate/meso-level and municipal controls over political, fiscal and administrative elements of public authority. One track is premised on the predominance of continued decentralization and local control; the second is premised upon substantial recentralization to larger regional and national bodies. Moreover, precisely the mix of economic and political forces that has sustained Sweden and Finland in the first direction, while pushing Norway and Denmark in the second, is likely to strengthen rather than abate over the next years. Therefore, in practice, the Nordic region could find itself with two quite different health sector strategies for the foreseeable future.

This consolidation of two different approaches suggests that there may well be future opportunities to assess these two different strategies in terms of visible differentials in their outcomes. Will Norway and Denmark find that a stronger national role in fiscal and political matters produces greater equity of outcomes across geographical, socioeconomic and gender groupings? Will greater state control generate broader cost-efficiencies in the use of available funds? Will Norway's 'state enterprise' hospitals out-perform the traditional directly managed institutions in the other three health care systems in terms of timeliness and quality of care? Will Denmark's new emphasis on increased responsibilities for prevention on the part of municipalities and GPs begin to demonstrate better long-term upstream outcomes?

More broadly, over time, will Sweden and Finland feel increasing pressure from their citizens to shift away from traditional decentralized steering methods for political and fiscal decisions if the more centralized systems in Norway and Denmark do, in fact, demonstrate better outcomes and service quality? Alternatively, will the debate over recentralization fade as more fundamental issues – for example rising demand for expensive new technologies and pharmaceuticals – pressure all four health systems to introduce and/or strengthen what will be essentially similar cost-containment measures? At a more conceptual level, will decentralized control, local participation and multilevel democracy come to be seen as less-necessary processes for managing health services in an era when sophisticated electronic information systems and comparative information about patient outcomes from other countries are available?

Several possible health system scenarios can be developed, depending on the answers to these and similar questions. One possibility would be that national governments in Sweden and Finland feel strong pressure to intervene more forcefully to push lower levels of government to merge into larger units, and to surrender more political and fiscal control to the national government. An alternative scenario could see the decentralized authority of Swedish counties and Finnish municipalities strengthened if recentralized national efforts in Norway and Denmark appear *not* to have had a major impact on service costs or outcomes, or if, quite differently, local governments gain additional leverage politically over national decision-making. The varying impact of the seven factors detailed above suggests that the policy calculus could differ significantly in different national contexts. Recent reports that the Finnish Government, facing a growing shortage of primary care physicians, has decided to close a number of publicly operated primary health centres, potentially expanding private provision, provides an example of the differing effects these factors can have (J. Vuori, personal communication, January 2009).

There appears to be, however, little likelihood that either Norway or Denmark will return to their prior, more decentralized, policy-making or fiscal arrangements. In Norway, while there is concern about what critics refer to as the 'autocratic' power of the state in the health care arena, and although one can point to the belated decision to appoint local politicians to the boards of the regional health enterprises, there has been no discussion about returning the hospital sector to the county councils. Most speculation has centred on an even larger state role emerging if current arrangements prove inadequate. The only concession to local authority currently mooted has been the possibility of strengthening the role of the municipalities, perhaps by combining them into larger/fewer units and then giving them needs-based budgets. While such a change would give municipalities a larger role in administering health services – mirroring in certain administrative respects the role of the primary care trusts in the United Kingdom – these newly empowered municipalities would, like the the primary care trusts, receive their funds from the state, and, therefore, would be expected to defend their local decisions to an ultimately responsible national government.

The Danish picture is not too dissimilar. Although the new regions currently have board members who are elected, there also is a widespread expectation that poor performance of the reformed system would lead to more, not less, state intervention and control. The real battleground has been over the relative power and authority of the municipalities and regions on the one hand, and the national government on the other. One part of the 2007 reform required cooperation agreements between municipalities and regions in order to improve prevention initiatives. Once negotiated, these agreements must be approved by a state-appointed committee of experts. As mentioned above, the first round of these plans was rejected, suggesting that a new balance of power between national and local levels has yet to be stabilized.

One notable development in both Norway and Denmark has been the growth of private provision. As noted above, the number of private hospital clinics has grown considerably in both countries over the last few years. This expansion, in turn, has been driven by a similar growth in voluntary private health insurance in Denmark and by public contracts triggered by the introduction of tighter waiting-time guarantees in both countries. In Finland, there are a small but growing number of municipalities that have either contracted out management of their primary health centre or that now staff their health centre through a private agency (Chapter 9). In Sweden, there also has been growth of privately run primary health centre and home-care services.

This expansion of private provision (and in Denmark, private insurance) has led to discussion about its likely impact on Nordic health systems in the short and medium term. To the extent that this upsurge has been fuelled by private insurance, it remains to be seen whether premiums will continue to be paid during and after the current recessionary period. In a previous expansionary period during the 1980s, many Finns bought private health insurance for their children. These previously popular policies largely disappeared once the serious recession of 1990–1992 began.

However, much of the increased private provision is being fuelled by public funds, tied to implementation of waiting-time guarantees. In Finland, growth in the usage of occupational health services reflects the 55 per cent subsidy that these services receive from the Social Insurance Institution, along with a corporate tax deduction for the remaining 45 per cent of the cost. While public funds could also decrease with the recession, the reforms that led to these private contracts almost certainly will continue, being both popular with patients and also necessary in response to decisions in the European Court of Justice regarding the timely provision of care.

The broader question is whether and/or at what point a growing private sector could begin to undermine solidarity and public control. This issue has been debated since the early 1990s, with the advent of the purchaser–provider split and patient choice (Saltman and von Otter 1995). Based on past experience, there would appear to be two key aspects. First is the extent to which public sector services provide the same quality of care and outcomes as the private sector. It is important that public policy-making does not allow too visible a gap to open up between the two sectors (de Roo 1995). Second is the degree to which a separate, private stream of funding becomes available. As long as private providers remain largely dependent on public funders, public sector values and objectives are likely to remain paramount.

An additional, related factor is the social acceptability of seeking and receiving private health services among the broad middle class. This differs among the four countries. At present, it is not particularly acceptable behaviour to seek private health care in Norway or Sweden; however, it is reasonably acceptable in Denmark (which also has publicly funded private GPs and specialists, and private schools) and also in Finland (where private provision is partly reimbursed by public funds through the Social Insurance Institute).

Taking all these aspects into account, the current picture is one of small but growing private provision, mostly in primary health care and elective procedures, rather than in the core acute activities of Nordic health systems, and mostly funded publicly or out of pocket by patients. Consequently, while the present picture may be volatile, it would appear to remain within the confines of a diverse publicly operated system rather than becoming a two-tier public–private system. How this relationship progresses over the next few years remains a decision in the hands of public policy-makers and, in that sense, remains consistent with the objectives of equity and public (democratic) participation that sit at the core of the traditional Nordic approach.

An additional set of issues for the future character of Nordic health systems will be ongoing developments in the external economic and political contexts within which they are embedded. Economically, the continuation of export-led growth, and the ability to maintain competitiveness vis-à-vis both the central European states of the EU and the rapidly changing global economy, will be crucial to the domestic fiscal framework within which Nordic policy-makers reach their decisions. An important underlying issue will be the degree to which domestic resource flows to the health sector can be reconfigured to be more stable even as European and global economic conditions continue under pressure.

Politically, a key issue will be broader societal decisions about the future scope and character of Nordic welfare states. While universality and equity will likely continue to underpin health sector values, the specific institutional arrangements through which these values are pursued, and the alternative health sector strategies that might be adopted to fund and deliver services, will necessarily reflect hard decisions about how to transform an industrial era configuration of social programmes for a very different, postindustrial economic and political environment. As part of this rethink, a number of factors will have increasing impact, including the ongoing melting of public–private boundaries in the health sector (Saltman 2008), efforts to extend funding and provision across national boundaries both within and beyond the EU and the growing emphasis in countries like the Netherlands and the United Kingdom on innovative strategies that span both public and private arenas (Saltman et al. 2008). These pressures will be even stronger if recessionary conditions prevalent in 2009 do not abate.

Conversely, future developments in the health sector will have an important impact on the overall development of the broader Nordic welfare state. To the extent that core objectives concerning equity and democratic participation in health systems reflect a more general set of objectives for social democratic style welfare states, the health sector will continue to reinforce the universal character of the Nordic welfare state. If, however, these core objectives weaken, that too will be felt in the overall capacity of welfare state activities. To date, changes in the Nordic health sector fall within the boundaries of a 'recalibration' (Pierson 2000) of welfare state programmes rather than representing a fundamental shift in the core purpose of these programmes.

Beyond their influence within the four Nordic countries, the lessons and outcomes from Nordic health reform can provide a useful comparative lens on the likely future direction of health policy in other countries in Europe. How the interplay among the seven key factors evolves both within and between these countries, through such changes as the growing diversity of providers within a publicly funded system and the expanding demand for patient influence over both logistical and clinical decisions about their care, can provide useful information to policy-makers in western and especially central Europe as they grapple with a similar set of policy dilemmas in both tax-funded and (to a lesser degree) social health insurance systems. How the Nordic countries address difficult structural issues such as sustainable finance and integrating multiple service lines will be watched with particular interest, and the strategies that are selected may well become influential as all health systems across Europe seek better answers to these problems. Lastly, with regard to the impact on EU policy of Nordic health system development, emerging Nordic preferences and responses, when translated through the deliberative bodies of the EU, may also help to steer the development of health system change in the other countries of the Union.

Exactly how the next developmental stages will play out within the Nordic health sector is contingent upon the usual caveats and will depend on the particular mix of economic, political, social and cultural factors impinging on health policy-making within each country. However, it seems fair to conclude that, overall, the effort to articulate more fiscally efficient and more clinically effective health systems, which are simultaneously more responsive to patient needs and preferences, will likely continue for some years to come.

References

Adler-Karlsson, G. (1967) *Functional Socialism: A Swedish Theory for Democratic Socialization*. Stockholm: Prisma.

Anell, A. (2005) Swedish healthcare under pressure, *Health Economics* 14(Suppl 1): S237–54.

Anell, A. (2008) *Vårdval in Primärvården*. Lund: Institutet for Ekonomisk Forskning.

Axelsson, R., Marchildon, G.P. and Repullo Labrador, R.R. (2007) Effects of decentralization on managerial dimensions of health systems, in Saltman, R.B., Bankauskaite, V. and Vrangbaek, K. (eds) *Decentralization in Health Care: Strategies and Outcomes*. Maidenhead: Open University Press/McGraw-Hill Education, pp.141–66.

Bruce, A. and Jonsson, E. (1996) *Competition in the Provision of Health Care: The Experience of the US, Sweden, and Britain*. Aldershot: Arena, pp. 39–70.

Byrkjeflot, H. and Neby, S. (2008) The end of the decentralized model of healthcare governance? Comparing developments in the Scandinavian hospital sectors, *Journal of Health Organization and Management* 22: 331–49.

Coulter, A. and Magee, H. (2003) *The European Patient of the Future*. Maidenhead: Open University Press.

de Roo, A.A. (1995) Contracting and solidarity: market-oriented changes in Dutch health insurance schemes, in Saltman, R.B. and von Otter, C. (eds) *Implementing Planned Markets in Health Care*. Buckingham: Open University Press, pp. 45–64.

Esping-Andersen, G. (1990) *The Three Worlds of Welfare Capitalism*. Cambridge: Polity Press.

Figueras, J., McKee, M. and Menabde, N. (eds) (2008) *Health Systems, Health and Wealth*, Copenhagen: WHO Regional Office for Europe.

Glenngård, A.H., Hjalte, F., Svensson, M., Anell, A. and Bankauskaite, V. (2005) *Health Systems in Transition: Sweden*. Copenhagen: WHO Regional Office for Europe on behalf of the European Observatory on Health Systems and Policies.

Harrison, M.I. and Calltorp, J. (2000) The re-orientation of market oriented reforms in Swedish Healthcare, *Health Policy* 50: 219–40.

Kagan, R. (2008) *The Return of History and the End of Dreams*. New York: Knopf.

Kaye, R. (2007) Report on Long Term Care to Association International de Mutualités, Brussels, mimeo.

Kjellberg, J., Søgaard, J. and Andreasen, M.N. (2009) *Privat/offentligt samspil i sundhedsvæsenet*. Copenhagen: Danish Institute for Health Services Research. http://www.laeger.dk/nyhed/download/docs/F10345/Privat-offentligt%20samspil%20i%20sundhedsv%C3%A6senet,%20DSI.pdf (accessed March 2009).

Lagergren, M., Batljan, I. and Zavisic, S. (1998) *The Welfare State and the National Economy*. Stockholm: Cabinet Office and Ministerial Publications.

Maino, F., Blomqvist, P., Bertinato, L., Bohigas Santasusagna, L., Urbanos Garrido, R.M. and Shishkin, S. (2007) Effects of decentralization and recentralization on political dimensions of health systems, in Saltman, R.B., Bankauskaite, V. and Vrangbaek, K.

(eds) *Decentralization in Health Care*. Maidenhead: McGraw Hill/Open University Press for the WHO European Observatory, pp. 120–40.

Mossialos, E. and McKee, M. (2002) *The Impact of EU Law on Health Policy*. Brussels: PIE-Peter Lang.

Mossialos, E., Permanand, G., Baeten, R. and Harvey, T. (2009) *Health Systems Governance in Europe: The Role of EU Law and Policy*. Cambridge: Cambridge University Press.

OECD (2008) *OECD in Figures 2008*. Paris: OECD.

Olsson, S.E. (1990) *Social Policy and Welfare State in Sweden*. Lund: Arkiv.

Pedersen, K.M. (2005) The private–public mix in Scandinavia, in Maynard, A. (ed.) *The Public–Private Mix in Health*. Oxford, UK: Radcliffe, pp. 161–90.

Pierson, P. (ed.) (2000) *The New Politics of the Welfare State*. Oxford: Oxford University Press.

Rehnberg, C. (1995) The Swedish experience with internal markets, in Jerome-Forget, M., White, J. and Weiner, J.M. (eds) *Health Care Reform Through Internal Markets*, Washington, DC: The Brookings Institution, pp. 49–74.

Saltman, R.B. (2008) Decentralization, re-centralization and future European health policy, *European Journal of Public Health* 18: 104–6.

Saltman, R.B. and Bankauskaite, V. (2006) Conceptualizing decentralization in European health systems: a functional perspective, *Health Economics, Policy and Law* 1: 127–47.

Saltman, R.B. and Bergman, S.E. (2005) Renovating the commons: Swedish health care reforms in perspective, *Journal of Health Politics, Policy and Law* 30: 253–76.

Saltman, R.B. and von Otter, C. (1992) *Planned Markets and Public Competition: Strategic Reform in Northern European Health Systems*. [*State of Health* Series]. Buckingham: Open University Press.

Saltman, R.B. and von Otter, C. (eds) (1995) *Implementing Planned Markets in Health Care: Balancing Social and Economic Responsibility*. [*State of Health* Series.] Buckingham: Open University Press.

Saltman, R.B., Dubois, H. and Chawla, M. (2006) The impact of aging on long-term care in Europe and some potential policy responses, *International Journal of Health Services* 36: 719–46.

Saltman, R.B., Bankauskaite, V. and Vrangbaek, K. (eds) (2007) *Decentralization in Health Care: Stategies and Outcomes*. Maidenhead: Open University Press.

Saltman, R.B., Allin, B.S., Mossialos, E.A., Wismar, M. and Kutzin, J. (2008) Assessing health reform trends, in Figueras, J., McKee, M. and Menabde, N. (eds) *Health Systems, Health and Wealth*. Copenhagen: WHO Regional Office for Europe, pp. 125–50.

Scott, F.D. (1977) *Sweden: The Nation's History*. Minneapolis, MN: University of Minnesota Press.

Shapiro, R. (2008) *Futurecast 2020: A Global Vision of Tomorrow*. London: Profile Books.

Tilton, T. (1991) *The Political Theory of Swedish Social Democracy*. Oxford: Clarendon Press.

Tremonti, G. (2008) *La Paura e la speranza – Europa: la crisi globale che si avvicina e la via per superarla [Fear and hope – Europe: Global Crisis Approaching and the Way to Overcome It]* Milan: Mondadori.

Valtonen, H. (2008) The Finnish welfare state meets the consumer society, *Eurohealth* 14: 12–13.

Vohlonen, I., Pekurinen, M. and Saltman, R.B. (1989) Re-organizing primary medical care in Finland: the personal doctor program, *Health Policy*, 13: 65–79.

Vuorenkoski, L., Mladovsky, P. and Mossialos, E. (2008) Finland: Health System Review. *Health Systems in Transition*, 10(4): 1–168.

Part II

Nordic health systems: key issues

chapter five

The changing political governance structures of Nordic health care systems

Terje P. Hagen and Karsten Vrangbæk

5.1 Introduction

The health care systems of the Nordic countries share basic features with the National Health Service (NHS) models in the United Kingdom, New Zealand and southern Europe: Funding is tax based; most services are free of charge and the main actors, both purchasers and most suppliers, are public. In contrast to these centralized NHS models, the health care systems of the Nordic countries give a more pronounced role to local and regional governments in allocation and localization decisions and base parts of their legitimacy on broad elements of local political participation. Multilevel democratic governing processes are thus a key feature of all the Nordic health systems. The central state establishes the basic legal framework and has key roles in terms of financing, coordination, education, licensing and control. The decentralized levels are largely responsible for the delivery of services and thus for allocation, organization and management of services.

A commonly used perspective for analysing decentralized governance of local services has been developed by Tiebout (1956), Musgrave (1959) and Oates (1972). In this perspective, the assumptions are that local government takes care of local public goods such as utilities and local roads; goods are financed mainly by local taxes and mobility is high to induce homogeneity in preferences. This perspective is too simplistic for understanding the Nordic context. The Nordic local and county governments, although having important differences between countries, are designed by the central state and take care of welfare services with redistributive characteristics; financing is to a high degree centralized to the state and mobility is low, leading to heterogeneous preferences over services (Rattsø 2003). Both financing of welfare services and decisions on the service levels are, therefore, subject to negotiations and conflicts of interests both within decentralized units and between governance levels. Rather than autonomous decentralized governance, there is a multilevel governing structure. Such multilevel governing structures typically face challenges and dilemmas with regards to coordination and division of responsibilities.

This chapter will explore and compare developments in the formal multilevel governing structures of the Nordic health systems, discuss possible explanations for the observed changes in the four countries and present some preliminary evidence of how different models work.

5.2 The changing governing structures of Nordic health care

Changes since the early 1990s have been radical in two of the Nordic countries, Denmark (Vrangbæk and Christiansen 2005) and Norway (Hagen and Kaarboe 2006) (see also Chapter 3), and moderate in Finland (Hakkinen 2005; Hakkinen and Lehto 2005) and Sweden (Saltman and Bergman 2005). The main governance structure and steering processes in existence around 1990, and before these changes were implemented, are first described in terms of six variables: responsibility, local political participation, financing, cooperation and planning, and patient choice. Then follows a description of the major reforms subsequently implemented.

5.2.1 Governing structure in existence around 1990

Responsibility

With the exception of Norway, primary and secondary care was integrated at the same governmental level in all Nordic countries. In Finland, health care was the responsibility of local governments (452 units in 1990), but with the hospitals owned and managed by 20 hospital districts organized as associations of local governments.[1] In Denmark and Sweden, the responsibility for health - care was at the county level (15 amts, including two cities in Denmark and 24 landsting, including three cities, in Sweden). The Norwegian model implied separation between primary and secondary care, with the responsibility of primary care placed at the local governmental level (435 units in 1990) and the responsibility for specialist care placed at the county level (19 fylkeskommuner in 1990).

Coordination and planning

In all countries, the central state was responsible for legislation, supervision, parts of health care planning and resource allocation at a general level. As already stated, the Finnish model implies cooperation between local governments through 20 hospital districts. Norway was divided into five health regions in 1974 with three to five counties within each region. Each region was set up with a university hospital and the main aim of the regionalization was to facilitate patient flow between hospitals with different specialties, in particular to increase flow into the specialized university clinics. Voluntary horizontal network arrangements could also be found in Denmark (five regions) and Sweden (six regions), although the models for county cooperation were less formalized here (Calltorp 1995). Annual budget negotiations between the government and the decentralized authorities became an important mechanism for coordination of policy developments in Denmark during the 1990s. Similar arrangements can be found in Sweden, and to a lesser extent in Norway and Finland. The agreements provide an example of a semi-informal negotiations based 'multi level governance' structure, which is typical for the Nordic countries.

Local political participation

Participation could be characterized as broad in all the four countries, as local politicians not only made up local and county councils but also the standing committees for health and, in some countries, hospital boards. In addition, local politicians in Finland made up the boards of the health districts. The underlying principle was that decentralized democratic participation would lead to solutions that were customized to the preferences of the population in each area, and thus increase the legitimacy of the health care system. Local democratic participation was generally seen as a value in itself, but also as a mean to improve responsiveness, accountability and efficiency through the short 'distances' between politicians and the voting population.

Financing

Main revenues to local and county government came from general and earmarked grants from the central state and local/county income taxes. Finland's grant system was more fragmented than in the other Nordic countries, with a higher share of revenues coming from earmarked grants (Hakkinen and Lehto 2005). In Denmark and Sweden, tax discretion for both local and county government was temporarily reduced during the first part of the 1990s by limits (Sweden) or agreements (Denmark) because of the difficult economic situations. In Finland, local government tax rates were stable in this period but with local variations. The Norwegian model diverged from the others as income taxes were only allowed to vary up to an upper level fixed by the central state. This made the Norwegian financing system very centralized.

Inpatient activities in hospitals were mostly funded by global budgets based on negotiation and soft contracts with the counties, while outpatient activities were funded by fee for service and capitation. Finland was a special case since hospitals collected their revenues by invoicing the local government. Primary physicians in all countries were paid by combinations of salaries and/or fee-for-service and capitation-based payments.

Patient choice

The right to choose a hospital in other regions/hospital districts was restricted in all Nordic countries at the start of the 1990s. Choice of GPs was restricted in Sweden and Finland while patient choice of GPs and practising specialists was an option in the Danish system since the 1970s (choice of practising specialists involved co-payment). Also in Norway, choice of GP had been practised for a considerable time.

5.2.2 Major reforms implemented during the 1990s and early 2000s

The Nordic health care reforms started in Sweden in the early 1990s with the introduction of internal markets and amalgamations of counties into regions. While the internal market reform in Sweden was gradually reversed, even more radical reforms were implemented in Norway and Denmark, although based on somewhat different principles and policy models.

Sweden

Sweden was a pioneer in the introduction of market-oriented reforms in publicly funded health care systems (Harrison and Calltorp 2000). Starting with local initiatives around 1990, several county councils introduced internal markets within the health sector by introducing a split between purchaser and providers (Anell 1996). The most radical experiment was probably represented by the county of Dalarne, where 15 local boards with close ties to primary care clinics became fundholders. The city of Stockholm represented another model, with districts boards without close ties to primary care institutions, being the fundholders. The purchaser–provider split was accompanied by a national patient choice reform and care guarantee that aimed to increase the access to hospital care. These led most counties to introduce models where 'moneys were to follow the patients', meaning that county councils had to finance hospital care outside their formal organization. Thus, a weak form of competition between hospitals was introduced. An increasing number of counties also introduced diagnosis-related group (DRG)-based financing of hospitals. Most county councils combined DRG-based financing with global budgets. Stockholm was an important exception as the district boards developed activity-based financing (ABF) contracts, first for internal medicine (1993), later also for other parts of the hospitals' activities. A measure for cost control remained as the reimbursement rates were to decrease as activity exceeded target levels.

However, within just a few years, the county councils abandoned the internal market models and turned to a more diverse set of reform initiatives (Harrison and Calltorp 2000). First, nearly all counties that had introduced a purchaser–provider-spilt chose to consolidate the decentralized purchasing bodies. For example, Stockholm introduced a single board that coordinated purchasing from 1996. Later on, concerns for fragmentation in the chain of care replaced cost-efficiency concerns and a more consultative and negotiation-based process replaced competition between hospitals. Second, by the mid-1990s, regional planning became an alternative to county-based reform initiatives. County politicians facing tight county budgets increasingly viewed regional regulation as a mean to contain cost and at the same time supply patients with high-quality care. Far-reaching moves towards regionalization got underway and several counties both in the western and southern part of Sweden were amalgamated into two larger county regions.

The proposal of creating larger county regions was further developed by the National Committee on Public Sector Responsibility (Ansvarskomiteen), which delivered its proposal in February 2007 (SOU 2007). The Committee's main suggestion implied reduction in the number of county councils and creation of larger county regions and thereby larger health care authorities. The proposals are at the time of writing in a process of deliberation in the Swedish political system. The counties are, however, free to form larger regions on a voluntary basis. Currently, voluntary amalgamation seems more likely than a major amalgamation reform implemented from the top.

Norway

Four major reforms were implemented at the turn of the century: ABF for hospitals (1997), a list patient system in primary care (2001), free choice of hospitals (2001) and the central state takeover of hospitals (2002).

During the 1980s, counties and hospitals were given annual global budgets based on risk-adjusted capitation payment. The introduction of ABF from 1 July 1997 implied that a fraction of the block grant from the state to the county councils was replaced by a matching grant depending upon the number and composition of hospital treatments measured in DRG equivalents. The counties were expected to pass on the matching grants to the hospitals. This also happened, and by 1998 close to 90 per cent of the acute hospitals was financed by contracts where 45 per cent of the expected revenues came as DRG-based reimbursement (Biorn et al. 2003). The share of ABF peaked in the years 2003 and 2005 (60 per cent) but subsequently reduced (2006–2009: 40 per cent). Free choice of hospitals was introduced through the new Patients Rights Act, which was implemented in 2001. Implementation of choice of hospitals at national level came after a period of experimentation with choice within the five health regions that started in the early 1990s.

There were three main elements in the list patient reform in primary health - care: (1) every citizen became listed on a specific GP's list and the GP became responsible for a share of the population; (2) the reimbursement system changed from a combination of global budget and fee for service to a combination of capitation and fee for service; and (3) most GPs changed their organizational form from being local government employees to being self-employed. The main idea behind the reform was to reduce turnover among GPs in primary care and introduce more stability in the GP–patient relationship (Fjermestad and Paulsen 2000; Iversen 2004).

The hospital reform implemented on 1 January 2002 had four main elements (Hagen and Kaarboe 2006; Magnussen et al. 2007). First, the central government took over responsibility of all public hospitals and other parts of specialist health care from the counties. Second, the Minister of Health was given responsibility for the overall general management of specialist care and would stand surety for the hospitals in the event of bankruptcy. Third, the central government maintained the five health regions established in 1974 as the organizational unit for coordination and steering and established five regional health authorities (RHAs) with the responsibility for acquisition of health care from public or private providers.[2] Combined, these three elements can be said to imply centralization. The fourth element of the reform represented elements of decentralization, as both the RHAs and the hospitals were organized as health enterprises or trusts. These bodies were set up as independent legal subjects with their own responsibilities for personnel and capital. The enterprises both at regional and local level were to be governed by professional boards with state-appointed representatives, preferably with business experience, assuming the role of stock-holder representatives in private firms. This particular element of the reform was, however, reversed from 2006 as local politicians appointed by the Minister of Health were reinstated as board members.

Denmark

Several important changes have been implemented in Denmark starting in the early 1990s. Free hospital choice was introduced in 1993 and expanded to certain private facilities for patients who are facing waiting times of more than two months from examination to treatment.

A DRG system has gradually been introduced and has become an important part of the governance structure. Patients crossing county lines are fully reimbursed on a DRG basis, and many counties used the DRG system to introduce limited ABF schemes. The central government also used the DRG system to develop incentive schemes for specific extra funding to the hospitals (2002–2004), and to measure and compare productivity developments. However, the level of ABF to counties and hospitals has been far below the Norwegian levels.

A major structural reform was implemented in 2007. As of 1 January 2007, the responsibility for hospital care in Denmark was moved from the existing 15 counties to five newly created regions. The counties ceased to exist as political and administrative entities. The new regions are governed by generally elected councils of 42 members, which maintain responsibility for managing the hospital services. Tax financing of the system is removed from the regional level. Municipalities gain a stronger role in prevention and health promotion. They also get a new role in financing of hospital services as they pay both ABF and a basic capitation fee to the regions for their citizens. Approximately 12 per cent of all regional hospital expenses will be financed this way. The idea is to create incentives for municipalities to develop prevention and rehabilitation services and generally put pressure on the regions.

Regions and municipalities are mandated to coordinate efforts via special regionally based coordination councils. The National Board of Health is intended to take a stronger role in planning and coordination of decentralized activities. The implementation of a national quality assurance programme will standardize treatment programmes and generally facilitate monitoring of regional health system performance.

The structural reform maintains the governing of primary care at the regional level. The GPs also remain private, albeit strongly integrated in regional planning structures and with a continued strong role as gate keepers to the system. New linkages between GPs and the municipalities have been introduced as the municipalities get more responsibility for rehabilitation, prevention and health promotion. Many municipalities are setting up health centres but the exact coordination with GPs is unclear as yet. The ambiguity is reinforced by the fact that the reform creates incentives for municipalities to reduce the flow of patients to hospitals (through the co-payment), while the actual referral decisions in most cases are made by GPs.

Finland

The most important reform in the Finnish health care system during the 1090s occurred in 1993 as part of a reform of the grant system between the central state and the local governments (Hakkinen 2005). The essential element of the reform was to reduce the number of earmarked grants based on actual costs and to increase the share of the grants coming as global budgets derived from need-based capitation formulae. In health care, the reform was intended to give local governments a more active role as purchasers of health care, in that local governments were given more discretion in organizing, regulating and administer the service production.

In parallel to the state subsidy reform, several central state regulations of the local health system, such as control of capital spending and control of user fees, were abandoned. It is, however, a mistake to see only deregulation (Hakkinen and Lehto 2005). Parallel to the deregulation of some policy measures, there is the development of softer regulations and information guidance, such as improvement of statistic gathering and development of guidelines for technology assessment. A consequence of the greater autonomy at local level has been projects and experiments with quite different purposes. The experiments include strategies for merging hospitals into larger units, utilizing the non-profit private sector as providers and formalizing the purchaser–provider split. At the time of writing, several hospital districts are planning experiments with more integrated health and social care organizations. The integration implies both closer cooperation between the municipalities within a hospital district and closer integration between primary and specialist care.

Since 1997, the DRG-based financing has gradually replaced per diem-based financing. At first, a few hospital districts started to use DRGs as the basis for invoicing local governments. By 2005, almost half of the hospital districts based their invoice system on DRGs. However, the system is not activity based in the sense that it prospectively signals the price per unit of activity. Rather it is used to allocate hospital district costs between participating municipalities and as a tool in negotiations at the hospital district level with local politicians whenever there is a discrepancy between the actual and agreed cost/volume.

5.2.3 Summary of major changes

Returning to the five variables that were used to describe the health care system, we can conclude that major changes have been implemented.

Responsibility

The Norwegian hospital reform of 2002 represents the most radical change, as the central state took over responsibility for specialist care. The organizational changes in Denmark created larger regional and municipal units, moved responsibility for prevention and health promotion to the municipalities and strengthened central level competencies. Reforms in Sweden have not yet implied changes in responsibility between the tiers of governments. However, in respect of *coordination and planning*, the conclusion is that the reforms implemented in both Norway, Denmark, and partly in Sweden, represent major restructuring of the system. In all three countries, coordination and planning are now performed within greater regions. New types of formal coordination between regions and municipalities have also been introduced in Denmark. Coordination between state and decentralized levels in terms of general agreements has gradually been strengthened in Denmark and Sweden. In Denmark, the National Board of Health has gained stronger formal powers to influence coordination processes at the regional and municipal level. In Finland, work is presently underway with the ambition of both simplifying the system of intergovernmental transfers and encouraging a higher level of between-municipal cooperation. This means that there are financial incentives for municipalities that merge, and the stated ambition is that primary health care and social services should be organized by municipalities or joint organizations of municipalities with a minimum of 20,000 inhabitants.

The role of *local politicians* has changed, most notably in Norway where indirectly appointed boards have replaced directly elected politicians at the regional level. The same structure was considered as part of the negotiations for the structural reform in Denmark, but the decision-makers finally settled on a model with directly elected politicians in the reduced number of regions.

Financing

The financing of health care has changed markedly. This is particular the case in Denmark where regional (county) taxation has been removed and municipalities have become co-financers of hospital care for their citizens. The Norwegian hospital reform also implies that taxation at the regional level has been removed. However, since tax rates were also fixed by the central state before the reform, this hardly changed regional discretion. All four countries have introduced DRG-based financing of acute hospitals. In Norway and Denmark, DRG-based financing is combined with ABF at various levels, although with important differences. *Patient choice of hospitals* was introduced in Denmark, Norway and Sweden at the beginning of the 1990s and gradually formalized (Vrangbaek and Christiansen 2005). Choice was introduced via national legislation in Denmark (formalized in 1993) and Norway (formalized in 2001), while in Sweden it is based on an agreement between the county councils.

5.3 Explaining changes and reforms

In the case of the Nordic health care systems, objectives have been fairly stable over time, although the relative weight given to each may have differed. In all four countries, equality and efficiency are main objectives, while service quality, patient choice and legitimacy are just some of numerous additional goals. The means to achieve these goals have, however, changed over time. In this section, we try to explain the reforms since the early 1990s by identifying some underlying policy beliefs.

5.3.1 Size and scale effects as means to increase efficiency and quality

All four countries have believed that efficiency can be increased by more emphasis on large-scale hospital production. Investments, particularly in university hospitals and high-technology equipment, have been extremely expensive for the former Finnish hospital owners as well as the traditional counties in Sweden, Denmark and Norway. This led to larger hospital districts in Finland from 1990, as well as the present trend to merge municipalities into larger units, amalgamation of counties in Sweden from mid-1990s, the establishment of five RHAs in Norway from 2002 and five regions in Denmark from 2007.

In Sweden, regional planning was proposed as an alternative to county-based reform initiatives during the mid-1990s. County politicians facing tight county budgets increasingly viewed regional regulation as a means to contain cost and at the same time supply patients with high-quality care (Harrison and Calltorp 2000). The arguments were clearly spelled out by the Swedish National Committee on Public Sector Responsibility that recommended amalgamation of counties into regions (SOU 2007).

The belief in scale effects as a mean to increase efficiency was not clearly spelled out in the proposal for central government takeover of the acute hospitals that was forwarded to the Norwegian parliament by the spring of 2001 (Ministry of Health and Care 2000–2001) although this had been an argument for centralization of the hospital sector in commission reports leading up to the reform (NOU 1996, 2000). However, as documented by Nerland (2007), the RHAs were granted discretion in the choice of organizational structure and discussed two main options: (1) an integrated model with large health enterprises and integration (no purchaser–provider split) between the RHAs and the health enterprises, and (2) smaller health enterprises that competed for contracts from the RHA (purchaser–provider split). The analysis indicates that the primary goals of the RHAs were cost-efficiency and clinical quality. The RHAs gave less weight to goals such as patient choice and proximity to hospitals as they selected organizational models. The belief that cost-efficiency and clinical quality could best be realized by large-scale production led to the implementation of the integrated model.

In Denmark, there has been a general growth in the development of horizontal coordination across counties in the form of national agreements and coordinative efforts by the Association of County Councils and in the form of voluntary regional integration of functions. This has led to a de facto reduction in county variation in delivery of health services and possibly to scale effects for highly specialized medicine. The belief in scale effects was pronounced in the final report from the Government Commission for Structural Change (Ministry of Health 2004). The report argued that both efficiency and quality benefits would be the result of centralizing and thus specializing hospital delivery. The general argument was that larger and more specialized units would provide broader experience and better specialist training through larger volume.

5.3.2 Prospective payment systems as means to increase efficiency

The belief in prospective payment systems as a mean to increase cost-efficiency has led all four countries to utilize the DRG systems in a financial setting. The DRG system has served as a platform for various types of financing scheme, both ABF, as in Denmark, Norway and Sweden's capital Stockholm, and global budgets based on benchmarking and per-case payment, as in several Swedish counties and parts of Finland. However, in most countries, the belief in prospective payment systems as a mean to increase efficiency was combined with a belief that it would also increase activity. As stated by Anell (1996) for the Swedish case: 'The focus on per-case payments can be explained by the fact that the major problems discussed in the late 1980s were first of all, the long waiting times and the lack of incentives for high productivity'.

Similar thinking can be found in Norway (Hagen and Kaarboe 2006). Long waiting times for elective treatment was a central political issue in the late 1980s and during the 1990s. A waiting-time guarantee, increased global budgets at the beginning of the 1990s and the introduction of ABF from 1997 were all reforms that were directed towards addressing this problem. However, the former two initiatives did not successfully bring down the number of patients on waiting lists or the number of violations of the waiting-time guarantee. The main reason was that the county councils responded to the increased funding by reducing their expenditure on specialized health care. For example, while total real expenditure on specialized health care increased by 6.3 per cent from 1991 to 1994, the county councils' share of expenditure fell by 1 per cent. In addition, some hospital departments strategically chose to maintain long waiting lists since these were interpreted (by the counties) as a signal of excess demand. In this manner, long waiting lists in one year were often followed by increased budgets in the following year. The use of ABF can be viewed as a solution to these problems as revenues are tied to the hospitals' activities.

5.3.3 Patients' choice of hospital as a mean to higher efficiency, better quality and service

Patient choice is linked to several of the underlying objectives for the Nordic health systems (Vrangbæk and Østergren 2006). The political rhetoric around choice has emphasized that the introduction of contestability via choice will put pressure on hospitals to deliver better quality and service. The availability of information is an important prerequisite for this, and all Nordic health systems have introduced internet-based declarations of quality and expected waiting times. Yet, issues of interpretation may reduce their usefulness.

Another underlying belief is that choice leads to increased mobility and that increased mobility leads to higher efficiency through the utilization of spare capacity. As patients become aware of differences in waiting times, they are expected to travel to facilities offering the shortest waiting times as they have spare capacity (Vrangbæk 1999). Choice has been combined with waiting-times guarantees in Denmark and Norway. The guarantees offer access to treatment in a number of private facilities when the public system is unable to secure treatment within particular time limits (one month for all non-acute treatment in Denmark). The belief is that this type of choice will provide more flexibility for the patient and make the public hospitals work harder to improve service quality since they will otherwise have to pay for patients seeking treatment in private facilities. Assessment of the results is complicated by the fact that few patients have used choice, and many other changes have been introduced at the same time. Finland introduced a waiting-time guarantee in 2005, covering both primary and specialized health care. The legislation was accompanied by a substantial increase in funds, primarily to reduce the backlog of patients waiting. Notably, Finland also published national guidelines for non-elective care; such guidelines were not a part of the Norwegian process, and the result was substantial geographical variations in the interpretation of the patient rights legislation.

5.4.3 Stronger hierarchical governance as a means to increase equality, quality and (macro-) efficiency

Stronger regulatory ambitions of the central state seem to be a common trend in all four countries, but this trend is more pronounced in Norway and Denmark than in Finland and Sweden. Standards for quality and waiting times have been introduced in all countries, and monitoring systems are currently being implemented to follow these up. Waiting-time guarantees have been combined with other elements of a rights-based health system, such as right to information, right to second opinion and right to choice of hospital, as can be found in the Norwegian Patient Act.

Another indication of stronger hierarchical steering ambitions is a gradual intensification of vertical coordination between state, county and municipal actors. This has been the case in Denmark in particular, where annual budget agreements specify targets for municipal taxes and expenditure and increasingly also include details on other performance targets and organizational and management measures to reach these targets. These negotiations have thus developed into an important arena for steering and streamlining efforts in the sector. The position of the state in these negotiations has been backed by overt or latent threats of legislative intervention. It is, therefore, a form of forced self-regulation in the shadow of the state hierarchy. National legislation has supplemented agreements, for example on choice, waiting-time guarantees (extended free choice) and the introduction of special schemes with ABF. Further, at least in Denmark, it has been an explicit purpose of the structural reform to strengthen the role of the National Board of Health in regards to placement and planning of specialty services. This reflects a reduced trust in decentralized authorities with regard to self-governance and voluntary horizontal coordination. Steering through standards, vertical coordination and more formal planning power invested in state institutions are all policy means aimed to create more equitable service levels across geographical regions. Monitoring performance with regard to standards is supposed to raise quality and service levels, via benchmarking and implicit threats of intervention in performance failure.

5.3.5 Country-specific explanations

Apart from these instrumental beliefs in policy means to achieve common objectives, explanations of reforms seem country specific. This has been the case in Denmark and Norway, in particular, which have implemented the most radical reforms.

Norway

The fact that Norway ended with a model with hospitals owned by the central state can be explained by two mechanisms. First, Norway can be characterized by a strong resistance against amalgamations of local and county governments. This made the reforms at the local level difficult as problems of high costs in specialized hospitals materialized during the 1990s. Second, the introduction of ABF in 1997 increased the number of patients treated, as a consequence of both higher technical efficiency and general increases in funding. From 1999, the number of waits and waiting times started to come down. However, this is overwhelmed by what Hagen and Kaarbøe (2003) call three dysfunctional effects concerning the management of the health care sector. First, county councils became more financially dependent on the central government, with the share of county council own spending on acute-care hospital services decreasing from more than 72 per cent in 1996 to less than 44 per cent in 2001. Second, since the ABF did not fully cover marginal costs (only 40–50 per cent of the standard national cost per DRG-point was actually reimbursed in this period), increased production led to deficits and claims for supplementary funds during the budget years. In general, the minority government cabinets from this period responded positively to these claims and the counties were bailed out. Finally, and as a consequence of the increased dependence on central funding and bailouts, the transparency of the governance system was reduced and a 'blame game' was initiated between the central state and the counties over responsibility for increasing deficits. This eroded the trust between the central authorities and the county councils.

By June 2000, Prime Minister Stoltenberg (Labour Party) hinted that radical changes in the hospital sector were under way, and during the autumn of 2000 the central committee of the Labour Party approved the main elements of the 2002 hospital reforms. The reform proposal was sent to the parliament in

January 2001 and was passed with votes from the Labour Party and the right-wing Progressive Party, a party that had favoured central government takeover for a long time. The Conservative Party also voted for central government takeover of hospitals, given the reform a comfortable majority, but preferred an organizational model with a purchaser–provider split.

Denmark

A rare window of opportunity for large-scale structural reform opened with the election of a new centre-right government with relatively fixed majority support from 2002 and onwards (Bundgaard and Vrangbæk 2007). This basic condition was combined with a number of other more or less coincidental factors. The opposition was weak and divided, as the Social Democrats were in a leadership transition. An opinion poll in the summer of 2002 showed weak support for the county institution. A coalition of industry representatives, media and younger, more ideologically oriented, politicians in the two government parties served as policy entrepreneurs and agenda setters. The policy change was facilitated by a general normative shift from support of 'local democracy' as a means of ensuring legitimacy to a strong belief in 'benefits of scale', partially inspired by the wave of mergers and fusions in the private sector. In other words, the legitimacy focus shifted from input and process dimensions to output dimensions (Vrangbæk 2007). The interest organization for Danish municipalities (Local Government Denmark) supported the reform, as it became clear that they would gain more responsibilities at the expense of the counties. The government support party and the minor government coalition party strongly favoured the reform. Both parties had been critical of the counties for a long time, and both had weak representation in the county councils. The largest government party (Venstre (Liberals)) and the largest opposition party (the Social Democrats) both had strong representation in the counties. Venstre also had a large number of mayors in small municipalities, but within the parliamentary group it appeared that the younger and more centralist members had gained power at the expense of more traditional decentralist voices. The structural reform reflected several of the policy beliefs presented above. It created larger regions with the explicit purpose of scale and scope benefits. It also strengthened the national steering competencies, and weakened the position of the regional governance structure.

5.3.6 Summary

Health care has become more important on the national political agenda in all four countries. This has led to a process where national and decentralized actors have sought policy responses to emerging challenges for meeting underlying goals. A number of general policy beliefs have emerged in all countries. In particular, it appears that beliefs in size and benefits of scale, prospective payment systems, choice and stronger hierarchical steering by the state have fuelled a number of gradual institutional changes in the governing structure for the Nordic health systems. Stronger national-level steering ambitions and less faith in decentralized democratic solutions have, therefore, been common in all four countries. Another general trend has been to emphasize incentives, surveillance and sanctions as key instruments in state control over decentralized health services. Two of the countries, Denmark and Norway, have embarked on major structural reforms that are based on a combination of beliefs and related institutional changes. The specific timing and design of the institutional changes have differed between the countries according to specific conditions and strategic situations.

5.4 Effects of the reforms

We commence with some speculations on the effect of the reforms in terms of the general health policy goals, and in terms of the inherent dilemmas of coordination, division of labour in governing processes and maintaining legitimacy. Before starting, it should be emphasized that in many cases it is still premature to evaluate the results of the reforms, and that some of the studies referred to are flawed by confounding factors: in many cases, different changes were occurring at the same time. Effects on outcome and service quality are even more difficult to measure and relate to the reforms.

5.4.1 Equality

Nordic countries are known for their egalitarianism. However, cross-national analysis indicates that income-related inequality in health is also present within the Nordic countries and in the elderly in particular (van Doorslaer and Koolman 2004). Furthermore, access to medical care does not seem completely without an income gradient (van Doorslaer et al. 2006). However, only one study has been identified that explicitly addresses the effects of a reform on equality of access. One of the main goals related to the Norwegian hospital reform of 2002 was to achieve a more equitable access to specialist health care. The analysis by Nerland and Hagen (2008) indicates that waiting time, travel distance and primary care supply, as well as hospital-specific effects, have significant effects on the use of specialist care, even after controlling for need. However, estimation of Gini coefficients for the distribution of the non-need-related consumption indicates that the inequality has been stable over time and, therefore, the objective of a more equitable access has not been achieved. Consequently, a definitive conclusion as to whether there has been an increase in inequality after the 2002 hospital reform cannot be drawn.

5.4.2 Cost-efficiency

Effects of the reforms on cost-efficiency have been analysed more systematically. A study of the purchaser–provider-split in Sweden (Gerdtham et al. 1999) concludes that the switch from budget-based allocations to output-based allocations led to a 13 per cent decrease in costs among Swedish hospitals. The study utilized data from two years, 1993 and 1994. Later analyses, such as that of Charpentier and Samuelsson (1999), have studied productivity changes in the county of Stockholm in the period from 1992 to 1997 and find productivity gains in 1993 and 1994 followed by productivity reductions in subsequent years.

A test of efficiency gains through the introduction of ABF in Norway has been performed by Biorn and co-workers (2003). Efficiency indicators were estimated using data envelopment analysis with multiple inputs and outputs. Using a variety of econometric methods, the finding is that the introduction of ABF improved efficiency when measured as technical efficiency but the results were less uniform with respect to the effect on cost-efficiency. Danish studies have given the same inconclusive picture. Although cost-efficiency is supposed to have increased, it is unclear exactly what is the linkage to the reforms being implemented. Some studies indicate that the introduction of the DRG and the experiments with limited ABF have had some positive impact. However, the same studies also strongly emphasize that the effects depend on the institutional choices and management reactions in each case (Pedersen et al. 2006).

A project comparing Norway and Finland (Linna et al. 2006) reveals marked differences in efficiency, both within country and across countries. According to preliminary results, there was more variation in cost-efficiency among Finnish hospitals, and the average level of cost-efficiency was 17–25 per cent lower in Norwegian hospitals. A follow-up study utilized a similar Nordic dataset and tested the efficiency effects of the Norwegian hospital reform of 2002 (Kittelsen et al. 2007). The analysis indicates a positive and significant effect of 3–4 per cent for the reform.

Another, more or less explicit, aim with the reforms has been to increase cost-efficiency by increasing the size of the hospitals. A recent analysis of hospital mergers in Norway during the 1990s (Kjekshus and Hagen 2007) indicates that mergers involving radical restructuring of the treatment process may have improved efficiency as intended, as positive effects on both cost and technical efficiency were found in a merger where more hospitals were involved, and where administration and acute services were centralized. However, most mergers did not have the intended effects. In general, the mergers showed no significant effect on technical efficiency and a significant negative effect of 2–2.8 per cent on cost-efficiency.

5.4.3 Governance dynamics, coordination and division of labour

The 2002 Norwegian hospital reform had as its most important goal to stop the 'blame game' between the regional actors (counties) and the central government. It was argued that removing such gaming was a necessary condition for hardening the budget constraint, and a harder budget constraint was seen as a means to increase efficiency. At the time of writing, evidence indicates that this has not happened. Hospital activities still exceed production targets and since reimbursements through ABF do not cover marginal costs, the hospitals produce deficits (Tjerbo and Hagen in press). Neither has the reform performed well in the restructuring of the hospitals. The removing of politicians and the introduction of professionals into the process were seen as instrumental to this aim. As demonstrated by Tjerbo (2007), the new professional leaders at first acted in accordance with the intentions of the hospital reform and proposed numerous plans for structural reorganizations, but these were overturned by the parliament and the central state as the proposals went forward to be implemented. The evidence indicates that the removal of formal political organization locally did not necessarily increase the decision-making capacity for issues that are considered politically controversial. From 2006, the government reintroduced local politicians into the decision-making process at RHA level and fewer plans for restructuring have been discussed.

In Denmark, a comprehensive planning process is now taking place in the new regions. This involves significant structural changes, where treatment functions are combined and hospitals and departments are closed down. A new hospital infrastructure, including several new hospital facilities, is being planned. The establishment of new facilities and the restructuring of old facilities imply new investments which must be covered from the central (state) level. So far, there has been agreement on a general increase in health care spending, but this is unlikely to be sustainable in the longer term. The regional demands and the national signals of willingness to pay are quite far apart. The most likely future development is towards a situation as in Norway, with ongoing political conflicts between regions and state on the financial situation of the sector.

The political structure in the regions is somewhat problematic. They have lost their financing responsibility, which leads to incentives for pressuring the national government. They are also structurally constrained as they are not allowed to create specialized standing committees. This means that all health issues must be discussed in the plenary sessions of 42 members. This is likely to change the dynamics of policy-making from detailed, pragmatic and expert based to more general (party) political interaction. The new powers of the National Board of Health and the implementation of a national quality assessment programme with standards and accreditation will reduce the scope for regional variation in service delivery.

It is uncertain as yet whether efficiency or service improvements will be the outcome of the reform. So far, it seems that transition costs are high and that the structure may lead to ongoing pressure for expenditure increases and political conflicts. This has led some observers to conclude that the current regional structure is unstable and most likely a temporary design, which may be replaced by either more regional power or state-run enterprises.

5.4.4 Maintaining legitimacy?

Have the reforms brought closure to the political debates over the public health system? Are there indications that the population is more supportive of the public system now than before? Health care has continued to be high on the political agenda in all countries. Rather than targeting the new regional governance structures or issuing demands for local democratic participation channels, the general population appears to be focusing on the national political forum. This provides part of the explanation for the increased steering ambitions from the state, as national politicians are held responsible for health system performance but have relinquished direct management power.

Private health insurance is increasing in all four countries. Although fuelled by other factors such as the tax structure, this is an indication of reduced faith in the delivery level of the public system. On the more positive side, the population in each country appears willing to pay taxes when they are directly linked to health care. This may change as larger part of the population pay double via private insurance. Patient satisfaction ratings also continue to be high in all the Nordic countries, although with slightly declining trends.

5.5 Conclusions

The reforms implemented in the Nordic health care systems since the early 1990s have striking similarities but also important differences. The shared policy beliefs include the benefits of scale and incentive systems as pathways to increase efficiency and higher national steering to increase equality. Alongside these beliefs, there is less faith in decentralized democratic solutions. However, the dissimilarities are even more striking. While reforms in Sweden and Finland are grounded in a decentralized model, elements of the Norwegian model for specialist care and possibly also the Danish model point towards a more centralized NHS-style model with less local representation and stronger hierarchical governance. The balance of power in health policy-making, therefore, seems to have shifted towards the state level in regard to financing, planning and quality/ service dimensions, although regional and municipal authorities have retained a strong role in the actual implementation and management of services for two of the Nordic countries. How these changes affect the legitimacy of the models remains to be seen and will depend upon several factors, including the degree of rationing of health care, the effect of patient choice and a more pragmatic view of the supply from private sector. It can be concluded that the reforms have not brought closure to the legitimacy debate for the public health system.

Notes

1. The islands of Åland constitute a demilitarized and neutralized, Swedish-speaking region within Finland with an autonomy guaranteed through international treaties. Åland's autonomy is significant in all matters related to public service production, including health and social care.
2. The number of RHAs was reduced to four from 1 July 2007 as the eastern and southern RHAs were amalgamated.

References

Anell, A. (1996) The monopolistic integrated model and health care reform: the Swedish experience, *Health Policy* 37: 19–33.

Biorn, E., Hagen, T.P., Iversen, T. and Magnussen, J. (2003) The effect of activity-based financing on hospital efficiency: a panel data analysis of DEA efficiency scores 1992–2000, *Health Care Management and Science* 6: 271–83.

Bundgaard, U. and Vrangbæk, K. (2007) Reform by coincidence? Explaining the policy process of structural reform in Denmark, *Scandinavian Political Studies* 30: 491–520.

Calltorp, J. (1995) Swedish experiments with fixed regional budgets, in Schwartz, F.W., Glennerster, H. and Saltman, R.B. (eds) *Fixing Health Budgets: Experience from Europe and North America*. London: Wiley.

Charpentier, C. and Samuelsson, L. (1999) *Effekter av en sjukvårdsreform: En analys av Stockholmsmodellen*. Stockholm: Nerenius and Santérus.

Fjermestad, T. and Paulsen, B. (2000) List patient system: straitjacket or a tool for developing general practice? General practitioners' experiences from a pilot project in Norway, *Scandinavian Journal of Primary Health Care* 18: 21–4.

Gerdtham, U.G., Lothgren, M., Tambour, M. and Rehnberg, C. (1999) Internal markets and health care efficiency: a multiple-output stochastic frontier analysis, *Health Economics* 8: 151–64.

Hagen, T.P. and Kaarbøe, O.A. (2006) The Norwegian hospital reform of 2002: central government takes over ownership of public hospitals, *Health Policy* 76: 320–33.

Hakkinen, U. (2005) The impact of changes in Finland's health care system, *Health Economics* 14: S101–18.

Hakkinen, U. and Lehto, J. (2005) Reform, change, and continuity in Finnish health care, *Journal of Health Politics Policy and Law* 30: 79–96.

Harrison, M.I. and Calltorp, J. (2000) The reorientation of market-oriented reforms in Swedish health-care, *Health Policy* 50: 219–40.

Iversen, T. (2004) The effects of a patient shortage on general practitioners' future income and list of patients, *Journal of Health Economics* 23: 673–94.

Kittelsen, S. Magnussen, J. and Anthun K. (2007) *Sykehusproduktivitet etter statlig overtakelse: En nordisk komparativ analyse*. Oslo: Health Economic Research, University of Oslo.

Kjekshus, L.-E. and Hagen, T.P. (2007) Do hospital mergers increase hospital efficiency? Evidence from a National Health Service country, *Journal of Health Service Research Policy* 12: 230–5.

Linna, M., Hakkinen, U. and Magnusen, J. (2006) Comparing hospital cost efficiency between Norway and Finland, *Health Policy* 77: 268–78.

Magnussen, J., Hagen, T.P. and Kaarboe O.M. (2007) Centralized or decentralized? A case study of Norwegian hospital reform, *Social Science Medicine* 64: 2129–37.

Ministry of Health [Indenrigs- og Sundhedsministeriet] (2004) Betænkning nr. 1434. Strukturkommissionen. Copenhagen: Government of Denmark.

Ministry of Health and Care (2000–2001) *Ot. prp. nr. 66: Om lov om helseforetak, m.v.* [*Proposition to the Odelsting No. 66: Act considering Health Enterprises, a.s.o.*] Oslo: Ministry of Health and Care.

Musgrave, R.A. (1959) *The Theory of Public Finance: A Study in Public Economy*. New York: McGraw-Hill.

Nerland, S.M. (2007) *Effekter av sykehusreformen: Fire essays om mål og virkemidler i styringen av spesialisthelsetjenestene*. Oslo: Faculty of Medicine, University of Oslo.

Nerland, S.M. and Hagen, T.P. (2008) Forbruk av spesialisthelsetjenester: Ble det større likhet etter sykehusreformen? *Tidsskrift for samfunnsforskning* 49: 37–72.

NOU (1996) *NOU 1996: 5. Hvem skal eie sykehusene?* Oslo: Ministry of Health and Care Services.

NOU (2000) *NOU 2000: 22. Oppgavefordelingen mellom stat, region og kommuner*. Oslo: Ministry of Health and Care Services.

Oates, W.E. (1972) *Fiscal Federalism.* New York: Harcourt Brace Jovanovich.

Pedersen, K.M., Beck, M. and Hansen, M.B. (2006) *Incitamentsstyring i Sygehusvesenet.* Odense: Syddansk Universitetsforlag [University Press of Southern Denmark].

Rattsø, J. (2003) Vertical fiscal imbalance in a welfare state: Norway, in Rodden, J., Eskeland, G., and Litvack., J. (eds) *Fiscal Decentralization and the Challenge of Hard Budget Constraints.* Cambridge, MA: MIT Press.

Saltman, R.B. and Bergman, S.E. (2005) Renovating the commons: Swedish health care reforms in perspective, *Journal of Health Politics Policy and Law* 30: 253–75.

SOU (2007) *SOU 2007: 10. Hållbar samhällsorganisation med utvecklingskraft, Ansvarskommitténs slutbetänkande.* Stockholm: Slutbetänkande. Statens Offentliga Utredningar [Government Offices].

Tiebout, C.M. (1956) A pure theory of public expenditures, *Journal of Political Economy* 64: 416–24.

Tjerbo, T. (2007) *HORN Paper* 4: *Målkonflikter og styringsdilemmaer. Utviklingen av Sykehuset Innlandet etter etableringen.* Oslo: Health Organization Research Norway.

Tjerbo, T. and Hagen., T.P. (in press) Deficits, soft budget constraints and bailouts: budgeting after the Norwegian hospital reform, *Scandinavian Political Studies.*

van Doorslaer, E. and Koolman, X. (2004) Explaining the differences in income-related health inequalities across European countries, *Health Economics* 13: 609–28.

van Doorslaer, E., Masseria, C., Koolman, X. for the OECD Health Equity Group (2006) Inequalities in access to medical care by income in developed countries, *Canadian Medical Association Journal* 174: 177–83.

Vrangbæk, K. (1999) New public management i sygehusfeltet – udforming og konsekvenser, in Bentsen, E.Z. and Borum, F. (eds) *Når Styringsambitioner møder praksis.* Copenhagen: Copenhagen Business School Press.

Vrangbæk, K. (2007) Towards a typology for decentralization in health care, in Saltman, R.B., Bankauskaite, V. and Vrangbaek, K. (eds) *Decentralization in Health Care.* Maidenhead: McGraw Hill/Open University Press for the WHO European Observatory, pp. 44–62.

Vrangbaek, K. and Christiansen, T. (2005) Health policy in Denmark: leaving the decentralized welfare path? *Journal of Health Politics Policy and Law* 30: 29–52.

Vrangbæk, K. and Østergren, K. (2006) Patient empowerment and the introduction of hospital choice in Denmark and Norway, *Health Economics, Policy and Law* 1: 371–394.

chapter six

Meeting rising public expectations: the changing roles of patients and citizens

Ulrika Winblad and Ånen Ringard

6.1 Introduction

The relationship between patients and health care professionals has tradition-ally been described as hierarchical and paternalistic. On the one hand, patients have been subordinated by their lack of knowledge and vulnerability. On the other hand, health care personnel were assumed to know what was in the best interest of their patients and thereby entitled to make the treatment decisions (Kennedy 2003).

Today, increased patient involvement is often presented as a way to redress the power disparity between health professionals and patients. The main approach for strengthening the role of patients has been to enhance their involvement in decision-making and more generally to support a feeling of personal autonomy vis-à-vis the health care system. This, in turn, makes them more satisfied and more responsible for their own health. A growing body of literature has also shown that patient involvement in decision-making improves outcome of care (Rachmani et al. 2002; Arnetz et al. 2004; Coulter 2007). An involved patient is more motivated to comply with treatment plans and decisions. Engagement of patients in their health care is also seen as the best way to ensure sustainability of health systems as involved patients act in a more cost-efficient way.

In line with this reasoning, improving responsiveness to patients has been the primary aim of many health care reforms in the last decades in the Nordic coun-tries as well as in the rest of Europe. All Nordic countries have taken measures to strengthen the role of patients. For example, health care legislation in all four countries now dictates the responsibility of health care professionals to inform patients and involve them in decisions concerning care and treatment. Also, measures have been taken to introduce choice of provider in a health care system, where patients were previously bound to seek care at their nearest health care facilities.

The Nordic countries belong to what has come to be known as the 'social democratic welfare state regime' (Esping-Andersen 1999). The assumption underlying this classification is that the four countries share a common array of features, which, in turn, sets them apart from countries belonging to other regimes. This chapter will examine whether the Nordic countries are similar regarding the roles of citizens and patients in relation to the health care systems. More precisely, the intention is to investigate the prerequisites and formal possibilities for citizen/patient involvement provided by the institutional arrangements in each country. How are the influencing mechanisms formed in the Nordic countries? What, if any, are the main differences between the countries?

6.2 How can citizens and patients influence health care services?

Traditionally, the opinions of citizens have been channelled through the representative parliamentary system. In a Nordic context, this means that it is primarily through public elections, held every three to four years, where citizens are free to express their wishes and/or discontent with social welfare services. Explicit issues about health care are then often intertwined with other political opinions that a political party represents, and it is not uncommon for official party statements about health care to be negotiated or changed in the political process. Another difficulty is that decisions about health care are often divided between different political and/or geographical areas. Taken together, this means that it is often hard for an individual to influence health care decisions directly through the representative parliamentary system. Le Grand (2007, p. 31) addresses the issue in the following way: 'Voting, which could be called a collective mechanism of influencing, takes account of the interests of the community, but is a clumsy instrument for dealing with individual preferences'.

Another collective mechanism of influencing health care is lobbying by interest groups, such as patient organizations. When citizens participate in democratically organized interest groups, a way of influencing health care is created alongside the representative parliamentary system. Most commonly, these interest groups are non-profit and non-governmental; they are often involved in advocacy and representation and are considered to be an integrated part of the democratic civil society. All Nordic countries have a long corporatist tradition where interest groups have been established for reasons such as increasing the knowledge and power of the members. Olson (1965) mainly considered that individual gain was the motivating factor for joining an organization, but later research has shown that another reason could be a common interest in political and social change (Pestoff 1979). While health care interest groups, such as patient organizations, have predominantly been established around specific disease groups for supporting the members with information about the disease and available treatments, they are also involved with lobbying in the political arena in order to improve the conditions of their members.

Both collective mechanisms of influencing (voting and lobbying by interest groups) are effected through the traditional democratic process and are what Albert Hirschman (1970) called 'voice' mechanisms. Another more direct way of influencing health care services is when individuals through their own choices of providers are given powers to influence health care, what Hirschman called 'exit'. When choosing a specific care provider, and leaving another behind, patients are sending signals to the system about what kind of services they prefer. If the actual choice is connected to economic incentives, the power of the patient is strengthened even more.

In political–theoretical terms, the introduction of choice within the public sector implies a displacement from a society-centred democracy model, here called the collective model, to a more individual-based democracy model (Olsen 1990; Möller 1996). In the collective model, it is the political institutions that define needs and steer the service supply. In the individual-based democracy model, the citizens themselves influence the supply by choosing specific caregivers and punishing others by their 'exit'. Citizens using patient choice are acting more like customers in a free market. The demand for patient choice within health care can, therefore, be seen as the promotion of a more individualistic democratic ideal. The collective democracy model, by comparison, emphasizes the citizen's role as a member of society. It builds on solidarity between groups and the premise that every individual feels responsible for the whole. Olsen (1990) writes that this model has often been connected with social democratic politics and that it has been stronger in Swedish politics than elsewhere. During the 1980s and the 1990s, this ideal was more and more displaced by the individual-centred ideal, both by political parties and by the population in general.

To summarize, the two models described here have different perspectives on the individual. Within the collective, society-centred, model, the individuals are citizens with rights and obligations and their opinions are channelled through the political system. Thereafter, needs are allocated together on the aggregated level. In the individual model, decisions of allocation are made through the direct choices of the individuals. In the latter model, the role of the institutions is only to help individuals make the right choices.

The following sections will consider the different institutional factors, both at the collective and the individual level, that have enhanced the possibilities for involvement for both citizens and patients. The chapter is organized around the typology shown in Table 6.1.

Section 6.3 deals with patient involvement on a collective level, although the

Table 6.1 Organization of the discussion of institutional factors

Level at which influence is being exercised	Mechanisms	
	'Voice'	*'Exit'*
Collective level	Patient organizations	–
Individual level	Patient legislation, complaint procedures	Choice of provider

representative parliamentary system is not further addressed in the chapter. Instead, the chapter addresses the possibilities available to citizens and patients to influence the collective level by looking at the role of patient organizations in each country. Questions addressed in this part of the chapter include how well these organizations manage to influence health policy issues and if their role has changed over time.

Section 6.4 considers an institutional factor, on the individual level, that might affect patients' possibilities for influencing their health care; this is the varying legal arrangements in the Nordic countries. The topic of patient rights legislation has been under discussion in all Nordic countries during the last decades. From a European perspective, the Nordic countries have been particularly active in the development of such rights. In addition, the formal complaint procedures are described since they give patients a clear 'voice' in cases of discontent.

Section 6.5 deals more explicitly with policy initiatives that have increased patients' possibilities to influence their health care services through the development of exit-mechanisms. More precisely, the opportunities offered to patients to choose their health care provider will be studied. Sweden, Norway and Denmark have all introduced different rules and legal arrangements to provide for greater patient choice: both for GP and for hospital care. In Finland, patients so far have no formal right to choose. Yet, in practice, private alternatives and a developed occupational health sector offer substantial choices for patients. It is shown that diverse institutional arrangements create different incentives for caregivers to promote patient choice.

Finally, it has to be noted that one part of the typology will not be further investigated in the chapter. So far, we have not found any examples of initiatives/policies that aim to create exit mechanisms on the collective level that are distinct enough to study. A hypothetical example would be the collective ability to opt out of health insurance schemes (e.g. for particular trade groups or regions). Also, the various extensions of patient choice through EU legislation are not addressed in this chapter (Chapter 14 has more on this topic).

6.3 Collective voice mechanisms: the role of patient organizations

The opinions of citizens and patients are in varying ways transferred through the lobbying of patient organizations. Collective action in this way is increasingly recognized as an important way of influencing health policy and service production (Baggott and Forster 2008). Many scholars have noted a serious gap in the literature concerning studies about the role of patient organizations (Baggott and Forster 2008; Söderholm Werkö 2008). In particular, there is a lack of comparative studies.

6.3.1 Increase in numbers and varying size

Looking across the Nordic countries, the number of patient organizations has increased in recent years. For instance, in Finland, scholars talk about the development as 'exponential' since the 1990s (Baggott and Forster 2008). Today, there are about 130–150 national patient organizations in Finland (Vuorenkoski et al. 2008). In Sweden, there are over 200 patient organizations, 92 of them receiving state subsidies and presenting themselves on a national website. In Norway, as well, the number of organizations has steadily increased. In two surveys carried out at the end of the 1990s, between 100 and 110 organizations representing health care users were identified (Glenton and Oxman 1998). In Denmark, there are approximately 200 active patient groups in the country (Strandberg-Larsen et al. 2007).

Another similarity in all four countries is that the size of the organizations varies considerably. In Sweden, for instance, the biggest organization (Reuma-tikerförbundet) has over 60,000 members, whereas the smallest has less than 300 members (Föreningen för Neurosedynskadade). In Denmark, as well, there is a sizeable variation among the organizations, with respect to number of members, size of operating budgets and whether they have a professional staff or mainly rely on volunteers (Strandberg-Larsen et al. 2007).

In all four countries, there are examples of organizations that were founded in the beginning of the twentieth century. The Norwegian Association of the Blind and Partially Sighted can trace its roots back to 1901. Yet the development of Norwegian patient organizations is closely associated with the development of the Norwegian welfare state since the Second World War. The majority of the organizations were, as in the other three countries, formed around particular diseases or health problems, such as heart disease, cancer, arthritis, diabetes or multiple sclerosis. All four countries have also seen a more recent establishment of patient organizations around newly defined diagnose groups and new treatment techniques (Söderholm 2005).

6.3.2 Increased politicization

The Nordic patient organizations seem to work in roughly the same way irrespective of country. Traditionally, the most important aim for patient organizations in Sweden, but also in the other Nordic countries, has been to serve their members with information and support concerning their disease as well as information about new health policies (Ternhag et al. 2005). It is now evident that, in recent years, the patient organizations in all the Nordic countries appear to be more politically aware and have a tendency to take on the role of pressure groups against health care authorities and politicians. This is done by actively participating in public hearing processes, through lobbying national politicians in the parliament and by participating as members in publicly appointed boards and councils. In addition to these efforts, the biggest patient organizations in Sweden, Denmark and Norway act as consultative bodies for new legislation. Finally, the organizations in all Nordic countries have activities aimed at influencing society as a whole, for example through broad information campaigns focusing on either questions of particular interest to their members or on broader public health issues.

A recent Swedish study shows that lobbying and influencing public opinion in a more active way has become increasingly important for the organizations.

A survey sent to the chairpersons in the 60 biggest patient organizations showed clearly that they considered their most important aim to be to safeguard the interests of their members by influencing the decision-makers (Virdeborn 2006). This could be done through official hearings or informal meetings. In Finland, a high level of access to parliament was reported (Baggott and Forster 2008). In Denmark, increased politicization of activities is seen. At least since the mid-1990s, many of the Danish patient organizations can be seen to have taken on a more active role in the ongoing political debate. In addition to being policy advocates, the organizations also act as the voice of patients in the media to ensure that patients' views are not neglected. Some of the larger organizations have a strong track record of involvement in health policy. This is, according to Strandberg-Larsen et al. (2007), often achieved through the formation of coalitions with health care professionals or other patient groups. The smaller patient organizations, however, face far greater challenges when it comes to navigating different decision-making structures. Participation within the corporative channel is not as common among the smaller organizations. This has most certainly led to collaboration in 'umbrella-organizations' that represent a range of different patient organizations.

6.3.3 How efficient are the patient organizations?

As shown above, there is considerable information available regarding the numbers and activities carried out by patient organizations; however, little is known about how efficient these organizations are in representing their members' views on the national political agenda. Few, if any, studies in the Nordic context have looked at the real impact of patient organizations on the policy process. Studies from the United Kingdom have shown that in most cases when patient organizations have been influential they have had support from either powerful professional or commercial interests, or from state agencies. When coalitions were created between patient organizations, drug companies and/or clinicians, they could be very influential (Baggott and Forster 2008).

Studies of 'real impact' are difficult, as patient organizations typically employ multiple direct and indirect strategies simultaneously, and also work with other patient organizations, medical associations or pharmaceutical companies to promote their cause. Consequently, it is hard to design an objective measure for the impact of each patient organization.

6.4 Individual voice mechanisms: patient rights

Section 6.3 described patient organizations, or what we have termed collective 'voice' mechanisms, in the four countries. In this section, the attention is shifted towards 'voice' mechanisms available for the *individual* patient. Since such mechanisms normally are introduced through different kinds of legal arrangement, the section begins with a short presentation of the reasons for the development of patient rights legislation in the Nordic countries.

6.4.1 Patient rights legislation

There are several *motives* for the introduction of patient rights legislation. A motive that is often presented in public debate is that sick patients are in a vulnerable situation because of their dependence on the health care system. It is difficult for patients in this situation to speak for themselves, so they need mechanisms to promote and protect their rights, which could be achieved by patient rights legislation (Perälä 1999). A second motive for such legislation is that patients as *subjects* have traditionally been quite invisible in the legal texts regulating health care. For instance, the Swedish Health and Medical Service Act focuses on the *duties* of health care personnel. The new patient rights laws in the Nordic countries more explicitly regard patients as subjects – and not solely as objects for caregivers' actions (Einevik Bäckstrand 2006). In addition, medical and technological developments have ethical implications that make patient rights legislation more important than previously. Patients of today are also often more demanding. Changes of preferences within the population and requirements for participation in the decision-making process of health care have led to higher demands for more explicit patient rights. International human rights conventions introduced in Europe during the years after the Second World War classified the right to health services as a human right (Kjønstad 1999). A more practical argument, particularly evident in the Swedish debate, has been that comprehensive patient rights legislation should be readily available for patients as well as for staff. Previously, in some of the Nordic countries, patient rights were found in different legal documents and were difficult for patients or staff to locate.

The following text examines patient rights legislation in the Nordic countries in more depth. The particular laws under consideration share certain similarities. Thus, the discussion will be structured according to a typology developed by Kjønstad (1999). The typology consists of three broad categories of rules: (1) those regulating the right to become a patient (e.g. the right to acute care when needed); (2) those regulating the rights patients have when they have attained the status of patients (e.g. the right to confidentiality or the right to refuse treatment); and (3) those providing patients with procedural rights (e.g. the right to appeal to court in case of malpractice). Kjønstad's third category is further examined in Section 6.5 under 'complaint procedure'. In addition to Kjønstad's model, a fourth (procedural) category is added, the 'time limits' offered in regulations that specify a time period for the patient to be treated. Waiting-time guarantees are an example of this category.

Sweden

Sweden, as opposed to the other Nordic countries, has no comprehensive law that regulates patient rights within health care. Different rights for patients, such as the right to a second opinion, patient choice or rules about confidentiality, are incorporated in various legislative acts, agreements and policy documents at state and county council level. Significantly, the Swedish laws regulating the health care field are mostly directed at regulating the behaviour of the personnel and only indirectly provide rights for patients. For instance, one section in the

Health and Medical Service Act stipulates that health care personnel are obliged to provide individualized information to the patient, but it is not stated that the patient has the *right* to receive such information.

Historically, the idea of introducing a formal patient rights act has been raised several times in Sweden but the main climate until 1999 was against formal patient rights legislation. A committee report from 1997 called *The Patient Is Right* is illustrative. The name was somewhat misleading since the report opposed new patient rights legislation. Instead, the committee considered precise patient rights too hard to specify within health care and also implied that explicit rights would require medical experts in court since these matters concerned medical issues.

The committee also argued that explicit individual rights would jeopardize the strong self-determination of the county councils and that the economic consequences for the county councils could be negative if a new patient rights law were introduced (SOU 1997). This whole discussion shows clearly that the committee considered local self-determination as more important than formal rights for the patients.

Still, the Swedish Parliament chose, in 1999, to add some paragraphs to the Health and Medical Service Act that formally reinforced the rights of patients. For instance, patients gained the right to choose treatment (in cases where treatments were equivalent and not too costly), to receive individually adjusted information and to a second opinion in cases of serious diseases. On the surface, these changes look significant; however, from reading the government and parliamentary documents that formed the basis of these changes, it is clear that the new rights were highly conditional. For instance, patients were only allowed to choose treatment when there was a reasonable relation between costs and benefits, and a second opinion could only be used by patients with severe illnesses and ailments. It is unclear who is to make this distinction. All in all, it is open to discussion whether the new additions are helpful in strengthening the position of patients.

In 2007, a new committee, the so-called Responsibility Committee (Ansvarskommittén) suggested that all different regulations about patient rights should be included in one comprehensive law (SOU 2007). Yet, it was emphasized the committee report that it would still be the *duty* of the county councils to provide health care and only a few of the proposed regulations contain individually enforceable rights for the patients. It seems that the issue is still ongoing.

In June 2007, the present Liberal-Conservative Swedish Government gave a new committee of inquiry the task of further developing the proposal for a patient rights act. So far, no final decision has been made based on the work of this committee. The present Government has, however, taken several other initiatives to strengthen the role of patients during recent years. For instance, a Government Committee Report (SOU 2008) was presented in December 2008 with several suggestions as to how patients could be empowered. A mandatory waiting-time guarantee was proposed, meaning that the county councils would be obliged to introduce time limits within which patients are examined and treated. However, the National Inquiry refrained from deciding on actual time limits but recommended that the county councils introduce a time limit maximum of 30 days for assessment by a specialist and 120 days for treatment. The county councils have, of course, the possibility of deciding on shorter time limits. If the time limits are exceeded, the patient has a right to choose another caregiver with the cost being borne by the home county council. Also, the report suggests that patients should be given individually adjusted information about waiting times, their rights to choose a caregiver and the waiting-time guarantee. The report is now sent on referral to several institutions and the final decision will be taken during 2009. The new paragraphs will most probably be included in the forthcoming Patient Rights Act but also in other legal acts, such as the Health and Medical Service Act and the Act outlining professional responsibility. To sum up, many initiatives are currently in place in Sweden to strengthen the legal role of patients. However, it seems likely that regulations concerning patient rights will still be spread across different legal acts in the future.

Norway

The Norwegian Patient Act came into force in 2001, after a preparatory phase of more than 10 years.[1] It has been changed several times since then and now consists of nine chapters and is by its length and contents the most comprehensive patient rights act among the four Nordic countries.

The first part of the act is concerned with the right to become a patient (i.e. regulates patient rights to health care services). The 434 municipalities are supposed to provide care to help patients in acute situations. The municipalities are also responsible for providing primary health care: basic types of treatment, preventive care and rehabilitation. Access to specialist care, for example hospital care, is also regulated by this law. A patient that is referred to specialist care has the right to be assessed within 30 days. Patients are then prioritized by a doctor into two groups according to the patient's need. Patients in the high-priority group have the right to an individual care-plan with a fixed *time limit* regulating when the care/treatment will be provided. The time limit is *individual* and is set by the patient's doctor. If the time limit is exceeded, the patient has the right to seek care at private specialists or abroad at the expense of the home regional health authority.

In December 2008, the Directorate of Health responded to concerns regarding unwanted geographical variation in individual time limits by issuing a number of 'priority-setting guidelines', which are recommended to be used by doctors when they decide on the individual time limits. When finished, the project aims at producing guidelines for 30 different medical specialities. Each guideline contains information about how long a patient with a specific diagnosis has to wait in order to receive specialist care. The suggested waiting time has been decided by taking into account the severity of the illness, the expected effect of treatment and the cost-effectiveness of the treatment.

Norwegian citizens also have many explicit rights when accepted as patients. These rights are based on the principle of patient autonomy (Kjønstad 2007). For instance, patients have the right to participate in the process of treatment, to be informed, to make their own decisions and to have access to their written health records. In addition, the act also includes rules dealing explicitly with issues of consent, the rights of children and incapable patients.

Concerns that the act will make the relationship between patients and providers more bureaucratic have been expressed by health care professionals on several occasions (Molven 2002). In contrast to Sweden and Finland, the Norwegian Act also includes specific regulations on choice of hospital provider. This will be discussed further below.

Finland

Finland was the first Nordic – and European – country to pass a comprehensive act on patient rights in 1993.[2] The act consists of five chapters and is mainly built on regulations from existing laws and policies. The first part of the act regulates Finnish citizens' rights to health care in the same way as the Norwegian Act does. The act sets out that every person living permanently in Finland is entitled to the medical care required by his or her mental or physical state, within the limits of the resources available (Partanen 1994; Vuorenkoski et al. 2008).

Other parts of the act regulate the rights citizens have when they are admitted as patients. For example, the act covers patient rights to information about their health status and information about different treatment alternatives and risks, the right to self-determination and informed consent, the status of under-age patients and rules about confidentiality. A distinctive feature of the act is that Finnish patients on waiting lists have the right to be informed when the treatment will take place, and also about possible causes of delay and its estimated duration.

Many patient rights in Finland, as in Sweden, are covered by other legal acts. For example, a waiting-time guarantee that regulates the time period within which a patient must be treated was implemented in 2005. This change had its background in the state's increasing concerns about geographical inequalities in access to health care (Vuorenkoski et al. 2008). From 2005, it has been mandatory for health centres to provide immediate contact by telephone the same day as the patient calls. If treatment is required, a visit to the health care centre within three days must be offered. At hospitals, an assessment of the patient must be made within three weeks from the day the referral arrives. After that, treatment must take place within six months. If the hospital cannot provide treatment within that time period, the hospital must pay for care somewhere else in the country.

Denmark

Several laws have strengthened the position of patients in Denmark in the last decades. The most explicit Patient Rights Act came into force in 1998 and regulates different areas such as patients' right to information and informed consent. In January 2007, a comprehensive Healthcare Act was introduced in Denmark.[3] This act builds on regulations from existing acts and policies and includes most of the patient rights from these previous laws.

One of the first parts of the Healthcare Act states that persons living permanently in Denmark have legal rights to health care. Danish patients have several explicit rights when they are accepted for care; for example, they have the right to informed consent before initiating any kind of medical examination or treatment in order to promote patients' self-determination and a right to receive appropriate information prior to the examination, treatment or operation. The information must be adjusted to the individual person's capabilities in terms of age, maturity, experience and so on.

Moreover, with regard to secrecy and confidentiality, the patient has to give his or her consent for the transfer of information between doctors and health - care personnel. In a Nordic context, this is quite unique. Consent can be given verbally or in writing; however, forwarding information is allowed without consent from the patient under some circumstances, such as when it is absolutely necessary for acute treatment of the patient.

Another interesting feature of the new act is that different time limits for treatment are set out. For example, the National Board of Health has set out specific time limits for life-threatening diseases. If these time limits are not upheld by the regions, the patients are allowed to seek care in other regions, abroad or at private facilities.

For elective care, a specific waiting-time guarantee is also included in the new Healthcare Act. A general two month waiting-time guarantee was introduced in Denmark in 2002. From October 2007, the time limit was lowered to one month. If the hospitals in one region fail to provide treatment for a patient within one month, the patient has the right to seek treatment at private facilities or at hospitals in other regions with the patient's home region paying the costs. The one-month guarantee was temporarily suspended from the fall of 2008 to June 2009 owing to increased waiting times caused by a strike among nursing staff in 2008, but has now been reintroduced.

As in the Norwegian act, the Danish act includes specific regulations on choice of hospital provider. This will be discussed further below.

6.4.2 Complaint procedures

Complaint procedures are an important means of influencing health care. Fallberg and MacKenny (2003, p. 343) state that: 'The existence of an effective complaints mechanism is fundamental in any social arena as a means for administrative bodies to respond to the feelings, emotions and reactions of the citizens in a country'. Patient complaints can be divided into two categories: one for complaints regarding patient rights (e.g. waiting times, information, consent) and another for complaints regarding malpractice or patient damages.

Complaints are commonly handled by different types of judicial and administrative bodies in the Nordic countries. In some cases, a complaint can be brought to a judicial body. Complaints can also be handled by public complaint-handling authorities, for example a committee, board or similar at regional or national level. In addition, ombudsmen often play an important role in the complaint process, sometimes merely as counsellors for patients but also with a more active role in the complaint process.

Sweden

When a patient feels that a doctor or nurse has caused harm through medical negligence, he or she can lodge a complaint with the Medical Responsibility

Board (Hälso- och sjukvårdens ansvarsnämnd, HSAN). This board is a national authority that has the ability to give disciplinary penalties (an admonition or a warning) to health care staff if they have not fulfilled their medical responsibilities. The Medical Responsibility Board does not, however, have the ability to change a health care decision or intervene in the actual health care of a patient. Patients cannot receive any compensation from the board if their rights have been violated (Socialstyrelsen 2008).

Swedish patients have no formal right to appeal to judicial or administrative bodies concerning violations of their rights such as access to information or a second opinion or waiting-time guarantees. Instead, each Swedish region has a patients' advisory committee (patientnämnd). Its main responsibility is to give patients information and assist them in safeguarding their rights by discussing the problem with the involved health care personnel; however, the advisory committee has no disciplinary mandate and is merely consultative. Some county councils also have a patient ombudsman in addition to the advisory committee and with similar duties (Socialstyrelsen 2008).

All health care institutions must participate in a patient insurance scheme. If a patient receives physical or psychological injuries through malpractice in health care, the patient is entitled to compensation from the scheme (Patientförsäkringen).

Norway

If a Norwegian patient feels that any of his or her rights as a patient have been violated, the patient may submit a complaint to an administrative body, the county medical officer (fylkeslegen). The county medical officer has a supervisory function with the purpose of withdrawing any decision by health care institutions that is not in accordance with the Patient Rights Act (MacKenney and Fallberg 2004).

The decisions made by the county medical officer can be appealed to the Norwegian Board of Health Supervision (Helsetilsynet). The county medical officer's decision is also admissible in civil court, which can compel hospitals and physicians to comply with patient rights law (Molven 2002; MacKenney and Fallberg 2004).

According to the Patients' Rights Act, every Norwegian county must also have a patients' ombudsman whose purpose is to safeguard patients' legal rights and interests in relation to specialist health care services. The ombudsman can, to a reasonable extent, provide information to anyone who requests it (Johnsen 2006). In addition, the ombudsman can also give advice and guidance on matters that are in the remit of his/her position. The ombudsman alone determines whether or not a request provides adequate grounds for investigation. Recently, an initiative has been launched to expand the ombudsman's area of responsibility to include the primary care sector.

In January 2003, the Patient Injury Act came into force in Norway. This act regulates claims for injuries sustained by a patient who has been treated in the public part of the health care system. To be covered by the law, a physical or psychological injury must have occurred during an encounter with a health care provider. The complaint is handled by a neutral public body assessing patient compensation (Norsk Pasienterstatning). Patients have the right to appeal decisions of this body to the Patient Injury Compensation Board (Pasientskadenemda), which is a public body under the Ministry of Health (MacKenney and Fallberg 2004)

Finland

If a Finnish patient is dissatisfied with the provided care, he or she can submit a complaint to the director of the health care institution. The director has, in accordance with the Patient Rights Act, the duty to rectify the situation without delay (Ministry of Social Affairs and Health 2005). If the health care director does not agree with the complaint, it is still possible for the patient to submit the complaint to a county administrative board (länsstyrelsen). If it is a more complex complaint, it will be transferred to a National Authority for Medicolegal Affairs (*Rättsskyddscentralen*) (Ministry of Social Affairs and Health 2005).

A patient ombudsman system was introduced in Finland in the Patient Rights Act in 1993. The act decreed that all health care authorities must have a patient ombudsman. The ombudsman's duty is to inform patients of their rights and assist them in submitting complaints concerning treatment, or claims for indemnity caused by malpractice (Ministry of Social Affairs and Health 2005).

The Patient Injuries Act, which came into force in 1987, covers a range of injuries that patients may have sustained in connection with health care. All claims are sent to the Finnish Patient Insurance Centre, which is an institution with obligatory membership for all Finnish health care providers. If the patient is dissatisfied with the decision of the Patient Insurance Centre, the patient may refer the matter to the Patient Injuries Board. The board does not have the ability to change the decision made by the Centre but its recommendations are, in general, respected by the Centre (Ministry of Social Affairs and Health 2005).

Denmark

The right to issue a complaint about health care provided is regulated in the new Healthcare Act implemented in 2007. A national Patients' Complaint Board was set up with the role of facilitating patients' criticism of medical facilities and staff. The board deals with complaints regarding treatment and care as well as patient rights issues such as requirements for consent, confidentiality and right to information. If the case is particularly serious, the Complaint Board will submit the complaint to a public prosecutor with the purpose of taking the case to court (Nys 2007; Strandberg-Larsen et al. 2007).

In addition to this, every region has a patient office. Its purpose is similar to that of a regional ombudsman. The patient office is supposed to give guidance and information to patients regarding their rights. The office also assists in the process of making formal complaints and submits them to proper authorities. Complaints may also be submitted to the parliamentary ombudsman. The ombudsman's opinions are not legally binding but are generally accepted by the health care institutions (Nys 2007).

Claims concerning malpractice and injuries are handled by the Patient Insurance Association, which is financed by all health care institutions. The insurance scheme at first only covered patients treated at public hospitals but it was extended in 2004 to include private hospitals, GPs and dental care. It is also possible for patients to receive compensation for injuries caused by medical products. The size of the compensation is regulated in Danish law (Nys 2007; Strandberg-Larsen et al. 2007).

6.4.3 *Trends in the use of complaint procedures*

Studies from the Nordic countries show that patients' complaints have increased during recent years in all countries (Helsetilsynet 2007; HSAN 2007; Sundhedsvæsenets patientklagenævn 2007; Vuorenkoski et al. 2008). Since 2005, Swedish malpractice complaints have increased approximately 10–13 per cent annually. Increasing dissatisfaction of patients with the health services is considered the primary explanation for this increase (HSAN 2007). It is important to remember that these Swedish complaints mostly cover medical aspects of care. In Denmark, the number of complaints submitted to, and accepted by, the national Patients Complaint Board increased by 60 per cent from 1998 to 2007 (from 2003 to 3215 admitted complaints).

In Norway, there has also been a steady increase in the number of complaints made by patients based on the Patients' Rights Act during recent years. In 2003, the Board of Health Supervision (Helsetilsynet) recorded 142 complaints; in 2007 the number was more than 750 (Helsetilsynet 2007). The plaintiff received support in more than one-third of the cases. The number of complaints shows that patients have become more aware of the possibility of using the Patients' Rights Act. In addition, it may indicate an increased trust in the procedures or organs established. Only a small number of cases have reached the judicial system (i.e. the civil court).

6.5 Individual exit mechanisms: patient choice of provider

The following section focuses more explicitly on political initiatives that have increased patients' opportunities to choose health care providers. By using the 'exit' mechanism, patients are given a strong instrument to influence their health care. Richard B. Saltman (1992) has previously given an account of provider choice in three of the four countries under investigation in the early 1990s (Norway was not included). The aim in the following section is to provide a description of the formal opportunities that exist for patients to choose some 15 years later. In doing so, an attempt will be made to highlight both similarities and differences in choice policies adopted in the four countries. The tax-funded nature of Nordic health care systems implies that certain aspects of choice, such as choice between public and private insurers, or between public insurance funds, are less common here than in European social insurance countries (Thomson and Dixon 2006). This presentation is, therefore, restricted to choice of first-contact provider (i.e. GP) and choice of hospital.

Sweden

The Swedish Health and Medical Service Act from 1982 regulates the county councils' responsibility to provide all their citizens with high-quality health care services. At the end of the 1980s and beginning of the 1990s, several policies were introduced with the intent of allowing individuals greater freedom to choose where to seek care. Until then, patients had been restricted to using the nearest medical facility (Winblad 2008). The new choice policies were, however, not included in the national legislation. Instead, the most important choice policy was adopted by the Federation of County Councils (FCC) in 1989, leaving it up to each county council to decide on the framework and the extent of the policy. Based upon the agreements between the FCC and the county councils, Swedish patients were, from 1991, formally entitled to freely choose primary health care centres and hospitals within their home counties. Also, patients were free to seek inpatient care throughout the entire country.

In 2000, the FCC began work on updating and extending the patient choice policy. A few of the counties opposed this revision because they feared that they could not afford the extra costs associated with the expansion, and because of what they considered to be unfair consequences of the policy. The new, updated choice policy came into effect in 2003 (Winblad 2008). According to these regulations, the patient was now also given the right to choose ambulatory care at hospitals or specialists throughout the entire country, making an exception for highly specialized care. In general, the patient does not have to pay for hospitalization whether s/he has exercised the right to choose or not. However, travel expenses to a hospital outside the home county always have to be paid by the patient. The Swedish Government has not until now launched any national information campaigns about the patient choice policy. However, each county council provides information on its website about this right. In 2000, the county councils and the central government created a national database and a website for publishing expected waiting times. None of the county councils provides any additional information on waiting times on the Internet. Information regarding hospital quality is partly available to the public. In practice, however, the information has proved too technical and difficult for the patient alone to interpret (Vrangbæk et al. 2007).

At the moment, there is an intense political discussion about patient choice in Sweden. The Swedish conservative coalition government that came into power in 2006 has focused on legalizing and extending patient choice within health care. In 2007, a national committee of inquiry was appointed to look into regulation of patient choice within primary health care. The report, which suggested a legalization of patient choice within primary health care, was referred to several organizational and political bodies for consideration. Many of the county councils responded negatively to the proposal and felt that their self-determination was threatened by the proposed legalization. In spite of this, the government bill that was proposed in December 2008 suggests that patient choice within primary health care will be mandatory. The government has, however, modified the original proposal. It is, for example, up to the county councils to decide what will be included in the services among which patients can choose. The changes will come into force in January 2010.

Norway

Norwegian municipalities are, according to the 1982 Municipalities Health Service Act, responsible for providing primary care services to their residents. Norwegian patients have traditionally enjoyed a large degree of freedom when it comes to choice of first-contact provider (GP). The actual GP choice was, however, often restricted by the small number of doctors practising within the same area, or the large number of vacant GP positions in certain parts of the country. In 2001, the Regular General Practitioner (RGP) Scheme was introduced on a national basis. Through this system, all Norwegians were assigned to the list of a GP. One consequence of the RGP was that the patient's right to choose GP, at least formally, became more restricted. Participants in the RGP scheme were given the right to change GP only twice a year. However, the local authorities of some municipalities have hesitated to apply for new practice licences and, consequently, there is only one or no GP at all with an open list. In these municipalities, the inhabitants have no real option to choose a different GP. In 2005, it was found that approximately 2.5 per cent of the population changed GP in a given quarter (Sandvik 2006). The official web pages provide no information about differences in waiting times or quality for patients wanting to change GP.

Norwegian patients have until recently had little opportunity to choose hospitals. Where the patient received treatment was to a large extent determined by where the patient lived, as each hospital operated with strict geographical catchment areas. This rather rigid system was, during the 1980s and early 1990s, blamed for causing both long waiting times and geographical inequalities in access to hospital care. The situation paved the way for increased political interest in the introduction of patient choice in the beginning of the 1990s (Johnsen 2006). In 2001, the right for patients requiring elective somatic treatment to choose hospital was introduced on a nationwide basis through the Patients' Rights Act. Initially, the right was restricted to choice between public hospitals, and patients were only entitled to receive treatment at the same level of specialization. Since then, the law has been extended to include the option to choose between private for-profit hospitals under contract with one of the regional health authorities. In Norway, patients do not pay for inpatient hospital treatment. It was, however, acknowledged from the start that travel expenses could represent a financial barrier for patients' uptake of choice. In order to avoid problems related to income inequalities, the authorities established a maximum co-payment.

An interesting feature of the Norwegian system, at least compared with the Swedish system, is the fact that the right to choose private outpatient specialists has not yet been included in the choice scheme. This extension of the scheme was debated by the parliament together with the question of including private commercial hospitals in the 2003–04 session. At present, the question of whether private specialists will be invited into the arrangement remains unanswered.

Finland

In 1993, the Finnish Patients' Rights Act came into force. This law did not include any legislation on patients' right to choose either first contact provider or hospital. During the second part of the 1990s, a review of the functioning of the law showed that it had influenced practical functions within health care, but active participation and access for patients needed to be improved (Järvelin 2002). Recent policy developments have, therefore, focused on the introduction of a new maximum waiting-time guarantee in order to improve patients' access to health care services (Vuorenkoski and Keskimäki 2004; Vuorenkoski 2006).

The Finnish municipalities have great freedom to organize health care as they like; however, many of the municipalities have based their primary health care on a so-called population responsibility model, in which a team of doctors and nurses is responsible for the health care of a geographically specified population. The system offers limited opportunity for choice of provider (Vuorenkoski et al. 2008). Some of the municipalities do, however, offer the possibility for patients to choose their own doctor. Importantly, Finnish patients always have the option to choose among private physicians (Häkkinen 2005). In addition, a well-functioning occupational health sector also offers some choice for the patient. More importantly, the Finnish Government is currently planning to reform the legislation on health services, with one aim being to extend choice of health care centre to other municipalities.

Patients cannot normally choose where to receive treatment within the public hospital services as the country is divided into 20 hospital districts, each responsible for providing specialized care within a defined geographical area. In addition, each primary care health centre has guidelines on where patients with certain symptoms and diagnoses should be referred. The situation within the private part of the system is different, as patients have the option to make an appointment with the hospital of their own choice (Häkkinen 2005). Consequently, the opportunity for choice across hospital district boundaries appears, at least in the public system, to be limited. Long travel distances to alternative hospitals also contribute to the limitation of hospital choice (Järvelin 2002).

Denmark

General practitioners play a key role in the Danish health care system as the first point of contact and as gatekeepers to specialist care. Danish residents over the age of 16 have, since 1973, been free to choose between two GP options (public health plans) known as Group 1 and Group 2 (Vallgårda et al. 2001). The Group 1 health plan allows treatment free of cost in general practice. The patients in Group 1 must enlist with a GP and the choice of GP is limited to a restricted, geographically determined set of providers. Patients can change their GP enlistment any time for a nominal fee and with a process time of about one month. Members of this health plan need a referral from their GP in order to gain access to a privately practising specialist but can choose freely among available practising specialists. The Group 2 health plan, by comparison, allows immediate free choice of both GP and privately practising specialist. Payment of services is only partially reimbursed by the Public Health Insurance, and physicians are allowed to bill their patients on this scheme extra. Only a very small fraction of the population (less than 2 per cent in 2001) has chosen the Group 2 health plan (Christiansen et al. 1999). This means that the choice of first-contact provider in Denmark is confined within geographical limits for the majority of the population (i.e. Group 1 patients) (Thomson and Dixon 2006).

Until 1992, the hospital referral system was characterized by very strict referral rules, based on geographical location and treatment needs. From 1993, the dependency on geographical location was removed, thereby giving Danish patients the right to undergo treatment at any public hospital and a few privately owned hospitals (at the same level of specialization) in the whole country. Since then, several expansions have been made to the patient's right to choose a hospital. Since July 2002, an 'extended choice' has been in place for patients for elective procedures who face waiting times above a specified threshold. This scheme provides access to additional private facilities in Denmark and abroad. The right to choose a hospital is specified in the Healthcare Act of 2007.

In general, Danish patients do not pay for hospitalization regardless of whether they have chosen the hospital. The exception to this is for any travel costs beyond the nearest public hospital in the home county, which have to be borne by the patient. Whether this increased co-payment for travel expenses acts as a financial barrier for choice remains uncertain. It should be kept in mind that potential travel distances in Denmark are much shorter than in the other Nordic countries. Danish hospitals are obliged by law to inform patients about their right to choose. In addition, government-sponsored websites have been established in order to provide patients with the necessary information for making choices. These websites contain information on variations in the average expected waiting times for common elective surgical procedures.

6.6 Concluding remarks

This chapter has shown that within all four Nordic countries patients now, at least formally, have a range of collective and individual ways of influencing health care services. At the same time, there is still little comparative evidence about the extent to which patients make use of these opportunities and their relative impact on system performance.

6.6.1 *Patient organizations*

Collective actions by patients and others are increasingly acknowledged as an important means of influencing health policy and service production. This is investigated in this chapter by looking at the role of patient organizations. There are some studies on this theme (Baggott and Foster 2008); however, studies from the Nordic countries are rare and this is a serious gap in the literature. The existing research has shown an increase in the number of patient organizations in the Nordic countries; in Finland, the development is described as exponential. However, the size of the groups varies considerably. Initially, most organizations focused on self-help – they provided information to patients concerning the disease and informed members about new policies. What is being seen now, in all four countries, is that the patient organizations seem to be more politically aware and increasingly engaged in lobbying. For instance, a Swedish study demonstrated that the patient organizations themselves considered that their most important task is to safeguard the interests of their members by influencing the policy-makers, for example through official hearings or informal meetings. Unfortunately, studies of their real impact on the policy-making process are rare and it is difficult to assess how well they manage to influence health policy issues in the Nordic countries or if their role has changed over time in this respect.

6.6.2 Legal rights

Another mechanism for influencing health care – but on the individual level – is the legalization concerning patient rights. In the last few decades, there have been many examples of policies in which the individual's judicial rights have been more clearly emphasized than hitherto. This trend towards an increased emphasis on individual rights within the social policy area reflects an international trend, which is also expressed within the European Community where existing social rights are protected by the European Community Court, while a more comprehensive bill of rights concerning social issues has been discussed (Blomqvist and Green-Pedersen 2004).

The development of rights legislation within health care has been examined explicitly in this chapter. We have shown that three of the Nordic countries have introduced special patient rights acts. These acts are, in many respects, a strong instrument for empowering patients. The Finnish Patients' Right Act consists mainly of sections that already existed in former laws and policy documents, for example rules about patient consent and information. Norway and Denmark have chosen to introduce more comprehensive patient rights laws that also include sections about access-related issues such as waiting times for health care, specific time limits and choice of health care provider. One difference between the Danish and the Norwegian legislation is that the former sets out specific time limits for certain diagnose groups, whereas the Norwegian act sets out time limits that are individual for each patient. This makes Norwegian patients more dependent on the doctor's decision. Sweden is the only country without specific patient rights legislation; however, much of the same content (e.g. right to individualized information, patient choice or rules about waiting-time guarantees) is found in other legal or policy documents in Sweden. A problem in Sweden is that many of the rules regulating patient rights have traditionally been in the form of recommendations and agreements between the county councils and the national state, which does not give these rules the same legal status as if they were included in a more comprehensive law. This is probably one of the reasons why some of the counties in Sweden have been reluctant to implement the recommendations (Winblad 2007).

6.6.3 *Complaint mechanisms*

Another individual voice mechanism is each country's system for administering patient complaints: channels to articulate discontent with medical as well as service aspects of care. Looking through the regulations, it seems that all four countries have similar legal arrangements to deal with complaints in many regards. There are administrative bodies to which patients are supposed to submit their complaints. Furthermore, they also have patient ombudsmen or similar institutions that help patients to handle their complaints. One of the most important elements when comparing and measuring complaint procedures is the degree to which patient rights are enforceable. In Denmark and Norway, patients have the formal possibility of appealing to a judicial court when their patient rights have been violated. This is not the case in Finland or Sweden, which means that patients in these countries are in a weaker legal position than those in Norway or Finland. However, all the Nordic countries have established patient insurance schemes in order to regulate patient rights to economic compensation when injuries have been inflicted by medical staff.

6.6.4 *Choice*

One distinct type of patient right, on the individual level, that has been discussed in this chapter is the right to free choice of health care provider, or what Hirschman (1970) has termed 'exit'. Historically, patients in the Nordic countries have been restricted to seeking care at the nearest medical facility. Consequently, the flexibility for the individual patient has been limited, and patients have had few possibilities to influence the care-giving process. In recent decades, the health care authorities in the four Nordic countries have introduced polices that have extended the rights for patients to choose, but these policies have been shaped in different ways. The regulations range from explicit legislation (in Denmark and Norway) to a less-formal agreement between regional authorities (Sweden) to no regulation at all (Finland). When it comes to choosing first-contact provider, three of the countries (Denmark, Norway and Finland) have implemented rules restricting choice within geographic areas or limiting the number of times a patient can change between GPs. Sweden allows patients greater freedom to choose GPs independently of where they live. In addition, Swedish patients are mostly allowed to go directly to a hospital without a referral. It is worth noting that the Finnish government is discussing introducing more patient choice within primary health care.

Despite the different ways of regulating hospital choice in the four countries, patients in Sweden, Denmark and Norway have few formal barriers preventing them from selecting a hospital. In contrast, Finnish patients still have little opportunity to decide where to receive hospital care. When considering the overall picture, Swedish patients seem to have the least limits in the possibility of choosing a health care provider geographically, since they have the right to choose any hospital in the whole country – even though patient choice is only formalized through a recommendation and not a law.

To summarize, even if the Nordic countries have moved in the same direction when it comes to patients' formal options for influencing their own care, for example by introducing legal arrangements and different policies that provide patients with rights to choose their health care provider, there are still significant differences among the countries both in the shaping of the policies and the enforceability of rights.

6.6.5 Collective or individual influence mechanisms?

The investigation of the different influence mechanisms available to patients in the Nordic countries has shown that patients in all countries have several options available. The development of *collective* influence mechanisms seems quite similar among the countries; for instance, there is a growing role for patient organizations in all four countries. Looking into the future, however; varying size and experiences of the patient organizations will create different prerequisites for them to succeed in influencing policy-making at the national level. Many of the organizations are fragmented, small and organized around single conditions such as breast cancer or diabetes. They are often reliant on a small pool of members who are highly active. In addition, they are often dependent on state funding (Baggott and Forster 2008). This is a problem particularly for the Swedish organizations, since they are not allowed to receive sponsorship from commercial companies.

However, compared with other European countries, there seem to be fairly good prerequisites in place for further involvement of patient organizations in the national arena in the Nordic countries (Baggott and Forster 2008). First, there seems to be strong support for consumerist values in all countries. Second, health systems with multiple levels of governance, as in the Nordic countries, provide better opportunities for patient organizations to interact with decision-makers and thereby influence health policy. Third, national proposals for new legislation in the Nordic countries are referred to the largest patient organizations for consideration.

When it comes to influence mechanisms at the *individual* level, Sweden seems to be the exception among the Nordic countries in that it lacks distinct patient rights legislation and offers fewer opportunities to appeal to court for unsatisfied patients. Many of the Swedish rights for patients are, according to Westerhäll (1994), so-called goal-oriented rights. These rights are not legally binding and do not give patients the right to demand services or the possibility of appealing to court. Trädgårdh (1999) claims that this discussion is, nevertheless, important as it has the moralistic–normative function of setting the target for politicians and giving patients a guideline of what to expect. Important to note is that the present Swedish Government has taken several initiatives to legalize new patient rights in Sweden.

Nonetheless, we would still argue that it is somewhat misleading to talk about real rights in this context. First, none of the Nordic countries have individually enforceable rights to health care in the *legal* meaning. It is always the physician that decides whether the patient needs an examination, treatment or surgery. Second, there are no direct sanctions in cases where authorities neglect their responsibility of providing health care (for details on Norway see, for example,

Molven 2002). To our knowledge, it is rare for the national state in the four investigated countries to punish medical providers who have not provided sufficient health care for its inhabitants. There might be a risk that patients feel disappointed in cases where their rights are not individually enforceable (see Karlsson 2003). This Nordic model can be compared with the insurance-based model in central Europe, in which mandatory and voluntary insurance creates more legible rights for patients that are also enforceable in other ways than those avaialable in the Nordic countries.

6.6.6 *Future implications*

The differences among the Nordic countries will, in our opinion, most probably lead to different opportunities for patients to exercise their recently acquired rights. Several important questions remain unanswered. The most pertinent, perhaps, is the question of whether Nordic patients will make active use of either collective or individual influence mechanisms in the future. This question becomes important when considering that there is a tension between increasing patient choice and more collective forms of patient and citizen involvement. As Andersson and co-workers (2007, p. 10) have commented: 'In particular, the promotion of individual "patient choice" as the best way to ensure responsiveness and flexibility in services potentially undermines the argument for user involvement as a more egalitarian mechanism for securing these outcomes'.

The outline in this chapter of the current situation may serve as a point of departure for further investigations within this (somewhat neglected) topic of development of the Nordic welfare states. Most likely, patients of tomorrow will express greater demands for involvement in health care decision-making. They will want to take part in decisions concerning their treatments and the planning of their care and will also have higher expectations for the responsiveness of the system. Yet, it is also likely that there will be significant differences in the exercise of these rights depending on socioeconomic status, education level and diagnosis. The increasing demands for responsiveness represent an important challenge for all Nordic countries, as well as for other European countries. But it also represents new opportunities for developing health care services. A good starting point would be to identify the best practices in each country and then strive towards creating a health care system that really empowers patients.

Notes

1. Lov 2. juli 1999 nr. 63 om pasientrettigheter (pasientrettighetsloven).
2. Lag om patientens ställning och rättigheter 17.8.1992/785.
3. Lov om patienters retsstelling, nr 482 af 01/07/1998, Sundhetslov nr 546 af 24/06/2005.

References

Andersson, E., Creasy, S. and Tritter, J. (2007) Does patient and public involvement matter? in Andersson, E., Tritter, J. and Wilson, R. (eds) *Health Democracy: The Future of Involvement in Health and Social Care*. London: NHS National Centre for Involvement.

Arnetz, J.E., Bergström, K., Franzén, Y. and Nilsson, H. (2004) Active patient involvement in the establishment of physical therapy goals: effects on treatment outcome and quality of care, *Advances in Physiotherapy* 6: 50–69.

Baggott, R. and Forster, R. (2008) Health consumer and patients' organizations in Europe: towards a comparative analysis, *Health Expectations* 11: 85–94.

Blomqvist, P. and Green-Pedersen, C. (2004) Defeat at home? Issue-ownership and social democratic support in Scandinavia, *Government and Opposition* 39: 587–613.

Christiansen, T., Enemark, U., Clausen, J. and Paulsen, P.B. (1999) Health-care and cost containment in Denmark, in Mossialos, E. and Le Grand, J. (eds) *Health Care and Cost Containment in the European Union*. Aldershot: Ashgate.

Coulter, A. (2007) Patient engagement: why is it important? in Andersson, E., Tritter, J. and Wilson, R. (eds) *Health Democracy: The Future of Involvement in Health and Social Care*. London: NHS National Centre for Involvement.

Einevik Bäckstrand, K. (2006) *Patienträttigheter i Sverige och övriga Norden*. Stockholm: Vårdföretagarna.

Esping-Andersen, G. (1999) *Social Foundations of Postindustrial Economies*. New York: Oxford University Press.

Fallberg, L. and MacKenney, S. (2003) Patient ombudsmen in seven Europeans countries: an effective way to implement patients' rights? *European Journal of Health Law* 10: 343–357.

Glenton, C. and Oxman, A.D. (1998) The use of evidence by health-care user organizations, *Health Expectations* 1: 14–22.

Häkkinen, U. (2005) *The Impact of Finnish Health Sector Reforms*. Helsinki: STAKES, University of Helsinki.

Helsetilsynet [Board of Health] (2007) *Tilsynsmelding 2007*. Oslo: Government Publications.

Hirschman, A.O. (1970) *Exit, Voice, and Loyalty: Responses to Decline in Firms, Organizations, and States*. Cambridge, MA: Harvard University Press.

Hirschman, A.O. (1986) *Rival Views of Market Society: And Other Recent Essays*. New York: Viking.

HSAN (2007) *Årsredovisning 2007*. Stockholm: Hälso-och sjuvårdens ansvarsnämnd [Medical Responsibility Board].

Järvelin, J. (2002) *Health Care Systems in Transition: Finland*. Copenhagen: WHO Regional Office for Europe on behalf of the European Observatory on Health Systems and Policies.

Johnsen, J.R. (2006) Norway: Health System Review. *Health Systems in Transition*, 8(1): 1–167.

Karlsson, L. (2003) *Konflikt eller harmoni? Individuella rättigheter och ansvarsutkrävande i svenska och brittisk sjukvård*. Gothenburg: Gothenburg University Press.

Kennedy, I. (2003) Patients are experts in their own field, *British Medical Journal* 326: 1276–7.

Kjønstad, A. (1999) The development of patients' rights in Norway, in Molven, O. (ed.) *The Norwegian Health-care System. Legal and Organizational Aspects*. Oslo: University of Oslo Press.

Kjønstad, A. (2007) *Helserett*. Oslo: Gyldendal Akademisk.

Le Grand, J. (2007) *The Other Invisible Hand: Delivering Public Services Through Choice and Competition*. Princeton, NJ: Princeton University Press.

MacKenney, S. and Fallberg, L. (2004) *Protecting Patients' Rights: A Comparative Study of the Ombudsman in Healthcare*. Oxford: Radcliffe Medical.

Ministry of Social Affairs and Health (2005) *Rights of Patients*. Helsinki: Ministry of Social Affairs and Health.

Möller, T. (1996) *Brukare och klienter i välfärdsstaten. Om missnöje och påverkansmöjligheter inom barn- och äldreomsorg*. Stockholm: Publica.

Molven, O. (2002) *Helse og jus. Innføring for helsepersonell*. Oslo: Gyldendal Akdemisk.

Nys, H. (2007) *European Ethica–Legal Papers*, No 2: *Patient Rights in the EU*. Denmark: Leuven.

Olsen, J.P. (1990) *Demokrati på svenska*. Stockholm: Carlssons.

Olson, M. (1965) *The Logic of Collective Action: Public Goods and the Theory of Groups*. Cambridge, MA: Harvard University Press.

Partanen, M.-L. (1994) Finns defined patients' rights before Dutch, *British Medical Journal* 309: 130–1.

Perälä, M.-L. (1999) Advancing patients' rights in the Nordic countries, *International Journal of Nursing Practice* 5: 230–2.

Pestoff, V. (1979) *Research Reports 1979:1: Membership Participation in Swedish Consumer Cooperatives*. Stockholm: Department of Political Science, Stockolm University.

Rachmani, R., Levi, Z., Slavachevski, I., Avin, M. and Ravid, M. (2002) Teaching patients to monitor their risk factors retards the progression of vascular complications in high-risk patients with Type 2 diabetes mellitus: a randomized prospective study, *Diabetic Medicine* 19: 385–92.

Saltman, R.B. (1992) *Patientmakt över vården*. Stockholm: SNS.

Sandvik, H. (2006) *Evalueringen av fastlegereformen 2001–2005: Sammenfatning og analyse av evalueringens delprosjekter*. Oslo: Norges forskningsråd.

Socialstyrelsen [National Board of Health and Welfare] (2008) *Socialstyrelsen: din trygghet och säkerhet som patient*. http://www.socialstyrelsen.se/Amnesord/halso_sjuk/Din_trygghet_o_sakerhet_som_patient.htm.

Söderholm, J. (2005) Utvärdering av statens organisationsstöd till handikap-porganisationerna. [Socialstyrelsen, 2005–123–8.] Stockholm: National Board of Health and Welfare.

Söderholm Werkö, S. (2008) *Patient patients? Achieving patient empowerment through active participation, increased knowledge and organisation*. Dissertation. Stockholm, School of Business, Stockholm University.

SOU (1997) *SOU 1997: 194. Patienten har rätt*. Stockholm: Fritzes.

SOU (2007) *SOU 2007: 10. Hållbar samhällsorganisation med utvecklingskraft*. Stockholm: Fritzes.

SOU (2008) *SOU 2008: 127. Patientens rätt. Några förslag att stärka patientens ställning*. Stockholm: Fritzes.

Strandberg-Larsen, M., Nielsen, M.B., Vallgårda, S., Krasnik, A., Vrangbæk, K. and Mossialos, E. (2007) Denmark: health system review, *Health systems in transition* 9: 1–164.

Sundhedsvæsenets Patientklagenævn (2007) *Statistiske Oplysninger 2007*.

Ternhag, A., Asikainen, T., Giesecke, J. (2005) Size matters: patient organisations exaggerate prevalence numbers, *European Journal of Epidemiology* 20: 653–5.

Thomson, S. and Dixon, A. (2006) Choices in health-care: the European experience, *Journal of Health Services Research and Policy* 11 (3): 167–71.

Trädgårdh, L. (1999) *Patientmakt i Sverige, USA och Holland. Individuella kontra sociala rättigheter*. Lund: HSO Skåne.

Vallgårda, S., Krasnik, A., Vrangbæk, K. (2001) *Health Systems in Transition: Denmark*. Copenhagen: WHO Regional Office for Europe on behalf of the European Observatory on Health Systems and Policies.

Virdeborn, C. (2006) Patient organisation för paradontit–en god idé? *Tandläkartidnignen* 98: 54–8.

Vrangbæk, K., Østergren, K., Okkels Birk, H. and Winblad, U. (2007) Patient reactions to hospital choice in Norway, Denmark and Sweden, *Health Economics, Policy and Law* 2: 125–52.

Vuorenkoski, L. (2006) Ensuring access to public health-care: follow up, *Health Policy Monitor* 7 (April). http://www.hpm.org/en/Surveys/THL/07/Ensuring_access_to_health_care_-_follow-up.html.

Vuorenkoski, L. and Keskimäki, I. (2004) Ensuring access to health-care, *Health Policy Monitor* 3: (April). http://www.hpm.org/en/Surveys/THL/03/Ensuring_access_to_health_care.html.

Vuorenkoski, L., Mladovsky, P. and Mossialos, E. (2008) Finland: Health System Review, *Health Systems in Transition*, 10(4): 1–168.

Westerhäll, L. (1994) *Patienträttigheter*. Stockholm: Nerenius and Santérus.

Winblad, U. (2007) Valfriheten – en misslyckad sjukvårdsreform? in Blomqvist, P. (ed.) *Vem styr vården? Organisation och politisk styrning inom svensk sjukvård*. Stockholm: SNS.

Winblad, U. (2008) Do physicians care about patient choice? *Social Science and Medicine* 67: 1502–11.

chapter seven

The changing autonomy of the Nordic medical professions

Peter K. Jespersen and Sirpa Wrede

7.1 Introduction

Professional autonomy is an important theme in the reforming of health care in the Nordic countries and this is evident when it comes to medical management in hospitals. Many years of experience with 'new public management' (NPM) reforms in the Nordic states indicate that governments no longer accept traditional professional monopolies. Instead, a new societal ethos leads to attempts to restrict the professional autonomy of the medical profession. A variety of measures have been taken to influence the autonomy of doctors, including marketization of health care services; changes in the regulation of medical monopolies in health care; reforms in the management and structure of health - care organizations; introduction of standards, output measurement and clinical governance schemes; changes in the discourse of professionalism from occupational to corporate professionalism; and greater regulation of the relationship between doctor and patient.

These measures reflect the degree to which professionalism and professions have been seen as part of the cause of an inflexible, inefficient and producer-oriented public health care service (Broadbent et al. 1997; Exworthy and Halford 1999). More recently, professionalism *itself* and the ways it is institutionalized in different countries seems to be on the agenda. While this template is shared, the ways in which elements of NPM are mixed, the specific governance structures and the relation between state and health care professions vary between countries (Byrkjeflot and Neby 2004; Dent 2006). The four Nordic countries under consideration here (Denmark, Finland, Norway and Sweden) were grouped by Pollitt and Bouckaert (2002) among the 'modernizers', where governments continue to invest in a large (welfare) state but also recognize the need for fundamental changes, making them interesting cases for the analysis of changes in the autonomy of the medical professionalism.

This chapter focuses on the ongoing reconfiguration of the position and autonomy of the medical profession in the modernized Nordic health care systems and on the changes in the management of doctors. Section 7.2 presents how the sociology of professions has viewed the issue of professional autonomy. Section 7.3 presents an analytical framework for examining the changes in professional autonomy, after which the individual country case studies are given. The chapter concludes with a discussion of the dynamics of professional autonomy and accountability and suggests that new management regimes have altered the autonomy of the medical profession and that the old 'natural' model with doctors in undisputed positions has been changed towards multiprofessional models characterized by competing professional autonomies.

7.2 The theme of professional autonomy in the sociology of the professions

Within the early functional 'trait' tradition in the sociology of professions, the concept of professional autonomy referred both to the profession's official and legal monopoly over certain types of work and to the technical autonomy of individual professionals in work situations. The two kinds of autonomy were perceived as interrelated and mutually supportive. While the trait approach succeeded in emphasizing the role of abstract knowledge (Morell 2007), it failed to analyse the power of the professions, nor did it help the sociologist to understand the situation of the professions in contemporary societies or the discourse of professionalism (Evetts 2006).

The second classic approach in the study of professionalism focused on the actions and interactions of individuals and groups. In this perspective, the autonomy of the professional was to a large degree constructed locally through the practices of working communities. Freidson's (1970) formulation of a theory of professional dominance and professionalization became a key contribution to later interactionist analysis of occupations, which to a large extent denied the idea of professions as fundamentally different from other occupations. Instead, Johnson (1972, p. 45) defined professions as a 'way of organizing an occupation' and focused on how professional power and status were historically achieved and organized in the specific contexts of different countries. The 'power' approach (Macdonald 1995) further criticized the professions for trying to obtain 'social closure' and for their unjustified elitism (McKinlay 1973; Collins 1979; Murphy 1988). A second strand predicted the decline of the professions such as law and medicine following the rising intervention of managers in professional work (Braverman 1974). Both themes remain dominant in contemporary sociology of the profession, as demonstrated later in this chapter.

The power approach shifted the analytical focus to studies of professionalism, professionalization and particularly 'professional projects' (Larson 1977; Abbott 1988; Macdonald 1995; Freidson 2001). Larson (1977) defined the professional project as the coherent and consistent efforts by a profession to secure a market for the special knowledge of the professions, to ensure high status and social respectability and to secure the support of individual professionals. Through historical and comparative studies in European countries, the dominating Anglo-American conception of market-based professions was challenged, and it was highlighted that professions in European contexts (with the exception of the United Kingdom) are dependent on the interventions of the state (Brante 1988; Burrage and Torstendahl 1990; Bureau et al. 2004). Bringing the state into the analysis of professionalization illustrated the importance of the specific national and institutional contexts for the shaping of conceptions of professional autonomy at both collective and individual levels (Dent 2003; Degeling et al. 2006; Wrede 2008). Governance structures and the interaction between professions and the state in different countries determine the institutional and organizational framework within which the professions and professionals seek to maintain autonomy (Kragh Jespersen et al. 2002). The strategies of the professions were important also within organizations (Kirkpatrick and Ackroyd 2003), and successful professional projects secured for a profession a form of 'double social closure' whereby closure in the labour market was combined with control inside the organization (Ackroyd 1996). This is important because professionals are more than ever before being employed by large organizations where bureaucratic authority can conflict with codes of ethics, expert knowledge and the collegial influence inherent in professional projects.

Recent research has developed approaches to study professionalism in organizations through new perspectives such as collaboration (Montgomery 1997) and intra- and interorganizational transactions (Oliver 1997), suggesting ways through which professionals can contribute to new and efficient organizational forms. Broadbent and co-workers (1997, p.10) suggest that, in the interest of achieving strategic control of an organization, those who make organizational policy need to be prepared to accommodate to professional identities and professional standards of practice rather than demanding that experts assume organizational identity. So even if professional work becomes restructured, there might still be a fundamental rationale for professionalism in the organizational contexts of the modern public service organization.

Contrary to this ideal, Freidson (2001, p.197) describes what he identifies as an 'assault' on professionalism that reflects the economic interests of both private capital and the state, but also the lack of credibility of the professional ideology, resulting in reordering of jurisdictional boundaries as well as intensified employer control. In his view, a two-tier professional system with a small elite plus a large population of practitioners is in the making, resulting in deterioration of the quality of professional services, narrowing of expert knowledge as well as the loss of the spirit of professionalism. In Freidson's view, the survival of the institutions of professionalism presupposes a certain degree of monopoly and elitist social closure. Freidson touches upon themes important in the contemporary discussion: how to understand the 'assault' on the positions of the professions, the new strategies of the professions and the professionals, and whether the old contradiction between bureaucracy and professionalism can be reframed.

All of these questions can be better understood if Freidson's discussion on autonomy is expanded by considering professional accountability. The notion of accountability is often associated with economic and political arguments about the need for reform in the public sector. However, professional accountability in the health care system has also been proposed with reference to new forms of democracy and the need to make the medical profession more directly and democratically accountable to the public, not least in the European welfare states (Stacey 1989; Plant 2003). The British sociologist T.H. Marshall (1939) was one of the first to discuss the emergence of the welfare state as generating a shift into a new model of regulation of professional work. This model, termed *social service professionalism*, as applied to the National Health Service (NHS) in the United Kingdom, was framed by health policy but at the same time the welfare state recognized the claim for technical and neutral professional authority in matters concerning disease and curing (i.e. clinical autonomy).

This recognition of the autonomy of the medical profession was later questioned by the international reform movement that has swept western health care systems in recent decades. The restructuring of health care systems has been paralleled by a paradigm shift in the scholarship on professional groups. The claim on neutrality has been rejected and a further challenge to the idea of clinical autonomy has come from the emancipating idea of patient empowerment, involving the accountability of providers to the patients they serve (Saltman 1994).

Resulting from this paradigm shift, while the classic question of autonomy remains a central topic in the sociology of the professions, the focus of the analysis has been broadened to consider the positive and negative implications of professionalism for clients, organizations, organizational fields and society. Professions are seen as key actors in health care and as mediators between states and their citizens, who are more demanding than ever before (Kuhlmann 2006).

This change implies a return to professionalism as a normative value founded in communities of practice that might restrain excessive competition and tight hierarchical control, and give rise to new forms of organizations and cooperation. Public and professional interests are not necessarily in opposition, and professionalism is now seen as a possible and maybe also desirable way to develop and provide complex services to the public (Exworthy and Halford 1999; Evetts 2006). If professionals at the same time are becoming more accountable to the state and the citizens, this does not mean a simple alliance between the three.

In the Nordic context, the reconfiguration of professionalism has been deeply enmeshed in the welfare state and its redefinition (Henriksson et al. 2006; Wrede 2008). Such a focus on professionalism gives new directions and interests for sociologists that refocus on some of the classical questions but also focus on the new ways in which professionalism is discussed and used by states, the public, employers and managers and by the professions themselves. Healthcare reforms and new forms of governance and management do not only challenge and change the health care professions, they also change the state itself and the ways in which the public interacts with professionals (Hewitt and Thomas 2007).

Summing up, the evidence from analysis of recent research demonstrates the need to examine emerging forms of professionalism through context-sensitive studies. Recent research further suggests that the reactions of health professionals in organizations vary depending on the content and strategy of the NPM reform, the institutional structures and governance traditions and also the strategies of the professions. First, there seems to be a role for the reactions of the professionals whether the reform strategy confronts their profession or not (Degeling et al. 2006; Kragh Jespersen 2006; Kirkpatrick et al. 2009). Second, reforms requiring collaboration across professions are likely to be retarded or decoupled (Ferlie et al. 2005; Fitzgerald and Dopson 2005) and top-down initiated reforms requiring changes in professional beliefs and culture, and the use of extraprofessional output measures, are difficult to implement even if they are sustained for long periods (Kirkpartick et al. 2004; Ackroyd et al. 2007). Third, management models and the interplay between professional groups and local management seem to be important for strategic change in complex and pluralistic organizations (Denis et al. 2001; Pomey et al. 2007), and increased control frequently became the answer.

7.3 Professional autonomy in eras of change

This section develops a conceptual framework for the analysis of professional autonomy and then applies it to the analysis of the Nordic countries. Three different notions of professional autonomy can be suggested to help in assessing changes in professional autonomy over time. The reconfigurations of professional autonomy are also related to different conceptualizations of professional accountability. *Traditional professional autonomy* corresponds to the position of the health care professions before the era of new public management and implies double social closure and accountability for providing an equitable social service (Henriksson et al. 2006; Wrede 2008). Traditional professional autonomy can, however, be curtailed by the effects of reforms stressing efficiency, hierarchy and market mechanisms. A second form of more limited autonomy can be termed *framed autonomy*. Here the aim of the 'performance movement' is to increase the accountability of doctors and other publicly funded professionals, particularly to include the cost of the service. A third new situation seems to be emerging, with several competing kinds of expert knowledge and a greater role for the public, which can be called *competitive autonomy*. The legitimacy of the medical monopoly has been eroded even more. While the emphasis on the economic performance of the health sector continues to be a core policy concern, the idea of a public service ethic and associated accountability emerges and further threatens medical autonomy. The three different kinds of autonomy are described in Table 7.1.

The classification scheme is based on the literature and empirical studies of relations between the state, the professions and the public. It reflects the way professional autonomy is conceptualized, examined and discussed in the sociology of professions. As the sociology of professions historically has been dominated by Anglo-American approaches, often without adequate theoretical attention to the welfare state, we have chosen to complement our theoretical discussion on autonomy with a consideration of how the issue of accountability has been raised in more recent literature. From a Nordic perspective, this expansion is motivated with reference to the welfare state as a particular political project that 'compromised' medical autonomy since its conception (e.g. Marshall 1939).

This conceptualization can be fruitful in the empirical analysis of changes in

Table 7.1 Three kinds of medical professional autonomy

Dimensions	Traditional autonomy	Framed autonomy	Competitive autonomy
Degree of monopoly	Recognized monopoly over certain kinds of work and control with areas of abstract scientific knowledge	Monopoly disputed by demands for efficiency, i.e. market accountability	No monopoly but open competition between professions
Control of boundaries	Professions important in regulation and development of health care	Boundaries disputed; demands for coherence and flexibility	Boundaries disputed and changing
Control of management	Professionals active in management of health care organizations	General management and political decisions important	Joint decision-making; several professions involved
Control over problem definition	Professionals define and solve problems in relation to clients	Management define problems; active, top-down reforms prevail	Recognition of both managerial and professional knowledge
Kind of professional identity	Professional identities defined in monoprofessional communities of practice	Professional norms and identities are subsided to organizational norms	Professional identities are diverse and democratically oriented
Kind of accountability	In welfare states, accountability is related to health care's position as a public service (social service professionalism)	Professionals are framed by utility norms and accountable to market logics professionalism	New relations with patients and accountability to the public

the autonomy of the medical profession in the Nordic countries along the axes of professional autonomy and accountability. This chapter will, therefore, contributes both to empirical analysis and to theories about professionalism today and suggests that former, rather crude, analyses of the decline of medical dominance need to be adjusted.

7.4 The Danish case: a joint management model and the concept of unambiguous management

Up to 1970, the Danish health care system was governed almost exclusively by the National Board of Health (dominated by doctors) in close dialogue with the medical profession. The political parties played a reactive role, such that the Danish system represented an almost clear-cut case of traditional professional autonomy with double social closure (Kragh Jespersen 2002). Important questions about hospital planning, expenditure and the development of health care were left to the National Health Care Board and the scientific medical societies, while the Danish health care sector became institutionalized within a public welfare context. The period before 1970 has been labelled the 'great times' period (Vallgårda 1993), meaning that the position of doctors was so strong that medical development in itself became a force not to be disputed. A reorganization of hospitals in 1956 was described by the chairman of the National Health Board as 'the specialization within medical science has made the reorganization of hospitals necessary'. In 1969, an advisory political hospital board did not discuss the important guidelines for future hospital planning proposed by the National Health Board and the scientific societies (Vallgårda 1993, p. 195).

This period of 'technocratic change' (Klein 1989) lasted until the end of the 1960s, when the status of the medical profession became disputed. The rise in expenditure became a problem in itself, especially after the publication of the first long-term plan for the public sector in 1968 (Finansministeriet 1971). The expenditure forecast was alarming and triggered discussions about prioritization and the ability of doctors to manage hospitals (Finansministeriet 1969; Tørning 1970). Politicians and civil servants also criticized the quality of services and the lack of cooperation between doctors, nurses and administrators at the hospital level.

The local government reform of 1970 abolished local hospital boards, where the chief medical consultant had direct access and great power. The medical profession lost its monopolistic position in relation to health care policy in general and hospital development and governance in particular. But the reform did not change the dominating medical logic in the field, and the medical profession maintained their power in relation to important questions such as guidelines for hospital structure and planning (Pedersen et al. 2005).

Management before 1970 was divided between three professional hierarchies. The council of consultants elected a chairman as head of the medical hierarchy, who was the most important manager in the hospital. Nurses had their own hierarchy with a head nurse at the top, and there also was an administrative hierarchy with a hospital administrator at the top. In this way, management in hospitals was divided between three parallel professional hierarchies (Mintzberg 1983). At the clinic level each (employed) consultant had their own clinic and was the clinic manager. There was a head nurse at each clinic, but her duties were related to nursing and she reported to the hospital head nurse. These management models had been institutionalized during a long period without interference from 'external' forces and were supported by the medical profession as the 'natural' way. The nursing profession controlled their own staff but had to recognize the doctors as the leading profession.

In the 1970s, there was a growing critique of the medical monopoly from politicians, hospital administrators and nurses. Since the early 1980s, the decentralized hospital arena has also been subject to NPM-inspired reforms, such as introduction of new management models, quality development and control, use of activity-based financing (ABF) for budgets, internal contracting, outsourcing, free choice of hospital and improved patient rights. The major reforms were prepared by central public commissions and implemented by the counties, often with great variations. This was also the case when it came to management models.

In 1984, a white paper about productivity in hospitals from a commission in the Ministry of the Interior recommended new management models (Indenrigsministeriet 1984). They wanted to improve productivity by decentralizing economic responsibility and recommended new management models, all with the participation of the medical and nursing profession. In this way, the *incorporation* of the two important professions in management became part of the official Danish NPM template. At hospital level, all counties later introduced the same troika model (with a doctor, a nurse and a general manager together responsible for hospital management) and different varieties of a joint management model at the clinic level (all with a doctor and a nurse in the management team).

The shift to a broader conception of the management agenda, including financial management, human resource management and strategic management, affected the position and strategies of the medical profession. At the hospital level, there was little conflict and the troika model quickly became dominating. However, clinical management became an area of conflict. The medical profession advocated for the old unitary model as the 'natural' model and never accept the joint management model at the clinic level. The Danish Medical Association stated (Gøtrik 1988): 'the leading consultant will be the natural person to perform unitary management'.

The implementation of the new models took place in a decentralized governance structure where county and local hospital interpretations became important. The Medical Association established local industrial conflicts in order to protect their jurisdiction within the new frames. A variation of the joint clinic management model in the County of Funen, where the head nurse and the leading consultant *together* became responsible for clinic management, was opposed by doctors in an industrial conflict that lasted for two years. The joint management model could not be implemented before it was agreed that the doctor in the management team alone was responsible for medical treatment. Then the joint management model was disseminated; and by the early 1990s, it was widespread in the Danish hospital field.

The interplay between a decentralized structure, the strategies of the medical profession and the content of the NPM reform is clear in this phase. The change in management models would probably never have been implemented without the formation of a general NPM management strategy. But the joint management model initiated in a top-down move could only be institutionalized at the clinic level through a local negotiated compromise where doctors kept control over treatment issues. The decentralized governance structure seems in this case to have helped the medical profession in securing the core of their professional project.

The long pathway of traditional unitary management by doctors could, however, no longer be maintained within the new frames. It became slowly deinstitutionalized, partly through public discourses and partly by the introduction of new management models initiated outside the profession. The medical profession succeeded in protecting their core knowledge, and control of treatment remained with the doctors, but they had to take responsibility for budgets, quality performance and human relations and to share it with nurses and general managers at the hospital level.

During the 1990s, there was a gradual shift in the NPM strategy, emphasizing stronger rights for patients (1988), new quality development schemes (1993), free choice of hospitals for patients (1992–93), standardized clinical guidelines (late 1990s) and the use of ABF and diagnosis-related group (DRG) rates (during the 1990s). Health care policy became more centralized and was accompanied by political criticism of the counties for not being effective in the governance of hospitals.

In relation to management models, the second hospital commission in 1997 (Ministry of Health 1997) pointed out that quality in hospitals was the main problem and suggested new management models as part of the solution. A new management concept called 'unambiguous management' was proposed for all levels, with total management responsibility held by one person. The joint management model did not, according to the commission, solve the question of accountability, and clinic managers were accused of leaving problems unsolved where there was disagreement. The principle of unambiguous management was adopted by the government in their own white paper in 1999. In the annual negotiations between the counties and the government in 1999, the parties agreed 'to encourage a principle of unambiguous management at all levels in the hospital sector' (Finansministeriet 1999). The implementation of the new concept was left to the counties, and the medical profession translated the new concept into unitary management by doctors even if the Minister of Health and the Head of the County Councils Association kept saying that no group had any monopoly in relation to management (Danish Medical Association 2000; Kragh Jespersen 2005). In the years after 1999, the medical profession was fast to take advantage of the new arena both in policy statements and, via local negotiation, to obtain local agreements reviving unitary medical management.

Management models have not been part of the central reform agenda since 2000. At the *hospital level*, the most important change since 2000 is the merger of hospitals under the same management team, and hospital mergers seem to continue after the formation of the new regions in 2007. The troika model is still the dominant model, in most cases with three members together responsible for management and with a hospital director having the last word. In this way, the NPM reforms in Denmark have effectively positioned doctors at the highest levels of hospital governance. Currently, doctors sit on the main board of all 30 hospital management teams in Denmark and are directors in four (Kragh Jespersen 2006). Most of the hospital management teams cover more than one hospital (from two to five).

At the clinic level, there are no general managers involved in the management teams but some can be found in staff positions in the bigger clinics. After the recommendations of unambiguous management, most counties have introduced a modified joint management model, with the leading medical consultant and the head nurse sharing the management of clinics – but usually the doctor has the final say. In most of the newer units in hospitals, such as clinical centres and function-bearing units (Borum 2004, p. 2005), the principle of unitary medical management has been reintroduced, but with nurses as vice-managers. Clinic managers are still responsible for treatment and care, budgets, human resource management and the development of the clinic.

Members of the clinical management teams can apply for management education but it is not a formal requirement. In 1999, 41 per cent of the leading consultants in clinical management had a formal management education lasting one to four weeks and only 34 per cent had more than four weeks management education. Of these, 29 per cent indicated that management education had permanent effects on their management practice, while 25 per cent indicated that training had little effect (Danish Medical Association 2000).

Summing up, the new concept of unambiguous management was indirectly inspired by the overall Danish NPM strategy in the 1990s. It was adopted by the central actors in the field, but implementation was left to the counties and the Danish Medical Association tried again to reinvent traditional unitary management. During recent years, doctors have improved their position in relation to clinic management, but the dominant model at the clinic level is still the joint management model, although in new varieties. In recent years, the position of doctors has been even stronger than in the 1980s and 1990s, backed by the Medical Association.

The NPM process in Denmark has been characterized by the incorporation of the professions in management at both the hospital and the clinic level, and no attempt has been made to introduce general management in *opposition* to the medical profession. The policy instruments in relation to management have been weak, and the specific implementation of new management models has been a matter for local decision. At this level, the medical profession has been able to make use of the new arenas created at the central level and has, to some degree, regained its position in management. It is important to note, however, that today they have to share management responsibilities with other professions.

7.5 The Norwegian case: developing unitary management while maintaining medical autonomy

Before 1970, the health care system in Norway was characterized as an extension of the medical clinic into the state (Berg 1987). The medical profession controlled the health system and penetrated the administration and policy system. It was personified between 1938 and 1972 by the doctor Karl Evang, former Health Director (Nordby 1989). After this period, the Norwegian health system was to a very high degree a public service organization based on principles of free access and tax financing. A very large percentage of total expenditure went to hospitals compared with the situation in other countries, and the governance structure was rather fragmented and decentralized with state, county and municipalities involved. However, the system was still 'depoliticized' and in fact the state and the medical profession were linked together to such a degree that it was labelled a 'profession-state' (Erichsen 1996, p.19). Until 1970, doctors were in the ascendency through their positions in the central state but also as the most important managers in hospitals and in local health boards. Some discussion about who should be preferred as managers in the hospitals occurred, and Karl Evang advocated that it should be doctors (Evang 1952). He was contradicted by nurses, who wanted to break with the monopoly of doctors in relation to management (Sommervold 1996).

In the late 1970s there was a growing critique of the 'medicracy' (Berg 1987) because of rapidly increasing expenditure and public perceptions of the health - care system as ineffective and not service oriented (Skaset 2003; Berg 2005). It was also pointed out that medical specialization had a negative impact on efforts to create coherent treatment and care for patients (Martinsen 1984).

In relation to hospital management, a nurses' strike in 1972 changed the position of the nurses. They had their own management hierarchy in relation to care and personnel but felt that they were not taken seriously. The Norwegian Nurses Association (Norsk sykepleierforbund) no longer accepted the full juris-diction of the doctors and wanted to keep their management position both in clinics and at the hospital level (Norwegian Nurses Association 2005, p. 6). After the strike, a system of divided management emerged from an informal division of work between nurses and doctors, but in reality there was no doubt about the domination of the doctors in relation to management.

In 1970, the counties (fylkene) took over responsibilities for hospitals. This represented a move away from the local orientation of the hospitals. The state refunded most of hospital expenses but also demanded that hospital services should be coordinated; a system of five health regional health authorities was established for planning purposes. The NPM wave also affected the Norwegian hospital system in the 1980s and 1990s, including state-initiated experiments with ABF, several reorganizations and new task distributions between primary and secondary care.

In 1995, the Norwegian Parliament made a decision about unitary manage-ment at all levels in the hospitals (Stortinget 1995) following a report from the Andersland Committee in 1990 (Andersland 1990). It was inspired by general management ideas, and managers from Norwegian companies participated in the committee and promoted the idea that management in hospitals should be professionalized (Kalleberg 1991; Byrkjeflot 1997). It was met with substan-tial resistance from doctors and the Norwegian Medical Association, and it was not implemented (Torjesen and Gammelsæther 2005). In 1996, a new public commission was appointed (the Steine Commission) to suggest new forms of management that could improve the running of hospitals in accordance with the 10 'patients first' principles stated by the Department for Social and Health Affairs. The patient perspective, together with pressure from the parliament and the earlier Andersland report, contributed to a continued pressure on the old divided management model.

In the Steine Commission's report, it was noted that hospital management had changed gradually into a system where the administrator had become hospital director and taken over management in nearly all respects (NOU 1997, p. 29). At the clinic level, management was still divided between head nurses and the leading medical consultant (NOU 1997, section 10.3).

The commission suggested that clinic management should be team based, with representatives from the relevant (health) professions; that one person in the team should be formal leader; and that personal qualities and management experience were important. They did not agree about the weight that medical background should have (NOU 1997, p. 154) but made a distinction between professional responsibility and what they called 'system' responsibilities. The clinic manager should take care of system responsibilities such as coordination, budgets and development issues, while health professionals should be responsible for treatment and care. This distinction is important because it directly questions the notion of full medical jurisdiction.

In 1999, the parliament passed a new law about specialist health services based on the proposals from the Steine Commission (Government of Norway 1999) and the principle of unitary management was to be implemented in all hospitals and clinics by 2001. Unitary management meant that the old system of divided management at the clinic level would be abolished and that only one person would have overall management responsibility.

These changes were implemented in 2001 before a broad hospital reform took effect in 2002 (Vareide 2002; Byrkjeflot 2005). The ownership reform removed ownership of hospitals from the counties and the Ministry of Health stated that it was 'essential that the framework for hospital management is clearly established . . . it is equally important to define and specify the responsibilities which will be placed with managers at different levels within the hospitals' (quoted from Torjesen and Gammelsæther 2004, p. 15).

Following the 1999 law, there was intense public debate about unitary management and how it could be interpreted. Especially in the clinic departments at the university hospitals, the medical elite opposed the new unitary principle because other health professionals could be appointed. It actually happened in Bergen, where a midwife was appointed unitary manager in a maternity department. The doctors fiercely opposed this, and the deputy for all consultants at the hospital stated that this decision would create a bad working environment and perhaps harm patient service, education and research (Mo 2006, p. 106). The President of the Norwegian Medical Association stated that:

> There is no doubt about the position of the Medical Association when it comes to management of clinics . . . We have supported the principle of unitary management, but we presuppose that it must be qualified management . . . We think it is necessary to place the medical management responsibility with an educated medical specialist in units which are engaged in medical diagnosis and treatment.
>
> (Bakke 2002, p. 2158)

However, doctors were heavily criticized for opposing national legislation, and the Ministry of Health and Care Service, after meetings with the Medical Association, had to issue a circular stating some important principles. The unitary manager should have total and overall responsibility for the unit he/she manages, but this does not interfere with the responsibilities of the individual authorized health professional. The unitary manager cannot change or reverse a decision of doctors in relation to treatment of individual patients (Helsedepartementet 2002, pp. 1–3). The department made a distinction between system and professional responsibility, and this made it possible for those other than doctors to be managers at the clinic level. This circular satisfied the medical profession and at the same time opened clinic management positions to other health professionals.

After the ownership reform, the unitary management model seems to disseminate quite fast. In 1999, only 14 per cent of hospitals had implemented the new model at the clinic level, while in 2003, one year after the law had come into force, all hospitals had implemented the new model. However, the implementation of unitary management had been demanding and conflict ridden (Kjekshus 2004, p. 19) and 20 per cent still used the divided model in some clinics. At the top hospital management level, the position of medical and nursing directors seems to be decreasing. They were represented in more than 90 per cent of hospitals in 1999 but only in 33 per cent in 2003. They are replaced by various kinds of general manager such as communication and organization specialists (Kjekshus 2004, p. 13). In another national survey and interview-based investigation of clinic managers in 2004, 67 per cent of the unitary managers were doctors and 28 per cent nurses, while 8 per cent had other professional backgrounds. In addition, 74 per cent of clinic managers reported that the introduction of unitary management had caused conflict to 'some' or 'high' degree (Gjerberg and Sørensen 2006, p. 1064). The conflicts were about responsibility for medical treatment, which were said to be unclear, and doctors simply not accepting other professions as unitary managers.

Two other studies should be mentioned here because another picture of the unitary manager reform emerges from these. First an interview-based investigation in two hospitals among clinic leaders from different kinds of unit and clinic showed that doctors thought of the position as temporary, a break in clinical career, and focused on the management of doctors and medical affairs (Johansen 2005). In another case study from a university hospital, 14 clinic managers, 4 clinical directors and the hospital director were interviewed (Mo 2006). Again, medical clinic managers stated that medical knowledge and clinical practice was needed in order to be a clinic manager with authority and legitimacy, but they also recognize that unitary management was something different from the old health professional management. Mo (2006, p. 244) interprets this as the contours of a new conception of management where clinic managers are more like general managers but with medical knowledge as an important element. These managers defined system responsibility as the balance between medical development and the 'orders of the profession' on the one side and the needs of the population and budgets on the other. This is different from the NPM-inspired conception of system responsibility as the efficient running of operations, and it points to new roles for the medical manage (Mo 2006, p. 246).

The Norwegian case shows a state that is constantly and with growing intensity engaged in hospital management at the central political level. It is no coincidence that the new management model of unitary management at all levels has been a matter of legislation and not left to decentralized authorities. The inspiration both from private management thinking and NPM strategies is very visible in the public commission reports in the 1980s and 1990s, and in harmony with the tradition of central regulation in Norway (Torjesen 2008). Management in hospitals is too important to be left to the health care enterprises even after the ownership reform, and while doctors criticized the unitary management they were themselves criticized in public by politicians and other professions. Doctors who hold positions as unitary managers have not left their profession and become general managers. They have interpreted the new role in their own ways and have not forgotten the clinic and the orders of the profession. Hybrid management roles are the result.

7.6 The Swedish case: from medical elite into a welfare state profession

In Sweden the depression in the 1930s paved the way for social democratic governments that favoured central decision-making based on scientific knowledge. This shift contributed to the creation of a medical hospital-based elite being advisers and policy-makers in relation to the state bureaucracy. The autonomy of the medical profession until the period after the Second World War, therefore, corresponds to the concept of double closure autonomy when it comes to medical work. Doctors could make autonomous decisions concerning content and processes without interference from outside, while the labour market for the medical profession was largely secured by the state.

The period immediately following the Second World War until the 1960s has been characterized as a time of hesitation (Garpenby 1989, p. 83). In this period, controversy emerged between the Swedish Medical Association and the state around the first social-democratically framed plan for the reorganization of ambulatory medical care (Riska 1993). Axel Höjer, then Director of the National Board of Health, was a key policy entrepreneur who actively campaigned for reform, introducing a unitary health service comprising hospitals, associated health centres and preventive activities. The Swedish Medical Association opposed these plans, remaining in conflict with Höjer throughout this period. Behind the conflict lay the interests of hospital physicians, who had grown into a powerful group in the profession. The Swedish Medical Association defended the existing labour market and the associated opportunities for private paid practice throughout the 1940s and the 1950s (Riska 1993; Dahlin and Kuuse 2005).

The opposition of the Swedish Medical Association hampered the reform of ambulatory care in the 1950s. Hospital expansion continued and solutions to the rigidity in ambulatory care were sought through institutional reform by change of principal for the provincial doctor system. In 1963, this system was transferred from the state to the county councils, and in 1969 the so-called Seven Crown Reform of the hospital sector was passed (Dahlin and Kuuse 2005, p. 160), which ended the power of consultants to collect fees from private patients in public hospital beds (Riska 1993).

After these reforms, the professional autonomy of the Swedish medical profession was curtailed by health policy, although medical expertise continued to be recognized. While the Swedish Medical Association in the 1950s opposed the expansion of the public health care system, in the 1960s it gradually became incorporated in the collective bargaining structure in the public sector (Riska 1993). In the 1970s, public planning reformed ambulatory care through the development of health care centres (vårdcentraler) (Dahlin and Kuuse 2006, p. 20).

At this point, early state-centred strategies were questioned as a result of growing awareness of the bureaucratization of the welfare state. This critical reflection led to more decision-making closer to the citizen (Allardt 1975). Reflecting such gradual change, the 1982 Act on Health and Medical Care formally decentralized the planning and production of health services, making the county councils the central arena. In 1985, the so-called Dagmar Reform continued the restructuring of the role of the county councils. Producer domination and lack of incentives for greater efficiency were seen to be the main problems (Saltman 1991, p. 615; Glennester and Matsaganis 1994, p. 244) and the reform aimed at a more personalized service and systematic cost containment.

These, and subsequent reforms, were implemented in a changed climate that reflected increased engagement with NPM ideas about the public sector. The decentralized system produced substantial variation in performance between county councils. Saltman (1991, p. 615) characterizes the situation in the early 1990s as a search for 'planned markets' that combine market-style incentives with residual planning. In terms of legitimacy of the welfare state, patient empowerment emerged as a response to rising pressures from groups of service users (Saltman 1994). Such pressures helped to call into question the command-and-control model of accountability, in which physicians and nurses were accountable not primarily to patients but rather to the elected authorities that administered the health care system at the regional level. When patient choice was put in place, providers also became directly accountable to the patients they served (Saltman 1994, p. 221).

In the 1990s, the complex restructuring of public health care delivery in Sweden resulted in the consolidation of health care governance focused on the regional level of county councils, with the Federation of County Councils emerging as a key actor on the national scene in contacts between the state and the county councils. The state, in turn, utilized the Federation of County Councils to enter a dialogue with the county councils. Garpenby (1999, pp. 409–10) argues that the state faced new economic challenges and a need to control public spending while the general public expected the state to offer an acceptable level of services. The state sought to intensify its dialogue with all actors in the health care sector, including the medical profession, and to introduce new logics, such as systematic quality improvement, without recognizing traditional claims on clinical autonomy (Garpenby 1999, p. 412).

The organization of managers as an interest group rapidly reflected the new legislation, and a new multiprofessional organization was founded in 1996 under the title Swedish Association for Adminstrative Medicine (Svensk Förening för Administrativ Medicin, SAM) which emerged as an arena for 'dialogues' between the state, the Federation of County Councils, representatives of the medical profession and other professionals and experts.

During the 1990s, the formal competence needed for managerial roles was constantly discussed, and in 1997, the Swedish Medical Association issued an action plan for defending medical leadership directed towards both policymakers and doctors themselves, reminding them that 'leadership is a part of professional identity' (Läkartidningen 1997, p. 1241). In recent years, doctors' interest in leadership roles has been smaller than the Swedish Medical

Association had hoped, as the *Swedish Medical Association Journal* includes numerous appeals such as: 'The medical profession must not disclaim leadership' (Widerström 2000), 'leadership in care is doctors' responsibility' (Grewin 2001) and 'you are needed as manager!' (Pernulf 2006).

According to the Health and Medical Care Act of 1991, the chief medical superintendants/medical managers in hospitals (chefsöverläkare) were no longer held responsible for the medical care of individual patients, instead they had holistic responsibility for their clinics and represented the employer towards other employees (Rhenman 2000). New legislation in 1997 transformed chief medical directors into health services managment positions (verksamhetschef) that no longer presupposed medical education. In this way, the multiprofessional model of health services management became legally based in Sweden. Indeed, the proportion of doctors in managerial positions has rapidly decreased, as new professionals have entered the scene. Medical leadership remains strongest in the hospital sector, where in 2005 70 per cent of managers were still doctors, but in primary care the proportion of doctors was only 42 per cent (Pernulf 2005).

In 1999, a national group for health management and organizational development (Nationella gruppen för vårdens ledar- och verksamhetsutveckling), coordinated by the Federation of County Councils, was established. The Swedish Medical Association struggled to redefine medical leadership in a situation where this new, multiprofessional meeting place had emerged. The new management ideology concerned leadership in dialogue with co-workers, politicians and administrators, and the tools were action plans, to be made in collaboration with co-workers, and development discussions (e.g. Grewin 2001). Through the Swedish Medical Association-initiated project 'Future Doctors' (*Framtidens läkare*), the medical interest group incorporated the idea of a 'balanced and respectful' dialogue with the other health care actors but emphasized the need for 'clarity' in terms of the long-term goals, division of responsibility and authority in care (Stenmark 2002). Indeed, in the professional discourse of the Swedish Medical Association, the call for 'clarity in terms of the division of responsibility and authority' seems to have replaced claims on professional autonomy (see also Sveriges läkarförbunds chefsförening 2000).

More recently, the Federation of County Councils has developed its leadership agenda on the basis of a redefinition of health care organizations. Health care is viewed as a complex, adaptive system consisting of multiple professional groups that all function independently while, at the same time, influencing each other (Berglund 2005). The new position further distances itself from classic hierarchical models to organize health care. Professionals are to work autonomously but as members in teams. The task of health care managers is to 'create enthusiasm, participation and willingness to improve' among co-workers (Berglund 2005).

Summing up, in the 1930s, the Swedish medical profession enjoyed double closure while the state was engaged in building up the welfare state. Relying on medical expertise, the state invested primarily in the expansion of the hospital sector. The goal to provide all citizens with equal access to health care supported the view of physicians as the key welfare state profession (Brante 1999). Gradually, the emphasis in health policy shifted from access to active promotion of health, and Brante (1999, p. 75) argues that in the 1960s a new type of 'political professional' emerged to administer what he calls 'governmental rationality'. In Sweden, 'political professionalism' was closely tied to the long period of Social Democratic rule.

Brante (1999) identifies the recent redefinition of professionalism in Sweden with reference to internationalization of the state. As has been demonstrated above, this entails competitive autonomy for the medical profession. More specifically, the medical profession, together with other professions, enters diverse 'dialogues' with the state (Garpenby 1999) that in the final instance can be identified as concerned with public accountability. Indeed, changes in the Swedish health sector can be associated with the deep-rooted institutional and cultural change in state governance, which Municio (1996, p. 6) has identified as the emergence of the 'rhetorical state' where the goals that the government pursues become formulated as a philosophy, often taking the shape of professional ideology. Leadership is a key theme within the rhetorical state, as it provides an organizational identity for those in management positions (Svedberg 2004). In the light of this discussion, the position of doctor-managers in the context of competitive autonomy is moving in a similar direction, where the organizational mission replaces the idea of a professional mandate.

7.7 The Finnish case: gradual interweaving of medicine and the state

From the mid-1930s onwards, as in Sweden, Finnish politics increasingly emphasized state-centred policy instruments. The building of a hierarchically organized network of public hospitals was implemented and a rural public health programme was outlined (Wrede 2000). The development of the medical profession from the 1930s onwards reflects these two orientations and their relative strength. The investment in hospitals was huge, creating a steady basis for the development of hospital consultants into a powerful group of specialist physicians (Pylkkänen 2002). General medical practice was not similarly emphasized, and, apart from public health activities, ambulatory medical practice remained in the sphere of private practice, reflecting a success for the actions of the Finnish Medical Association, as this largely corresponded to professional ideology of the day (Vuolio 1991).

The physicians' professional association was very strong in the early policy context. Similar to Denmark, the collaboration between the National Board of Health and the Finnish Medical Association was a case of traditional professional autonomy with double social closure and has been characterized as a 'cosy brotherhood' (Kauttu 1985, p. 129). Reflecting the power of the Finnish Medical Association, attempts to introduce compulsory public sickness insurance failed in the late 1920s and 1940s, and Finland was the last country in Europe to introduce a health insurance system, in 1963 (Kangas 1991). At that point, Finland had one of the highest numbers of hospital beds per capita in western Europe, but one of the least developed ambulatory care systems (Kuusi 1961). The situation resulted in unequal access for several categories of citizens. Furthermore, the payment system for hospital physicians, created in conditions of severe shortage of doctors, was out of the control of the state, with possibilities for substantial economic rewards especially for junior doctors (Pesonen 1974).

In the 1950s and 1960s, state policies and professional interests clashed as a result of the rapidly rising hospital expenditure (Pesonen 1974). The salary system for hospital doctors was renewed but the state took over the regulation of medical specialties and increased the number of medical graduates (Pesonen 1974; Kauttu 1985). These reforms strained the relationship between the Finnish Medical Association and National Board of Health, but medical expertise continued to be fundamental in the planning of the hospital sector (Wrede 2000).

The respect for the medical profession was also reflected in the design of the 1963 health insurance. All citizens can seek the services of private specialists without referral, provided that they pay a large part of the fee out of pocket. Thus free choice of doctor in this plan is likely to be limited to better-off patients (e.g. Kuusi 1964; Suonoja 1992). Despite constant criticism, the scheme persists as one of the core policy instruments in the Finnish health care system, in part because of lobbying from the Finnish Medical Association (e.g. Pylkkänen 2002).

The organization of ambulatory medical care was another core area of conflict between the National Board of Health and the Finnish Medical Association, beginning from the late 1950s. After 10 years of process and the work of three committees, the Primary Health Care Act of 1972 was pushed through by a social democratic government (Pesonen 1974; Suonoja 1992; Wrede 2001). The act aimed at greater equity and equal access in health care, creating a system of publicly provided primary health care for the entire population. In terms of professional autonomy of doctors, a key change occurred in that the physicians in primary health care centres were municipal employees, subordinated to the organizational charter of the primary health care system. Municipal physicians thus lost the far-reaching autonomy that the group had held prior to the Primary Health Act 1972. The reform was met with anger from the medical profession, and the contested reform was reflected in the public image of primary health care centres (e.g. Wrede 2001).

While the welfare state offered doctors continued economic rewards, its policies and institutions limited their autonomy. The constraint on medical authority was particularly salient in the context of the primary health care centres, where the clinical autonomy of rank-and-file doctors was curtailed (Riska 1993). However, the primary health care centres were managed by chief physicians, and, at the macro level, the medical profession could wield state power through the technocratic state bureaucracy and its policy-making (c.f. Rinne and Jauhiainen 1988; Julkunen 1994).

Neoliberal critiques challenged the 'profession state' in Finland in the mid-1980s, and the major institutional reforms that led to the restructuring of the welfare state occurred in the early 1990s the reforms resulted from the combined effects of international economic recession, the process of preparing Finland for membership in the EU in 1995 and changes in the welfare ethos, which reflected what can be called a rationality of efficiency (Wrede et al. 2008). Finland had received favourable international attention for its investment in primary health care centres, (e.g. WHO Regional Office for Europe 1991) and the policy-making of the early 1990s did not question this strategy. The first reforms aimed at continuity as well as quality of care and to make health care provision more effective (e.g. Sihvo and Lindqvist 1994) in the mid-1990s the pressures to control health costs dominated, forcing continued cuts in health care spending. Health spending in Finland is currently substantially below the OECD average (OECD 2007).

The reforms of the early 1990s shifted the responsibility for planning service provision to the municipalities, enhancing their role in health policy. Instead of earmarked state funding, block grants were introduced, making the municipality responsible for making decisions about primary health care services. In addition, the municipality was compelled to purchase specialized medical care services from a hospital district. Municipalities were encouraged to rationalize their service production by implementing models from the private sector, but they turned out to be rather cautious with their new liberty and 'marketization' of health services has remained limited (Torppa 2007). In recent years, the municipalities' reliance on private provision has slowly increased, often with reference to shortage of doctors, and the implementation of the so-called care guarantee in 2005 has substantially increased the use of private service provision by the municipalities. In spite of this, the overwhelming majority of medical services continues to be publicly provided (Pekurinen et al. 2008).

The decentralization of the health sector changed the role of municipal health administration, making it a central arena for the planning of health services. Until the 1990s, detailed steering from the central government left little room for the discretion of local policy-makers. Chief physicians were the key officials, but the emphasis in their leadership was on the content of services. The professional ideology depicted chief physicians more as 'senior colleagues' than as managers (Viitanen et al. 2002) and defined 'supporting' activities as administration, which was organized as a separate system (Finnish Ministry of Education 2004). Increased managerial concerns of the 1990s recast the framework and created pressure for larger municipalities (Torppa 2007).

As elsewhere, the managerial reorganization of the public Finnish sector has involved efforts to reduce the medical profession's claim on leadership positions. Policy-makers at different levels have wanted to change the competence requirements for positions as administrative directors of Finnish hospital districts and primary health centres so that medical education would no longer be required. In the early 1990s, a long-standing conflict in the City of Helsinki ended with a settlement where the city officials retreated from their efforts to promote nurses in management positions. In the compromise, services were divided into 'basic care' and 'active care', with managers for all of the active care units to be doctors (Anon. 1994).

The local settlement did not end efforts to introduce a new definition of management roles. The Ministry of Social Affairs and Health set up a committee in 1995 to prepare 'multiprofessional' educational programmes in health services management (Finnish Ministry of Education 2004, p. 17). In response, the Finnish Medical Association struggled to defend the administrative qualification included in the specialist physician programmes offered by the medical faculties. A transition period for doctors was declared until 2005, but after that time management training has developed according to the multiprofessional model outlined in 2004 (Finnish Ministry of Education 2004). The overall management model drafted in the recent committee report suggests a hierarchical structure where professional expertise only plays an important role for the lowest level of managers who supervise day-to-day practice, while the higher levels deal with management of multiprofessional organizations. The groups that can acquire such competences include, in addition to doctors, nurses and persons with a master's degree in health sciences (Finnish Ministry of Education 2004).

The Finnish Medical Association has opposed this new thinking by claiming that 'administrative power and clinical experience cannot be separated' (Kekomäki 2006) and by promoting the notion of professional seniority (e.g. Viitanen et al. 2002) rooted in the ideas of collegiality in early-modern medicine (Oker-Blom 1911 (facsimile 2000); Pesonen 1980; Finnish Medical Association 2005). Collegiality also survived the decentralization of specialized medical care in the early 1990s, in the shape of chief physician collegiums. Now, however, the chief physicians who manage the day-to-day activities of health care organizations appear to be in an untenable role. According to tradition, they should be senior colleagues but the new ideology assigns them the task of representing the goals of the organization. An example of current reforms challenging the positions of chief physicians in the hospital sector is the effort by the leaders of the Hospital District of Helsinki and Uusimaa to introduce multiprofessional leadership. After protests from the hospital doctors, this reform was waived, but it is likely that the trend towards multiprofessional leadership will continue. For instance, when the planned reconfiguration of local health centres into larger health care organizations is implemented, merging elements from specialized medical care with primary health care, it seems unlikely that the collegial model of organizing medical management will stay intact.

Summing up, from the point of view of the medical profession, managerialism has resulted in a major cultural transformation of public sector health organizations. Since the 2000s the medical leadership has been 'dethroned' from the level of policy design. Instead, a multiprofessional model is rising and it seems clear that the large-scale institutional restructuring underway implies a shift to a new management culture. In the new system, physicians in both the public and the private sector (Mattila 2006) will have to work in organizations led by persons with forms of expertise other than medical. Institutionalized forms of medical collegiality are likely to disappear gradually, being replaced by multiprofessional forms of governance. The developments described above suggest a gradual emergence of competitive autonomy for the Finnish medical profession.

7.8 Concluding remarks

We will now outline the pattern of changing autonomy for the medical professions. The point of departure will be the period where the medical professions in the Nordic countries came very close to the notion of double social closure. In Denmark and Norway, this period ended about 1970, when both countries experienced rapidly rising costs and public critique of the medical professions. In Sweden and Finland, the central state initiated rapid growth in the hospital sector until the 1960s and tried to establish state-governed ambulatory care. This led to conflicts in the 1950s and 1960s with hospital consultants. Before this period of open conflict, however, the relation between the central state and the medical profession in all Nordic countries was quite close. Some have described the period as medicracy (Berg 1987) or cosy brotherhood (Kauttu 1985), meaning that the medical profession and the state bureaucracy had merged to such a degree that distinctive new organizational forms had been created, differing from those existing in Anglo-American societies. The close relationship with the state put the medical profession in a strong position with a dominant jurisdiction (Abbott 1988, p. 59), meaning that they had a legal monopoly, an effective medical knowledge regime in relation to policy-making and public opinion, and control over workplaces. This strong position was not founded on the ability to establish and control a professional project independent of the state. It was more a result of a kind of 'social service professionalism' where the professions accepted political accountability related to the building of publicly governed health care as part of the Nordic welfare state. This is especially true in the hospital sector, dominated by professional elites in central bureaucracy and university hospitals. The only exception to this general picture seems to be the attempts to control primary care through the central state in Sweden and Finland, which was met by opposition from the medical associations.

During the 1970s and the early 1980s, two different but connected developments altered the relations between the state and the medical professions. First, rapid rising expenditure in hospitals became a problem, combined with political reactions against high and increasing taxes. Second, public debates stressed that hospitals were ineffective and not service oriented, and questioned the medical monopoly in relation to policy formation and management control in hospitals. Part of the answer to these developments was to decentralize ownership and responsibility for hospitals. This was the period where the so-called decentralized Nordic health care state was created (Byrkjeflot 2005; Vrangbæk and Christiansen 2005). The models and timing were somewhat different in the various Nordic countries, as was the degree of central regulation, but for a while the problems with prioritization, bureaucratization and efficiency were partly left to the counties (in Denmark and Norway) or to the health care centres in a regionalized hospital system (in Sweden and Finland). New arenas were created but the medical profession kept their management positions and still thought it was 'natural' that doctors should be managers in hospitals and public health care centres.

This period of transition was altered in the 1980s with the adoption of NPM strategies. New financial instruments were introduced; responsibilities were decentralized and a new conception of general management was introduced stating that management in itself is a profession. In Denmark, the troika and the joint management model meant that the medical profession had to share management with nurses and general managers. In Norway, the system of divided management had the same effect. In Sweden, doctors kept their position as clinic managers until 1997, but from 1991 the idea of general management was imposed by law and they had to take overall responsibility for the clinics. In

Finland, the chief physicians were key officials, but during the 1980s there were efforts to change the competence requirements for management and in some cases management was divided so that doctors were managers for all 'active care units' but that 'basic care units' could be managed by other professions.

There seems to be three dimensions in this NPM-inspired shift away from the 'natural' model of doctors as managers. First, economic budgets and the drive for efficiency of hospitals limited traditional medical autonomy. Second, physicians had to take overall responsibility for the units they managed (not only for treatment), including service quality and patient satisfaction. Summing up, the autonomy of the medical profession was reframed in ways that downgraded traditional professional autonomy to the goals of health care organizations; however, doctors still kept most of their managerial positions.

At the end of the 1980s, new agendas were triggered by growing waiting lists and the idea that patients' choice of hospital could improve quality and efficiency at the same time. The NPM strategies were renewed, with more weight on competition and market mechanisms, trying to make medical managers accountable not to state-based welfare projects but to the logics of the new quasi-markets and patients. During the 1990s, development in the Nordic countries seems to be more differentiated, partly as response to the new developments. In Denmark, the position of doctors in management was actually strengthened after 1997 because of the decentralized implementation of unitary management, with most counties preferring doctors as unitary managers at the clinic level. Norway and Sweden, quite differently, changed the management system by legislation in 1997 and 1999, following thorough commission work, professional debates and public deliberations. The Norwegian concept of 'system responsibility' and the similar Swedish notion of 'health business manager' (verksamhetschef) were stated in the legislation and it was made clear that no profession had a monopoly in relation to management position. This challenged the 'natural' model in a very direct way by the introduction of a new and competing regime. In Finland, it appears that the medical tradition has survived to some degree. The discussion about qualifications and education changed little, institutionalized forms of medical collegiality have survived and medical managers remain dominant. However, rapid change could follow any large-scale restructuring of hospital districts and municipalities.

Most interesting is the effect of central legislation in Norway and Sweden, where the number of management positions held by doctors changed dramatically in a rather short period. In 2008, approximately 70 per cent of managers at the clinic level in both countries are doctors, compared with nearly 100 per cent previously. Nurses and others have been appointed to positions as managers at the clinic level within the new politically created and NPM-inspired framework. This has created conflicts because doctors and their associations believe that management and medical responsibility belong together whereas the overall practice is to separate medical responsibility for treatment from management, making it possible for other professionals to manage at the clinical level.

The medical professions have tried to defend the traditional position, and in Denmark they seem to have succeeded at the clinic level but not in the hospitals. In Norway and Sweden, doctors seem to have lost the battle, at least when it comes to formal management positions. The Finnish case seems to be somewhat inconclusive at the moment, but it is expected that the multiprofessional model could potentially expand as fast as in Sweden and Norway.

The difference between Norway and Sweden on the one hand and Denmark and Finland on the other is that new conceptions of management have been institutionalized through public commissions and legislation in Norway and Sweden while no specific conception has emerged in Denmark and Finland and implementation has been decentralized. This again indicates that it is difficult for the medical profession openly to defend their monopoly in public debates about management but when implementation is decentralized, doctors appear to succeed in holding and even in expanding former managerial positions.

An important question is how the new unitary management models will work in reality. At least in Norway, it seems as if doctors are able to maintain substantial control of departments with a great deal of clinical treatment. It is also possible that the old parallel hierarchies can reemerge with an informal but powerful medical hierarchy within or beside unitary management by other professions. This is an open question, as doctors and the medical profession have not given up the idea that management and medicine belong together. This appears to suggest that management structures are much easier to change than institutionalized ideas and professional cultures (Ackroyd et al. 2007)

7.8.1 Summary

The concepts of traditional, framed and competitive professional autonomy seem to be adequate for the analysis of changing professional autonomy in the management of (hospital) health care in the Nordic countries. Empirically, the autonomy of the medical profession is changing with respect to management, which is an important element for medical professionalism. Traditional medical management with undisputed control as the 'natural' management model no longer exists in any of the Nordic countries. Instead, it has been framed since the early 1990s by NPM strategies and public debates, and the medical profession has lost its monopoly both in relation to the political and legal system and in relation to the public and the patients. This opens opportunities for competition with other professions for management positions, and doctors cannot be certain to win within the new legal framework, as is clearly demonstrated in Norway and Sweden in the years after 2000. Changing management autonomy in the Nordic countries shows that legal action from the central state can be effective.

It is, however, still an open question whether and to what degree new management models will, in fact, change the distribution of power in the health care system. The medical profession is trying to regain some of the lost territory. If doctors engage in management as recommended by the Danish Medical Association, or if they are able to establish the old parallel hierarchies, then they may regain a considerable measure of authority. This suggests that competition between professions regarding management is both intense and occurring in many different arenas simultaneously. It can lead to classic struggles among professions; however, it could also open up new professional roles as old monopolies disintegrate.

References

Abbott, A. (1988) *The System of Professions*. London: University of Chicago Press.

Ackroyd, S. (1996) Organization contra organizations: professions and organizational change in the United Kingdom, *Organization Studies* 17: 599–621.

Ackroyd, W., Kirkpatrick, I. and Walker, R. (2007) Public management reform and its consequences for professional organisation: a comparative analysis, *Public Administration* 85: 9–26.

Allardt, E. (1975) *Att ha, att älska att vara. Om välfärd i Norden.* Lund: Argos.

Andersland (1990) *Rapport fra Anderslandudvalget: Ledelse i sykehus.* Oslo: Department of Social Services.

Anon. (1994) Helsingin johtosääntökiista loppuunkäsitelty, *Suomen Lääkärilehti* [*Finnish Medical Journal*] 49: 50.

Bakke, H.K. (2002) Ledelse i sykehusavdelinger, *Tidsskrift for den norske legeforening* 122: 2158.

Berg, O. (1987) *Medisinens logikk.* Oslo: University of Oslo Press.

Berg, O. (2005) *Fra politikk til økonomikk: Den norske helsepolitikks utvikling det siste sekel.* Legetidsskriftets skriftserie. Oslo: Den Norske Legeforening [Norwegian Medical Association].

Berglund, I. (2005) *Sveriges kommuner och landsting. Ledarskap.* http://www.skl.se/artikel. asp?C=1150andA=1771; accessed 1 February 2008.

Borum, F. (2004) Means-end frames and the politics and myths of organizational fields, *Organization Studies* 25: 897–921.

Brante, T. (1988) Sociological approaches to professions, *Acta Sociologica* 31: 119–42.

Brante, T. (1999) Professional waves and state objectives: a macro-sociological model of the origin and developments of continental profession, illustrated by the case of Sweden, in Hellberg, I., Saks, M. and Benoit, C. (eds) *Professional Identities in Transition: Cross-cultural Dimensions.* Södertälje: Almqvist and Wiksell International.

Braverman, H. (1974) *Labour and Monopoly Capital: The Degradation of Work in the Twentieth Century.* New York: Monthly Review Press.

Broadbent, J., Dietrich, M. and Roberts, J. (eds) (1997) *The End of the Professions? The Restructuring of Professional Work.* London: Routledge.

Bureau, V. Henriksson, L. and Wrede, S. (2004) Comparing professional groups in health care: towards a context sensitive analysis, *Knowledge, Work and Society* 2: 49–68.

Burrage, M. and Torstendahl, R. (eds) (1990) *The Formation of Professions: Knowledge, State and Strategy.* London: Sage.

Byrkjeflot, H. (ed.) (1997) *Fra Styring til Ledelse.* [*From Government to Management.*] Bergen: Fagbokforlaget.

Byrkjeflot, H. (2005) *Working Paper 15-2005: The Rise of a Healthcare State? Recent Healthcare Reforms in Norway.* Bergen: Rokkansenteret.

Byrkjeflot, H. and Neby, S. (2004) *Working Paper 2-2004: The Decentralized Path Challenged? Nordic Health Care Reforms in Comparison.* Bergen: Rokkansenteret.

Collins, R. (1979) *The Credential Society: An Historical Sociology of Education and Stratification.* New York: Academic Press.

Dahlin, B. and Kuuse, J. (2005) *Öppen vård i Mittenälvsborg då, nu och sedan med fokus på Lerum. Del I Provinsialläkartiden.* http://www.bengtdahlin.se/HoSstoryn1/indexa. html; accessed 31 January 2008.

Dahlin, B. and Kuuse, J. (2006) *Öppen vård i Mittenälvsborg då, nu och sedan. Med fokus på Lerum. Del II Primärvårdstiden.* http://www.bengtdahlin.se/HoSstoryn2/indexb- .html; accessed 31 January 2008.

Danish Medical Association (2000) *DADL 'Lægernes arbejdsvilkår'.* Copenhagen: Danish Medical Association.

Danish Medical Association (2007) *Lægeforeningen debatoplæg til 5 debatmøde om kvalitets-reformen.* Copenhagen: Danish Medical Association.

Degeling, P., Zhang, K., Coyle, B. et al. (2006) Clinicians and the governance of hospitals: a cross-cultural perspective on relations between profession and management, *Social Science and Medicine* 63: 757–75.

Denis, J.L., Lamothe, L. and Langley, A. (2001) The dynamics of collective leadership and strategic change in pluralistic organizations, *Academy of Management Journal* 44: 809–37.

Dent, M. (2003) *Remodelling Hospitals and Health Professions in Europe: Medicine, Nursing and the State.* Basingstoke: Palgrave Macmillan.

Dent, M. (2006) Post-NPM in public sector hospitals? The UK, Germany and Italy, *Policy and Politics* 33: 623–36.

Erichsen, V. (ed) (1996) *Profesjonsmakt: På sporet av en norsk helsepolitisk tradisjon.* Oslo: Tano Aschehaug.

Evang, K. (1952) *Utviklingstrekk i sykehusenes funksjoner og administrasjon.* [[Progress in hospital organization and administration.] Oslo: Sykepleien [Norwegian Nursing Association].

Evetts, J. (2006) The sociology of professional groups: new directions, *Current Sociology,* 54: 133–43.

Exworthy, M. and Halford, S. (eds) (1999) *Professionals and the New Managerialism in the Public Sector.* Buckingham: Open University Press.

Ferlie, E., Fitzgerald, L., Wood, M. and Hawkins, C. (2005) The nonspread of innovations: the mediating role of professionals, *Academy of Management Journal* 48: 117–34.

Finansministeriet (1969) *Hovedtendenser i sundheds- og forsorgsinstitutionerne udvikling frem til 1985: Udgifter og personale.* Copenhagen: Finansministeriet.

Finansministeriet (1971) *Perspektivplan I: Betænkning af 10.3.1971. Perspektivplanlægning 1970–85.* Copenhagen: Finansministeriet.

Finansministeriet (1999) *Økonomiaftale 2000.* Copenhagen: Finansministeriet; www.fm.dk.

Finnish Medical Association (2005) *Lääkärin Etiikka,* 6th edn. Helsinki: Finnish Medical Association.

Finnish Ministry of Education (2004) Työryhmämuistioita ja selvityksiä 2004:30. Sosiaali- ja terveysalan johtamistyöryhmän muistio. Helsinki: Finnish Ministry of Education.

Fitzgerald, L. and Dopson, S. (2005) Professional boundaries and the diffusion of innovation, in Dopson, S. and Fitzgerald, L. (eds) *Knowledge to Action? Evidence-based Health Care in Context.* Oxford: Oxford University Press.

Freidson, E. (1970) *The Profession of Medicine.* New York: Dodd, Mead.

Freidson, E. (2001) *Professionalism: The Third Logic.* Cambridge: Polity Press.

Garpenby, P. (1989) *The State and the Medical Profession: A Cross-national Comparison of the Health Policy Arena in the United Kingdom and Sweden, 1945–1985.* Linköping: Linköping Studies in Art and Science.

Garpenby, P. (1999) Resource dependency, doctors and the state: quality control in Sweden, *Social Science and Medicine* 49: 405–24.

Gjerberg, E. and Sørensen, B.Å. (2006) Enhetlig ledelse-fortsatt en varm potet? *Tidsskrift for Den norske legeforening* 126: 1063–66.

Glennersteer, H. and Matsaganis, M. (1994) The English and Swedish health care reforms, *International Journal of Health Systems* 24: 231–51.

Gøtrik, J.K. (1988) Lægeforeningens mundtlige beretning, *Ugeskrift for Læger* 150: 2481–7.

Government of Norway (1999) Lov 2. juli 1999 nr. 63 om pasientrettigheter (pasientret-tighetsloven). Oslo: Government Offices.

Grewin, B. (2001) Ledarskapet i vården läkarnas ansvar (Editorial), *Läkartidningen* 98: 1753.

Helsedepartementet (2002) *Ledelse i sykehus*. Rindskriv I-9/2002. Oslo: Department of Health.

Henriksson, L., Wrede, S. and Burau, V. (2006) Understanding professional projects in welfare service work: revival of old professionalism? *Gender, Work and Organization* 14: 174–92.

Hewitt, J. and Thomas, P. (2007) The impact of clinical governance on the professional autonomy and self-regulation of general practitioners: colonization or appropriation? Paper presented at Critical Management Studies Conference, 11–13 July, Manchester University.

Indenrigsministeriet (1984) *Sygehusenes organisation og økonomi*. Betænkning fra. Indenrigsministeriets produktivitetsudvalg. Copenhagen: Direktoratet for Statens Indkøb.

Johansen, M.S. (2005) *Notat 16-2005: Penga eller Livet? Lederutfordringer i det reformerte norske sykehusvesenet*. Bergen: Rokkansentret,Bergen University.

Johnson, T. (1972) *Professions and Power*. London: Macmillan.

Johnson, T. (1995) Governmentality and the institutionalization of expertise, in Johnson, T., Larkin, G. and Saks, M. (eds) *Health Professions and the State in Europe*. London: Routledge, pp. 7–24.

Julkunen, R. (1994) Hyvinvointivaltiollisen professioprojektin katkos. *Tiede & Edistys* 19: 200–13.

Kalleberg, R. (1991) Kenning-tradisjonen i norsk ledelse, *Nytt Norsk Tidsskrift* 3: 218–44.

Kangas, O. (1991) *The Politics of Social Rights: Studies on the Dimensions of Sickness Insurance in OECD Countries*. Stockholm: Swedish Institute for Social Research.

Kauttu, K. (1985) Osallistuminen terveyspolitiikkaan, in Kauttu, K. and Kosonen, T. (eds) *Suomen Lääkäriliitto 1910–1985*. Helsinki: Suomen Lääkäriliitto [Finnish Medical Association].

Kekomäki, M. (2006) Johtaminen on muutoksen aikaansaamista, *Suomen Lääkärilehti* 61: 5007.

Kirkpatrick, I. and Ackroyd, S. (2003) Archetype theory and the changing professional organization: a critique and alternative, *Organization* 10: 739–58.

Kirkpatrick, I., Ackroyd, W. and Walker, R. (2004) *The New Managerialism and the Public Service Professions*. London: Palgrave.

Kirkpatrick, I., Dent, M., Jespersen, P.K. and Neogy, I. (2009) Medicine and management in a comparative perspective in the case of Denmark and England. *Sociology of Health and Illness*, Vol. 31.5.

Kjekshus, L.E. (2004) *INTORG. De somatiske sykehusenes interne organisering: En kartlegging av 50 somatiske sykehus i Norge i 2003*. Oslo: SINTEF helse.

Klein, R. (1989) *Politics of the National Health Service*, 2nd edn. Harlow: Longman.

Konttinen, E. (1991) *Perinteisesti moderniin: Professioiden yhteiskunnallisen aseman synty Suomessa*. Tampere: Vastapaino.

Kragh Jespersen, P. (2002) Health care policy, in Jørgensen, H. (ed.) *Consensus, Cooperation and Conflict: The Policy Making Process in Denmark*. Cheltenham: Edward Elgar, pp.144–66.

Kragh Jespersen, P. (2005) *Mellem Profession og Management*. Copenhagen: Handelshøjskolens.

Kragh Jespersen, P. (2006) Institutionalization of New Management Models in The Danish Hospital Field: The Role of the Medical Profession. Paper presented at the 22nd EGOS Colloquium, 4–6 July, Bergen.

Kragh Jespersen, P., Nielsen, L.L. and Sognstrup, H. (2002) Professions, institutional dynamics, and new public management in the Danish hospital field, *International Journal of Public Administration* 25: 1555–75.

Kuhlmann, E. (2006) *Modernising Health Care: Reinventing Professions, the State and the Public*. Bristol: Policy Press.

Kuusi, P. (1961) *60-luvun sosiaalipolitiikka*. Helsinki: Sosiaalipoliittinen yhdistys.

Läkartidningen (1997) Konkret om ledarskap. Programförslag preciserar moment och mål. (Editorial), *Läkartidningen* 14: 1241.

Levay, C. and Waks, C. (2005) Professions and the pursuit of transparency, two cases of professional response. Paper presented at the 21st EGOS Colloquium, July, Berlin.

Macdonald, K. (1995) *The Sociology of the Professions*. London: Sage.

McKinlay, J.B. (1973) On the professional regulation of change, *Sociological Review Monograph* 20: 61–84.

Marshall, T.H. (1939) The recent history of professionalism in relation to social structure and social policy, *Canadian Journal of Economics and Political Science* 5: 325–40.

Martinsen, K. (1984) *Freidige og uforsagte diakonisser: Et omsorgsyrke vokser fram 1860–1905*. Oslo: Aschehaug.

Mattila, P. (2006) *Toiminta, valta ja kokemus organisaation muutoksessa*. Helsinki: University of Helsinki.

Ministry of Health [Sundhedsministeriet] (1997) *Udfordringer i sygehusvæsenet: Betænkning fra Sygehuskommisionen*. Betænkning nr. 1329. Copenhagen: Statens Information.

Mintzberg, H. (1983) *Structure in Fives: Designing Effective Organizations*. New York: Prentice Hall.

Mo, T.O. (2006) Ledelse til begjær eller besvær. Om reformer, fag og ledelse i sykehus. PhD thesis Trondheim University.

Montgomery, K. (1997) New dimensions of professional/organizational relationships. [Introduction to special issue.] *Sociological Inquiry* 67: 175–81.

Morell, K. (2007) Re-defining professions: knowledge, organization and power as syntax. Paper presented at the Critical Management Studies Conference, 11–13 July, Manchester.

Municio, I. (1996) Den retoriska staten. Organisatorisk turbulens och diskursiv makt, *Häften för kritiska studier* 4: 3–18.

Murphy, R. (1988) *Social Closure*. Oxford: Clarendon Press.

Nordby, T. (1989) *Karl Evang en biografi*. Oslo: Aschehaug.

Norwegian Nurses Association [Norsk Sykepleierforbund] (2005) *Sykepleier med lederansvar. God på fag og ledelse*. Oslo: Norsk Sykepleierforbund.

NOU (1997) *NOU 1997: 2. Pasienten først! Ledelse og organisering i sykehus*. Oslo: Ministry of Health and Care Services.

OECD (2007) *OECD Health Data 2007*. Paris: Organisation for Economic Co-operation and Development.

Oker-Blom, M. (1911; facsimile edn 2000) *Lääkärintoimi ja sen etiikka*. Helsinki: Otava.

Oliver, A.L. (1997) On the nexus of organizations and professions: networking through trusts, *Sociological Inquiry* 67: 227–45.

Pedersen, K.M., Christiansen, T. and Beck M. (2005) The Danish health care system: evolution or revolution in a decentralized system, *Health Economics* 14(Suppl 1): 41–57.

Pekurinen, M., Mikkola, H. and Tuominen, U. (eds.) (2008) *Raportteja 5/2008: Hoitotakuun talous. Hoitotakuun vaikutus terveydenhuollon menoihin, toimintaan ja sairausvakuutuskorvauksiin*. Helsinki: STAKES.

Pernulf, A.-M. (2005) Vill vi axla chefsansvaret? [Editorial.] *Läkartidningen* 102: 3193.

Pernulf, A.-M. (2006) Du behövs som chef! [Editorial.] *Läkartidningen* 103: 3999.

Pesonen, N. (1974) *Lääkärinä ja virkamiehenä. Lääkintöhallituksen pääjohtaja muistelee*. Porvoo: WSOY.

Pesonen, N. (1980) *Terveyden puolesta, sairautta vstaan: Terveyden- ja sairaanhoito Suomessa 1800- ja 1900-luvuilla*. Porvoo: WSOY.

178 Peter K. Jespersen and Sirpa Wrede

Plant, R. (2003) A public service ethic and political accountability, *Parliamentary Affairs* 56: 560–79.

Pollitt, C. and Bouckaert, G. (2002) *Public Management Reform: A Comparative Analysis.* Oxford: Oxford University Press.

Pomey, M., Denis, J.L., Champagne, F., Gyslaine, T. and Préval, J. (2007) The pluralistic view of governance within healthcare organizations. Paper presented at the EGOS Colloquium, 5–7 July, Vienna.

Pylkkänen, K. (2002) Erikoislääkäriprofession sata järjestäytymisen vuotta. *Suomen lääkärilehti* 57: 1819–23.

Rhenman, K. (2000) Nytt från Chefsläkarföreningen, *Läkartidningen* 97: 2000.

Rinne, R. and Jauhiainen, A. (1988) *Koulutus, professionaalistuminen ja valtio.* [Education, Professionalism and the State.] Turku: Faculty of Education, University of Turku, Series A, p. 128.

Riska, E. (1993) The medical profession in the Nordic countries, in Hafferty, F.W. and McKinlay, J. (eds) *The Changing Medical Profession: An International Perspective.* New York: Oxford University Press.

Saltman, R.B. (1991) Emerging trends in the Swedish health system, *International Journal of Health Systems* 21: 615–23.

Saltman, R.B. (1994) Patient choice and patient empowerment in Northern European health systems: a conceptual framework, *International Journal of Health Services* 24: 201–29.

Sihvo, T. and Lindqvist, M. (1994) *Raportteja 135: Muutossuunnat kunnissa.* Helsinki: STAKES, University of Helsinki.

Skaset, M. (2003) Reformtid og makredsgløtt: det offentlige helsevesen etter 1985, in Schiøtz, A. (ed.) *Det offentlige helsevesen i Norge 1603–2005*, Vol 2: *Folkets helse – landes styrke 1850–2003:*. Oslo: Oslo University Press.

Sommervold, W. (1996) Ledelse i sykepleien: forståelsesmåter i endring, in Erichsen, V. (ed.) *Profesjonsmakt: På sporet av en norsk helsepolitisk tradisjon.* Oslo: Tano Aschehaug, pp.198–216.

Stacey, M. (1989) The General Medical Council and professional acountability, *Public Policy Administration* 4: 12–27.

Stenmark, S. (2002) Läkares ledarskap: mål och visioner. *Läkartidningen* 99: 729.

Stortinget (1995) *Stortingets vedtak av 21. november 1995 om ledelse i sykehus.* Oslo: Stortinget.

Suonoja, K. (1992) Kansalaisten parhaaksi: yhteistuntoa ja politiikkaa. Sosiaali- ja terveys-ministeriö 1939–1992, in Haatanen, P. and Suonoja, K. (eds) *Suuriruhtinaskunnasta hyvinvointivaltioon. Sosiaali- ja terveysministeriö 75 vuotta.* Helsinki: Ministry of Social Affairs and Health, pp. 323–739.

Svedberg, L. (2004) Rhetorical resources for management: the leading words, *Educational Management Administration and Leadership* 32: 423–38.

Sveriges läkarförbunds chefsförening (2000) Överenskommelse angående medicinskt ledaransvar. Sveriges läkarförbunds chefsförening and Svenska Överläkarföreningen. http://www.slf.se/templates/AssociationPage.aspx?id=3154; accessed 1 February 2008.

Torjesen, D.O. (2008) Foretak, management og medikrati. En sektorstudie av helsefore-taksreform og ledelse i den norske spesialist-helsetjenesten. PhD thesis, Unversity of Bergen.

Torjesen D.O. and Gammelsæther, H. (2004) *Working Paper No.1: Management Between Autonomy and Transparency in the Enterprise Hospital.* Bergen: Rokkan sentret.

Tørning, J. (1970) Sygehusplanlægning efter den nye sygehuslov, *Danmarks Amtsråd*, 1970/71, nr. 1.

Torppa, K. (2007) *Managerialismi suomalaisen julkisen erikoissairaanhoidon johtamisessa.* Oulu: University of Oulu.

Vallgårda, S. (1993) *Sygehuse og sygehuspolitik i Danmark: et bidrag til det specialiserede sygehusvæsens historie 1930–1987.* Copenhagen: Jurist-og Økonomforbundets.

Vareide, P.K. (2002) *Fra Fylkeskommunal til statslig eierskap av sykehusene. Et hamskifte i helsetjenestens styring.* Trondheim: SINTEF Unimed.

Viitanen, E., Wiili-Peltola, E. and Lehto, J. (2002) Osastonlääkäri lähiesimiehenä. Enemmän tämmönen seniorikonsultti, *Suomen Lääkärilehti* 57: 3755–7.

Vrangbaek, K. and Christiansen, T. (2005) Health policy in Denmark: leaving the decentralized welfare path? *Journal of Health Politics Policy and Law* 30: 29–52.

Vuolio, V. (1991) *Lunastettu vapaus. Kunnanlääkärin ammatillisen autonomian muotoutuminen.* [Publication 49.] Jyväskylä: Department of Sociology, University of Jyväskylä.

WHO Regional Office for Europe (1991) *Health for All Policy in Finland.* Copenhagen: WHO Regional Office for Europe.

Widerström, M. (2000) Läkarkåren får inte avsäga sig chefskapet! *Läkartidningen* 97: 2041.

Wrede, S. (2000) Suomalainen terveydenhuolto: jännitteitä ja murroksia, in Kangas, I., Karvonen, S. and Lillrank, A. (eds) *Terveyssosiologian Suuntauksia.* Helsinki: Gaudeamus, pp. 189–205.

Wrede, S. (2001) *Decentering Care for Mothers: The Politics of Midwifery and the Design of Finnish Maternity Services.* Åbo: Åbo Akademy University Press.

Wrede, S. (2008) Unpacking gendered professional power in the welfare state, *Equal Opportunities International* 27: 19–33.

Wrede, S., Henriksson, L., Høst, H., Johansson, S. and Dybbroe, B. (eds) (2008) *Care Work in Crisis: Reclaiming the Nordic Ethos of Care.* Lund: Studentlitteratur.

chapter eight

Maintaining fiscal sustainability in the Nordic countries

Clas Rehnberg, Jon Magnussen and
Kalevi Luoma

8.1 Introduction

A system will be fiscally sustainable if it generates a sufficient revenue stream to finance the desired level of health expenditure. In the Nordic context, this revenue stream is needed to finance a basket of public services that are provided to all citizens under a system of universal coverage. The Nordic systems all belong to the family of publicly governed tax-based systems. In this grouping, fiscal sustainability is primarily related to the level of taxation that the system can bear, and also to what type of coverage that can be provided under the umbrella of a public health care system. There is, therefore, a duality in the notion of fiscal sustainability: the possibility of raising public funds depends both on the level of taxation that a society is willing to accept and on the contents of the benefit package that these funds help to deliver. In contrast to insurance-based systems, where the concept of insurance itself implies that coverage needs to be specified, the publicly financed Nordic systems have traditionally operated under the term 'universal coverage' without being particularly specific about what exactly is (not) covered. Furthermore, a central feature of the Nordic systems is the long tradition of decentralizing the responsibility of health care to regional and local governments, including the possibility to raise revenues through local taxation. This can create possible confusion concerning at what level the system is (not) sustainable as well as about inequitable distribution of resources.

Consequently, in the Nordic setting, a discussion of how to maintain fiscal sustainability must include a discussion of which level of government is going to bear the financial burden of the health care system; whether, and how, a publicly financed benefit package (or 'basket') should be defined; and whether, and how, supplementary private purchase/funding of health services could be an option. At the same time, the discussion needs to recognize that even when (if) a basket of services is defined, fiscal sustainability is not only a question of raising funds. Health systems also have several available options to limit demand for services and to make sure that the services provided are done so at the lowest possible costs. Therefore, we also need to discuss what policy measures are taken (at what level) to secure financial sustainability (and whether they are working).[1]

The aim of this chapter is to discuss these questions in the context of the changes in the Nordic countries since the end of the 1980s. Underneath the perception of Nordic countries as part of a common health care model, we find substantial differences both in the degree of fiscal decentralization and in the particular policy instruments aimed at limiting demand and containing costs. Although some of these differences have been there for a long time, recent developments also suggest that the Nordic countries may now be on different paths, and that these are the result of different strategies in the four countries in maintaining fiscal sustainability.

8.2 Fiscal sustainability, fiscal federalism and fiscal decentralization

As noted, a central characteristic of the Nordic countries is the devolution of power from the central state to elected local governments. Thus, the Nordic model has much in common with the logic of models of fiscal federalism. In these models, focus is on aspects such as the devolution of responsibility to local governments, the right to levy taxes and the structure of transfer payments between different levels of government. Other issues concern the assignment of tasks and vertical division of responsibilities. Hence, the discussion refers both to pure financial issues as well as the provision of goods and services. The latter is also referred to as the regionalization or decentralization of services.

The classical theory of fiscal federalism originates from Musgrave (1959), who elucidates the functions of government in terms of macroeconomic stabilization, distribution and allocation. The normative implication was that the first two functions are best handled by the central government while the allocation function and provision of goods and services can be placed at lower levels. The decentralization theorem developed by Oates (1972) contends that it will always be superior for a local government to provide goods and services when the consumption is limited to their own jurisdictions, compared with centralized provision across several local authorities. The theorem has been adopted by representatives from regional authorities and interpreted as a justification of regional responsibility of supply of goods and services.

A central but also controversial question concerns the financial aspects in terms of the best way to finance intergovernmental levels. Usually, systems exist of transfer payments or grants by which a federal government shares its revenues with lower levels of government. In addition, local levels may be able to raise locally determined taxes. In several countries, a conflict between the allocation function and the distributional aspects is observed. A far-reaching decentralization of the right to levy taxes ('fiscal decentralization') might lead to geographical inequities, which may well have to be corrected by the central government. The Nordic model, with its traditional focus on local governance, creates the possibility of large variations in service levels determined both by local differences in preferences and by differences in income levels. At the same time, the egalitarian principle is clearly expressed in all Nordic countries and so geographical inequities have been dealt with by compensation from the central government. Tax equalization grants (and corresponding transfers) are essential for a fair distribution and access to health services across regions. Still, the decentralized decision-making may lead to differences in prioritizing between treatment programmes and variation in the introduction of new medical technologies. At the same time, the autonomy created by regional taxes and the redistribution across regions is also a source for conflicts and tension between the levels of governments.

Even when taxes are raised locally, the overall fiscal control of a country's finances lies in the central government, with the overall responsibility for the national budget. A system where the central government has a tight control of taxes levied, and thus the overall government revenues, in principle puts it in a position to control public finances. However, when there is central funding but local provision, that is, when the central government controls both the tax base and the tax level but local governments are made responsible for the provision of services to its population, a *double common pool problem* might arise (Rattsø 2002). In this setting, an individual will tend to claim excessive levels of local government services as this incurs marginal costs since a higher tax burden will be distributed across the whole population. Also local governments, following the same logic, will tend to seek central funds from the common pool generated by general taxation. In such a situation, there will be extensive pressure on total costs, which is likely to result in soft budgeting (Kornai et al. 2003) as well as lower levels of efficiency. If, in addition, there is no benefit taxation[2] on the local level, as is the case in the Nordic context, these problems might be excessive (Lotz 1998; Rattsø 2002).

The possibility of local governments manipulating the system to obtain more than their fair share of the central funds depends on information asymmetry between the two levels of government about local production costs and local preferences. Intergovernmental transfers serve two purposes: they reduce income inequalities between local governments and they compensate for differences in risk and cost structures. In doing so, central governments balance on a fine line between exercising national control and allowing for local (preference based) variations. Gilbert and Picard (1996) argue that full centralization is optimal if central government has full information on production costs, whereas the reverse is true if the central government has full information on local preferences (including the value attached to spillovers). If there is imperfect information on both costs and preferences, ambiguity arises. This ambiguity is also reflected in the wide variety of health system solutions that can be observed.

Also in otherwise decentralized systems, the central government may be faced with a pressure to directly access and address local needs. Then restrictions can be placed on local authorities through legislation and regulation of task responsibility, and these may restrict the autonomy of local governments, even in a situation of presumably fiscal decentralization. This can also be done more loosely by stating national norms or goals that will effectively limit the local government's discretion on how to spend their money.[3] In many countries, the central governments have kept close control and monitoring of the taxes levied, but allocated resources and the responsibility of detailed tasks to lower levels of government. The regional and local government responsibility has then mainly been the provision of services, whereas the central government decides both the budget framework for the services and the types of service to be provided. In the Nordic countries, both functions have to some extent been decentralized, given regional governments an influence on both the scope and the size of the health - care sector and also on how to provide the service. There is a long tradition in the Nordic countries for giving regional governments the right to levy taxes. In the policy debate, this has been motivated by the importance of designing services to local needs, and also avoiding problems of fiscal gaps. The fear has been that lack of cost control will occur as the regional governments focus on one sector and resources are not weighted against other needs for public services. There has also been the argument that common pool problems may be avoided by combining fiscal autonomy with the responsibility of providing services, as regional governments assume a larger fiscal responsibility by matching revenues to expenditures. At the same time, the current development and discussions of larger regions or transfer of tasks to the national level arise from the observation of inequitable geographical variations in certain treatments.

8.3 Fiscal autonomy and fiscal sustainability in the Nordic countries

Fiscal autonomy is not an entirely clear concept, but rather one that ties in to the relationship between local and central authorities on several levels. Important aspects are the right to levy local taxes, the exclusivity of the tax base, the relative size of locally generated taxes and the degree of conditionality of transfers from the central government. The central government could also, as noted above, use its power to enforce national rules and standards, for example terms of equity or access. It could also target specific objectives and give incentives for specific types of activity. Such regulations could (but need not) be reflected in the financial transfers between governmental levels. There are two primary types of transfer: *conditional* and *unconditional*. A conditional transfer from a federal or a central government to a region is intended to provide incentives for local governments to perform specific tasks or types of activity. The lower level of government then has to agree and act according to these spending instructions. Conditional grants may be dependent on a matching (open or closed) of the grant from the local government. Unconditional grants, however, gives the receiving government considerable freedom in how to spend the resources. As the central governments in all Nordic countries have decentralized both the financial and the operational functions to regional levels, there are several examples on how they have exercised their power through transfer payments. The objectives for these payments concern cost containment, encouragement of certain activities and to secure a fair and equitable access and distribution of resources.

There is no uniform measure of the fiscal autonomy of local governments. One possible indicator is the share of autonomous local taxes to total tax revenue. Another indicator is autonomy in the use of intergovernmental grants. Both these are reproduced from Blöchliger and King (2006) in Table 8.1. Here we also present an average index of fiscal supervision as presented in Sellers and Lidström (2007).[4] This index is a weighted average of grants as a percentage of local revenue, degree of local tax autonomy and degree of supervision of local borrowing.

Sweden is characterized by a high share of autonomous taxes, a high share of unconditional intergovernmental grants and a low level of fiscal supervision. We would, therefore, be inclined to characterize Sweden as a country with a high level of fiscal decentralization. The same applies to Finland, even though the share of autonomous taxes is lower. This is, however, compensated by almost all central grants being unconditional. Norway stands out as the country with the lowest share of autonomous taxes, the highest share of conditional grants and the highest degree of fiscal supervision. The numbers presented in Table 8.1 for Denmark are somewhat misleading because they are from before the Danish structural reform in 2007, when the counties' right to levy local taxes was abolished. This meant an end to a system that involved annual negotiations between the state and the counties in order to reach an agreement about the rate of regional taxes.[5] The discrepancies in the tax base of different regions were handled through a compensation system, where additional resources were been distributed according to the size of regional tax revenues. Consequently, there has been substantial fiscal centralization in Denmark since these figures were published.

Another approach to the question of central versus local autonomy as applied to health care would be the share of public health care expenditure that comes from the local versus the central level. This is shown in Figure 8.1, based on data from the OECD system of health accounts (OECD 2007). To account for the effect of the Danish health reform, the numbers for Denmark have been stipulated by the authors for 2007, based on the budget agreement between the Danish regions and the Ministry of the Interior. Figure 8.1 presents a roughly

Table 8.1 Fiscal autonomy in the Nordic countries around 2004

	Share of autonomous taxes to total tax revenue (%)	*Share of intergovernmental grants that are unconditional (non-earmarked) (%)*	*Fiscal supervision*
Sweden	32.1	71.3	0.56
Finland	19.3	90.8	0.60
Norway	12.9	55.1	1.64
Denmark	32.3	56.3	0.75

Source: data taken from Blöchliger and King (2006) and Sellers and Lidström (2007).

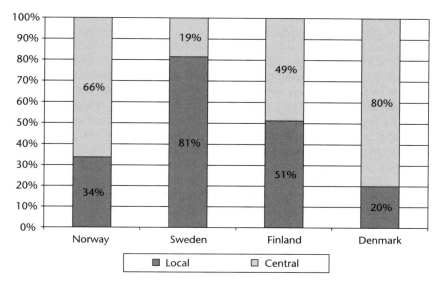

Figure 8.1   Share of central versus local financing of health care in 2006 (Denmark 2007).

similar picture of the four countries as seen in Table 8.1: Sweden bases most of its public financing on the local level, Finland splits 50/50, while both Norway and Denmark rely heavily on central state financing.

Although the Norwegian model before 2002 (i.e. with county ownership) did not include the right to levy taxes,[6] the 2002 state takeover of the hospitals was widely appreciated as a reform intended to enhance cost control. One consequence of the reform was that unconditional grants to counties were replaced with conditional grants to regional health enterprises in charge of running hospital service. In many ways, this was a logical consequence of a gradual increase in the share of state grants to the counties that was conditional. The introduction of partly activity-based financing (ABF) of somatic hospital services in 1997 replaced a share of the unconditional grants with a matching health-specific grant. Initially, the state contributed 30 per cent of average costs (as measured by diagnosis-related groups (DRGs)), but by 2001 this share had increased to 50 per cent. In terms of the framework laid out in Section 8.2, it could be argued that Norway recognized the need for a higher level of centralized control with overall spending and chose to exert that control through ownership rather than grapple with the common pool dilemma. The Norwegian reform, therefore, led to a fiscal centralization that was the logical consequence of a policy aimed at centralizing governance.

In Denmark, there is now an earmarked (8 per cent) share of income taxes that is allocated to health care. While municipalities may determine tax levels in principle, the present ban on tax increases ('skattestop') effectively limits the possibility to finance increases in service provision by tax increases. As for Norway, it could be argued that the abolishment of tax discretion on the regional level and the resulting fiscal centralization is the logical consequence of a centralization of governance that resulted from the Danish structural reform in 2007.

In Finland, municipalities finance their service provision by local income tax, property taxes, user charges and grants from the central government. Central government funding for municipal health care is passed on to municipalities in the form of unconditional block grants. These state grants are allocated to municipalities according to a weighted capitation formula designed to adjust the grants for differences in the need for services and differences in circumstances that affect local costs of providing services. Another component of the grant system is revenue sharing by a tax base equalization formula. The state share decreased radically during the recession in the beginning of the 1990s.

Before 1985, Sweden had a complex system with mainly conditional grants for the delivery of specific services. From 1985, the transfer payments from the state to the county councils were based more or less on unconditional grants, with the prime objective being to compensate for the variations in tax base across the counties. At present, a per capita grant calculated on the mean taxing power and certain population characteristics is used. However, recently, a conditional grant from the central government has been launched in order to give the county councils an incentive to reduce working absenteeism. The system of state subsidies for health care in Sweden has been discussed in terms of its stability and sustainability. The negotiations between the state and the regional county councils cannot be described as a system of partners with equal powers. The central government can always use its legislative power and the county councils are surrounded with regulations. One effect of the system has been a chronic deficit in the finances of the county councils.

In contrast to their Nordic neighbours, both Finland and Sweden seem to remain confident that a decentralized system based on a combination of local taxes, unconditional grants and low fiscal supervision is sufficient to keep the system fiscally sustainable. Table 8.2 provides a general description of the different strategies used in the four countries, and we note that all countries are either (leaning towards) centralized or (leaning towards) decentralized with respect to both financing and provision. The exception is Norway, which has chosen a mix, with a highly centralized hospital sector while decentralizing the responsibility for primary health care.

As all the Nordic countries historically have experience of far-reaching decentralization of financing and operational responsibilities, the concern for an inequitable resource allocation has been an issue. From a fiscal policy point of

Table 8.2 Financing and provision of services

Provision	Financing	
	Centralized	*Decentralized*
Centralized	Norway (hospitals), Denmark	Norway (primary health care)
Decentralized		Sweden, Finland

view, many other countries have avoided the right for local and regional governments to levy taxes because of the risk of adversely affecting an equitable distribution of financial resources across local jurisdictions. Yet, in international comparisons on the equity of finance, the Nordic countries show more equitable distribution of the financial burden of health expenditure than many other countries with national health systems (NHS) as well as countries with social health insurance (SHI) (van Doorslaer et al. 1999).

8.4 Health care spending in the Nordic countries

In this section we describe the development in health care spending in the Nordic countries in the 20-year period from 1985 to 2005. Looking at historical (differences) in spending patterns is useful when assessing the challenges the countries will meet in the future. Three commonly used indicators are presented: health care spending as share of gross domestic product (GDP), health care spending per capita in real terms and the share of health care spending that is financed by the public sector.

8.4.1 Share of gross domestic product

One way to put the development in health care spending in perspective is to compare the Nordic health care systems with countries with *centralized* NHS and countries with social health insurance systems. Table 8.3 shows this development from 1985 until 2005, comparing the Nordic countries with the United Kingdom and the average of seven SHI countries.[7]

Several observations can be made from this table. First, while the Nordic countries started out at a level above the SHI countries in 1985, they are now using a smaller share of GDP on health than their SHI counterparts. Overall, the growth in the share of GDP has been nearly four times as high in the SHI countries. The same development can be tracked in the centralized United Kingdom NHS, although they began at a substantially lower level in 1985. Another observation

Table 8.3 Health care expenditures as a share of gross domestic product, 1980–2005

	1985	1990	1995	2000	2005
Denmark	8.5	8.3	8.1	8.3	9.1
Finland	7.1	7.8	7.4	6.7	7.5
Norway	6.6	7.7	7.9	8.5	9.1
Sweden	8.6	8.3	8.1	8.4	9.1
Nordic mean	7.7	8.0	7.9	8.0	8.7
UK NHS	5.9	6.0	7.0	7.3	8.3
SHI mean	7.2	7.5	8.8	9	10.1

Source: OECD health databases.

UK, NHS, United Kingdom National Health Service; SHI, social health insurance system.

is the differences between the Nordic countries. While Norway and Finland initially spent a lower share of their GDP on health, Norway is now on the same level as its neighbours. Finland is still lagging somewhat behind, a possible consequence of the severe macroeconomic crisis of the early 1990s.

Figure 8.2 provides a clearer illustration of the development in this period. While Finland, Sweden and Denmark have had a moderate increase in their share of GDP spent on health care, Norway, the United Kingdom and the SHI seven countries all have increased their share by 35 to 40 per cent in this period.

The regional taxes in the Nordic countries have sometimes been regarded as earmarked taxes similar to the mandatory premiums in SHI systems. The argument concerning earmarked taxes and cost development has different strands. One argument states that earmarked taxes limit revenue for financing health care and will keep the costs down. The other argument is that citizens generally are more willing to pay taxes aimed at social and health services compared with other public duties and, therefore, these taxes are easier to raise. Still, a comparison with other tax-based countries or SHI systems shows that the Nordic systems do not show a diverging pattern. A comparison of the cost development using expenditure per capita as an indicator of cost development does not change the picture (Table 8.4).

The most expansive health system in the Nordic region since the late 1980s is the Norwegian. This is mainly explained by its strong economic growth, and the Norwegian spending on health as a share of GDP fits well into models of income elasticity. Even so, from 1990 onward, the health sector in Norway shows a drastic growth in real terms. Again looking at the overall change over this period (Figure 8.3) reveals dramatic differences.

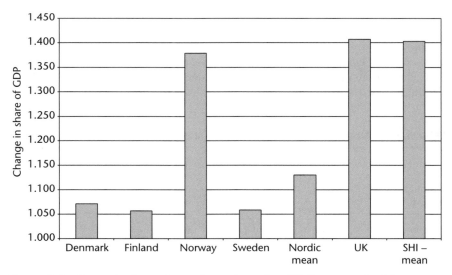

Figure 8.2   Change in share of gross domestic product (GDP) spent on health 1985–2005.

Source: OECD 2007.

Table 8.4 Total expenditure on health per capita, 1985–2005

Country	Purchasing power parity (US$)				
	1985	1990	1995	2000	2005
Denmark	1237	1521	1843	2381	3108
Finland	942	1392	1429	1717	2331
Norway	954	1392	1892	3082	4364
Sweden	1262	1581	1733	2272	2918
Nordic mean	1099	1472	1724	2363	3180
UK	712	989	1384	1859	2724
SHI mean	1099	1556	2113	2667	3772

Source: OECD health databases.

UK, NHS, United Kingdom National Health Service; SHI, social health insurance system.

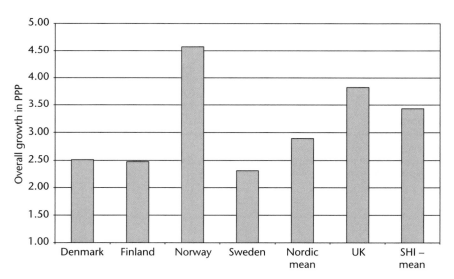

Figure 8.3 Overall growth in purchasing power parity (PPP, in US$) adjusted spending per capita 1985–2005.

Sweden, Denmark and Finland have all shown substantial growth but not to the extent of that of the growth in per capita spending in Norway. The Norwegian spending increase also exceeds that of the United Kingdom and the SHI countries by a large margin.

Theoretically, the increase in health care spending could come as a result of increased out-of-pocket payment or increased use of private voluntary health insurance. If this was the case, it could be argued that the fiscal pressure on the system is increasing and that further tax-financed expansion is unlikely. To explore this, the total cost for health care is split into public and private financing. Public financing constitutes different taxes and income-based mandatory premiums. The impact of health care on the fiscal policy depends on the public sector commitment to the sector. Public expenditure has in a historical perspective always been a large share of the total health expenditure in the Nordic countries (Table 8.5).

Sweden, historically the country with the largest share as public financing, is also the country with the largest decline in this share over this period (Figure 8.4). In Sweden during the macroeconomic turbulence of the 1990s, the intention was to spare the health sector compared with other public sectors (with the dental care as a clear exception). In spite of this, the health care sector clearly felt the burden of the worsening macroeconomic conditions and this is reflected in

Table 8.5 Public expenditures as a share of total health expenditures for the Nordic countries and mean values for European Union tax-based systems and social insurance systems, 1970–2004

	1985	1990	1995	2000	2005
Denmark	85.6	82.7	82.5	82.4	84.1
Finland	78.6	80.9	75.6	75.1	77.8
Norway	85.8	82.8	84.2	82.5	83.6
Sweden	90.4	89.9	86.6	84.9	84.6
Nordic mean	85.1	84.1	82.2	81.2	82.5
UK	85.8	83.6	83.9	80.9	87.1
SHI mean[a]	–	–	–	–	–

SHI, social health insurance system
[a] Data are not complete. The large differences between countries make between-year comparisons meaningless when data are not complete.

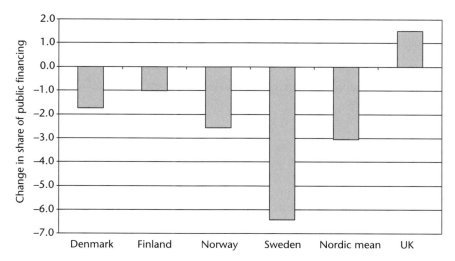

Figure 8.4   Per cent change in health care's share of public financing 1985–2005.

the decrease of public health spending as a share of total health spending from approximately 90 per cent in 1985 to less than 85 per cent in the 1990s. For dental care, the co-payment share increased from below 30 per cent to approximately 60–65 per cent during this period. The experience of the dental care sector in Sweden could serve as an example of the capability of the system to adapt to changes in the macroeconomic conditions. It also confirms the dependence of the health sector on the economic growth and the relationship between health expenditure and GDP.

The decline in the share of public financing in Sweden has meant that the country has the same level of public financing as Norway and Denmark. Finland, by comparison, has a substantially larger share of private financing of health - care. Because of worsening macroeconomic conditions in the 1990s and the inability to sustain recurrent government expenditure to provide free health - care to their population, the health system in Finland was also faced with severe constraints and real cuts in expenditure at that time. The contribution from the state to health care was mainly reduced during the recession in the beginning of the 1990s. Similar to the development in Sweden, the central government used its control and power over public expenditure to reduce subsidies to different sectors. Co-payments also lost their tax-deductible status, effectively increasing the burden on private finance.

The Nordic countries have a substantial higher tax burden than other countries in the OECD area; this, of course, partly reflects their tax-financed welfare systems. Denmark and Sweden, in particular, have a tax share of GDP that is close to 50 per cent. The increase in the overall tax burden has also been higher in Denmark and Sweden since the late 1980s than the corresponding increase in Norway and Finland. Although somewhat speculative, this could also contribute to the explanation of why the share of private financing has increased more in Denmark and Sweden over this period. However, it is noteworthy that Norway, with both the largest growth in share of GDP and the largest growth in per capita spending, has avoided a large increase in the tax burden and the share of private financing of health care. This reflects the overall oil-induced growth in the Norwegian economy but also highlights that Norway with its high level of expenditure is dependent on the oil to sustain spending at the present level.

8.4.2 The role of private supplementary insurance

Private supplementary insurance has played a minor role in all the Nordic countries apart from Denmark. One reason for this is the lack of links between public provision and private financing in legislation. Public providers (including private providers with public financing) are often prohibited from accepting additional payments beside stipulated patient fees. Hence private insurance is mostly linked to independent private provision. The Danish system is unusual as it combines a tax-financed health care sector with a high rate of private voluntary health insurance.

Finland has a tradition where employers have allocated funds to private insurance for rehabilitation services. This is a small share, estimated to be 2 per cent of the total health expenditures. Norway and Sweden have historically almost no traditions of private health insurance but in these two countries also, the private insurance companies have launched insurance products aiming at business leaders and other target groups (often through working/employment contracts). The number of insured, while relatively small, is increasing rapidly. Part of this increase can be explained by tax subsidies levied at voluntary health insurance. Recent estimates of insured citizens in Norway, Sweden and Denmark, as presented in Chapter 2, are 180,000, 450,000 and 800,000, respectively.

Private health insurance is most likely to play a minor role as a source of funding health care in the Nordic countries. However, the changes in demand for voluntary health insurances express dissatisfaction with the public services for certain segments of the population, who actually pay twice for health services. Therefore, voluntary health insurance is not an insurance against costs for services not covered by the public health care system but mainly provides a method of being able to jump the queue. In this respect, the amount of voluntary health insurance could be used as an indicator of the efficiency of the public health sector. There are some observations indicating that the demand for supplementary insurance increases during periods with long waiting time for treatment in the public health sector.

There is also a health policy issue regarding the extent to which supplementary health insurance should be encouraged to fill gaps created by priority criteria in the public sector. The rejection of subsidy for certain pharmaceuticals by the Swedish Pharmaceutical Benefits Board (LFN) raises this issue. Similar priorities have been made for non-pharmaceutical treatment within the public health care sector (in vitro fertilization is one example). A central question is if these types of low-priority treatment should be financed entirely through out-of-pocket expenditures or if voluntary insurance should play a role. The following question will inevitably arise: should public providers accept private payment for non-priority services?

In all countries (apart from Denmark), the policy has been to keep voluntary health insurance out of public provision; public hospitals and primary health - care are not allowed to accept private payments from voluntary health insurance (apart from overseas patients for highly specialized care, mainly in university hospitals). Therefore, none of the Nordic countries has turned to supplementary voluntary health insurance as a means of relieve the fiscal pressure on the health care sector. To do so would imply a fundamental deviation from the Nordic model of health care, and it would signal that the countries are not able to sustain the expected level of services within their public systems. Possible this would be a solution of the last resort.

8.5 Strategies to contain costs

While sustainability will depend on the bearable level of taxation, a parallel strategy will be to contain costs, by attempting to limit demand, by regulating supply or by increasing the efficiency of utilization of resources.

8.5.1 *Demand side measures*

With third-party payment, the subsequent problem of moral hazard has to be handled by the funding institutions within the public sector. The mechanisms used for controlling overall costs and handling the moral hazard problem differ across the Nordic countries. The demand pressures derived from a third-party payer system will inevitable involve different rationing mechanisms. The most used mechanisms at hand are cost-sharing, waiting lists and gate keeping.

From an insurance perspective, the use of cost-sharing through *patient fees* is a classical strategy. From a cost-containment perspective, patient fees are attractive because they limit demand – presumably by increasing the threshold, and thus turning away unnecessary demand – and also raise revenue. In the Nordic setting, however, user fees tend to be politically controversial, owing to their distributional effects. For example, the Danish system has for a long period worked without cost-sharing policies in the primary and the specialist sector whereas Finland, Norway and Sweden have all used patient fees for GPs and out-patient specialist care for many years. In all the Nordic countries, however, there are upper limits on total expenses that an individual can incur. In Denmark and Norway, inpatient hospital services are free, whereas Finland and Sweden charge low fees for inpatient care. All countries have co-payments for (out-of-hospital) pharmaceuticals, but again with an upper limit for expenses.

The Danish, Finnish and Norwegian systems rely on *gatekeeping* through the GPs for moderating access to hospital and specialist services. (In Denmark there is an exception for the 1 per cent of the population that have Group 2 insurance, who pay a small co-payment for direct access to specialists.) In Finland this holds true only in the case of patients who rely solely on municipal health services; in relation to private hospitals, occupational health and specialist services there is no GP gate keeping.) In Sweden, hospital specialist care can be sought without going through a GP. In all the systems, is it fair to say that the motivation for gatekeeping is explicitly fiscal but a major motivation for gatekeeping is also to limit demand for specialized services. Specialist health care is viewed as a limited commodity, and by using gatekeeping this commodity is believed to be more accurately distributed to those in greatest need.

Hospital waiting lists have been, and still are, a major political issue in the Nordic countries. A waiting list arises, of course, because capacity is limited, and as such is the result of policies targeting the supply side. Still the existence of waiting lists is also believed to deter some people from signalling demand: the belief is that the prospect of having to wait for a substantial time reduces some of what would otherwise be seen as unnecessary demand.[8]

Finally, there is also an increasing focus on patient *choice* and with it the strengthening of patient rights, which might have fiscal implications. In a positive sense, moving from the traditional model where a patient would be treated in the geographically closest hospital might increase system flexibility, capacity utilization and thereby efficiency. However, when choice is paired with a focus on an individual right to health services, as is the case in Norway, this may put increased pressure on the system and thus counteract the potential gain from increased efficiency.

8.5.2 Supply side measures

As an alternative to limiting demand, improving the utilization of resources thorough supply side measures has the advantage of being politically less controversial. Supply side measures include incentive-based payment systems, increased use of competition and limits on capacity through national regulation of capital and manpower. In addition, a more defined benefit package would contain costs through the exclusion of services from cover under the publicly financed health plan.

All Nordic countries have experienced long waiting lists, which also has been a topic in the health policy debate and an argument for more private provision and increased use of economic incentives. The fact that all countries directly address this question by some form of waiting-time guarantee or norms on maximal waiting time indicates that there are political problems with explicitly using capacity regulations to restrict costs. In this lies one of the deeper dilemmas of the Nordic health care model: in its distaste for private (presumably equity discouraging) solutions it does not allow surplus demand to spill over to a private sector. Yet, fiscal limits will necessarily lead to capacity constraints. These constraints are not, however, sufficiently acknowledged, and instead a backdoor is sought through a variety of waiting time policies.

8.5.3 Measures to improve the efficiency of resource utilization

Prospective payment systems based on, for example, the DRG system have been a prominent feature in Norway since 1997, and were introduced in a larger scale in Denmark from 2007. Prospective payment systems are widely believed to increase efficiency (e.g. Biørn et al. 2003) but have the unfortunate side-effect of being ill suited to limiting growth in costs. Furthermore, the introduction of an ABF system in Norway was motivated by a desire to increase activity and is widely believed to have contributed to the rapid growth in health care spending since the early 1990s (Hagen and Kaarbøe 2006). Denmark, by comparison, has mainly financed its hospitals through global budgets based on a firm belief that this was the best way to control costs, a strategy that seems to have been successful. Neither Sweden nor Finland has placed much emphasis on the use of payment systems as a means to increase efficiency. Sweden, after a period with competition and purchaser–provider split in the early 1990s, is also now mainly using a system of global budgets, although some county councils continue to rely on contracting and ABF systems based on DRGs. Finally Finland uses DRGs as a means of setting budgets and allocating costs between municipalities, but not systematically as an incentive to increase efficiency.

Competition as a policy measure has not been widely used in the Nordic countries. Sweden had its internal markets in the 1990s; Norway has a number of small, private hospitals, which has led to a somewhat competitive market for elective surgery, while neither Finland nor Denmark relies on competition to any extent to increase efficiency. Again, this is a policy measure that would collide with one of the basic principles of the Nordic model: the public provision of services. Instead, the strategy in the Nordic countries has been increased focus on management models, and the creation of quasi-markets thorough 'new public management' (NPM)-inspired reforms such as patient choice and separation of purchaser and provider.

8.5.4 Investment decisions

Finally we note that the four Nordic countries have different strategies when it comes to major investment decisions. In Norway, the decision as well as the financial responsibility is delegated to the regional health authorities. These are, however, unable to acquire loans from the private sector and must either finance new investments through reduced operating costs or through borrowing from the state. Denmark is presently (2009) discussing the recommendations from a committee concerning which investment projects should be realized and which should be put on hold. Also new investments are partially funded from a large central fund. In both Sweden and Finland, investment decisions are the responsibility of the local authorities, who also provide financing. Therefore, also in this area, there is a division between the more centralized funding and decision-making in Norway and Denmark, and the decentralized solutions of Sweden and Finland.

8.6 Future challenges

Predictions of future health spending are hard to find. Most previous estimates of the effects of ageing on health expenditure show small effects that explain 15–20 per cent of the total increase in health expenditure per capita. The results of analyses tend to be sensitive to the time period chosen, and for longer time series the effects are usually small and gradual. A clear trend, however, is the increasing concentration of health care expenditure to older age groups. Estimating the effects of new technologies involves major uncertainty. Even if some innovations are showed to be cost-effective and also cost-saving, the effect on total expenditure is an often an increase because of widened indications and an increase in the number of treated patients (especially in the older age groups).

The main features of demographic trends in the Nordic countries are similar. In all, the number of elderly will rise rapidly while the working-age population will start to shrink within next few years. This will lead to substantial increase in the old-age dependency ratio. All the Nordic countries will face the problem of how to meet the demand for rapid growth in public services in a time where the number of people in the age groups who are economically active will shrink. Therefore, it can be expected that the supply of an active workforce will seriously limit the possibilities for meeting the rising demand for public services without major wage rises for public sector workers.

The four Nordic countries are on different paths with respect to fiscal decentralization, growth in aggregate spending and the use of demand and supply side measures to contain costs. However, the responsibility for financing is broadly on the same level as the responsibility of providing services in all countries.

Therefore, the excessive use of common (central) resources by local authorities is unlikely to be a problem in the Nordic countries. Also, the objective of guaranteeing a fair and equitable allocation of resources has been achieved through central government grants aiming at compensating for differences in income, need and local cost structure. Nevertheless, we would expect increased fiscal pressure on a sector that provides services widely regarded as a citizen's right, yet with little consideration of the need to define exactly what is (not) included in the basket of public health care services. Whether the solution to this will be tougher prioritizing, more use of market style incentives, stronger regulation of capacity, increased use of a parallel private market or even increased taxes remains to be seen. It is fair to say, however, that the concept of the Nordic health care model as one of the core components of the Nordic welfare state will depend on how the countries choose to preserve the fiscal sustainability of the systems.

Notes

1. Another important issue, the relationship between macroeconomic conditions and the size of the health care system, is acknowledged but not discussed here.
2. That is, individuals being taxed based on the benefit they receive from local public goods.
3. As an example, in Norway it was for a long time assessed that 5 per cent of the population under 18 should receive psychiatric care. More general norms may be maximum waiting times, which also effectively will guide resources to areas where waiting times are longer. All Nordic countries have from time to time used this as a centrally imposed regulatory mechanism.
4. Note that these numbers reflect all tasks of the local governments, not only health care. The index of fiscal supervision is not clearly defined by Sellers and Lidström (2007) but ranges from 0 to 2, interpreted as 'no supervision' and 'full supervision'.
5. Note that budget levels are still negotiated.
6. Technically counties and municipalities may reduce the income tax level from 7 per cent (county) and 21 per cent (municipality), but the maximum rates are uniformly applied.
7. Netherlands, Belgium, Germany, France, Austria, Luxembourg and Switzerland.
8. While at the same time obviously making people with legitimate needs wait.

References

Biørn, E., Hagen, T.P., Iversen, T. and Magnussen, J. (2003) The effect of activity-based financing on hospital efficiency: a panel data analysis of DEA efficiency scores 1992–2000, *Health Care and Management Science* 6: 271–83.
Blöchliger, H. and King, D. (2006) *OECD Economic Studies No 43: Less Than You Thought: The Fiscal Autonomy of Sub-central Governments*. Paris: OECD.
Gilbert, G. and Picard, P. (1996) Incentives and optimal size of local jurisdictions, *European Economic Review* 40: 19–41.
Hagen, T.P. and Kaarbøe, O. (2006) The Norwegian hospital reform of 2002: central government takes over ownership of public hospitals, *Health Policy* 76: 320–33.

Kornai, J., Maskin, E. and Roland G. (2003) Understanding the soft budget constraint, *Journal of Economic Literature* 42: 1095–136.

Lotz, J. (1998) Local government reforms in Nordic countries; theory and practice, in Rattsø, J. (ed.) *Fiscal Federalism and State–Local Finance: The Scandinavian Experience.* Cheltenham: Edward Elgar.

Musgrave R. (1959) *The Theory of Public Finance.* New York: McGraw-Hill.

Oates W. (1972) *Fiscal Federalism.* New York: Harcourt Brace Jovanovich.

OECD (2007) *OECD Health Data 2007.* Paris: OECD.

Rattsø, J. (2002) Fiscal controls in Europe: a summary, in B. Dafflon (ed.) *Local Public Finance: Balanced Budget and Debt Control in European Countries.* Cheltenham: Edward Elgar.

Sellers, J.M. and Lidström, A. (2007) Decentralization, local government and the welfare state, *Governance: An International Journal of Policy, Administration and Institutions* 20: 609–32.

van Doorslaer, E., Wagstaff, A., van der Burg, H. et al. (1999) The redistributive effect of health care finance in twelve OECD countries, *Journal of Health Economics* 18: 291–313.

chapter nine
___

Harnessing diversity of provision

Unto Häkkinen and Pia M. Jonsson

9.1 Background

The major problems recognized in the Nordic health care systems in the 1990s concerned low productivity and efficiency in service production, and these problems were the main starting point for reforms. In the twenty-first century, there have been at least two general trends in health policy in all four countries. First, each country has implemented (Norway or Denmark), taken decisions on (Finland) or at least prepared (Sweden) health care reforms that were expected to improve the access to services and also might have far-reaching effects on the production of services. These reforms focused on the production side, mostly through centralization of decision-making by decreasing the number of local governments/authorities responsible for providing services. In addition, each country has implemented changes on the patient side and has tried to reduce waiting-time problems through the implementation of waiting-time guarantees. The topic has been at the centre of much political debate in Sweden, Norway and Denmark since the early 1990s (Siciliani and Hurst 2003). In the 2000s, it has prevailed as a central theme in the three countries and also arisen in Finland.

During the last few years, the shift of political power to centre-right wing coalition governments in Sweden and Finland has been associated with changing policies that have enhanced the situation of private health care providers. Much of the reform debate is taking place with reference to patient rights and increased consumer freedom of choice. In practice, this development also implies strengthening the possibilities for private providers to establish practices, attract patients and get funding from public finances.

This chapter focuses on how the latest health care reforms in the Nordic countries have affected the models of production of hospital and primary care services. It concentrates on four topics relevant for discussing the diversity of provision: scale and scope, vertical integration, public and private mix and payment structure for personnel. Each of the four topics has been widely discussed in all four countries but only the first has been a central theme in the reforms.

In the Nordic countries, the responsibility of health care has been decentralized to local or regional authorities, who usually both provide and produce health services. Many of the arguments for economies of scale and scope in the Nordic countries can be seen from this perspective. For example, decentralization may lead to a system of dispersed hospitals that fail to secure sufficient economies of scale and scope in producing services. Local authorities may also have aims that promote oversupply of services and inefficiency. Although these economic arguments seem to be prevailing in each country, at least in Norway (hospital reform in 2002), Denmark (structure reform in 2007) and Sweden (Committee on Public Sector Responsibilities set up in 2007), centralization to larger and more specialized units has also been supported by the belief in possible quality improvements. However, it should be noted that the economics of scale argument could also be applied to the size of local governments (i.e. providers) that usually produce (some) primary care services (as municipalities in Finland, Norway and Denmark).

It can be argued that the wider the range of services provided by the purchaser the better the possibilities for coordination. Therefore, vertical integration can be assumed to be more efficient if a purchaser of hospital services is also responsible for purchasing primary care, long-term care and even financing the use of drugs. The examples of the Veterans Health Administration (Evans et al. 2006; Perlin 2006) and Kaiser Permanente (Feachem et al. 2002) in the United States give some support to this argument, at least when applied in a competitive environment. Since a major part of health care in the Nordic countries is publicly owned and managed, the possibilities for vertical integration seem to be good. The differences between the countries in the degree of vertical integration can be seen to result from specific aspects of political, administrative and fiscal decentralization of public duties (not only in health care but also in other public services) between central government, regional authorities/governments and municipalities. In each country, voluntary measures have been tried in order to increase vertical integration.

In order to behave in an efficient way and to be able to respond to purchaser demands, producers (hospitals, GPs) must have flexibility and autonomy. Basically, this can be achieved through two mechanisms: by giving more autonomy to public providers, including contracting out some of the services; or by giving total responsibility for the production to a private producer. In the first option, the producers can be given decision rights in key areas such as hiring and firing, determining the number of staff and skill mix, financial management, determining the level and scope of activities and deciding on capital development, including the number of beds and the technology mix. Autonomy for producers does not automatically motivate increases in efficiency and may be combined with arrangements where 'leftover' resources remain with the producer. But this should be balanced to the extent that hospitals are placed at financial risk (Kirkman-Liff et al. 1997).

As in many other countries, the Nordic countries introduced the principles of 'new public management' (NPM) in the 1990s, including an ambition to increase competition by opening up the health care market for private producers of health services. The trend towards market orientation was most clearly seen in specialized hospital care, where elective surgery services in particular were relatively easy to compare and price, a process that is more difficult in primary health care services. Yet, despite the difficulties in describing, specifying and pricing the contents of primary care services, there has also been a shift towards more diversity of provision at this level of care. However, relatively small changes have occurred towards more involvement of private funding in terms of financing or provision (contracting out, private hospitals or private management of hospitals). Consequently, it has been claimed that the changes can be seen as evolution rather than revolution. More important are the changes in the way of thinking and managing the production and provision of care, which have led to changes in institutional organization (Pedersen 2005).

9.2 Scale and scope

There is a clear trend in all Nordic countries towards increasing the size of both producer and purchaser. Improving technical efficiency of hospital care by increasing the size of producers (economics of scale and scope) have been one of the starting points for the Norwegian and Danish reforms. In Norway the number of health enterprises (operated by regional health authorities) has been reduced from 43 in 2002 to 25 in 2008.[1] In Sweden, hospital mergers were a common strategy in the mid-1990s. The latest large-scale merger was between the Karolinska Hospital and the Huddinge Hospital in the Stockholm area, now forming the Karolinska University Hospital. The merger has been very much debated and an evaluation is presently being carried out of its consequences on hospital efficiency and, to a lesser degree, on the quality of care. In Finland also, centralization of hospital care to larger units has been under discussion and has been recommended by the Ministry of Health, but this has not been supported by legislation or regulation. Some centralization has happened on a voluntary basis. A current example is the merging of three hospitals (Helsinki University Hospital, Jorvi Hospital and Peijas Hospital) in the capital area in 2007 into one big unit, which provides approximately 25 per cent of all acute somatic care in the country (measured in monetary terms). The new unit is organized along the line of medical specialities so that the same specialties in the former three hospitals were merged.

Denmark

The structural reform in Denmark (2007) reduced the number of regional authorities from 14 counties to five regions and the number of municipalities from 275 to 98. The reform as such does not decrease the number of hospitals but there are plans for a significant rebuilding programme[2] driven by a political desire to concentrate activity in fewer, larger hospitals than at present.

Finland

In Finland many recommendations were made during the 1990s in order to increase the population base for units responsible for health services. As a response to the fact that municipalities did not seem to cooperate voluntarily, the Finnish Government established a project in February 2005 to restructure municipalities and services. The background was concern about the increasing financial difficulties faced by municipalities and the growing need for health and social services because of the ageing of the population. The project made three different proposals for organizing basic services: a model of basic municipalities, a regional model and a district model. The municipal model would merge the smallest municipalities into larger ones with a minimum population size of 20,000 inhabitants. The regional model would introduce 20 municipalities with a relatively large population size and responsibilities similar to those of the current municipalities. The third model would integrate primary and secondary health care as well as certain social welfare services into one and the same organization with a population size of 100,000–200,000 inhabitants, while leaving the responsibility for the remaining basic services to the current municipalities.

In January 2007, the parliament accepted a skeleton law governing how to continue the process. According to this act, the government will support mergers of municipalities financially. The act also states that primary health care and social services closely related to health services should be organized in geographical units covering at least 20,000 inhabitants. This would not necessarily require mergers of municipalities smaller than 20,000 inhabitants but could be solved by forming, for example, municipal joint federations. Currently, only about one in four health centres has a population base of 20,000 or more. Municipalities were obliged to make plans on how these goals could be achieved.

Although the issues of organizing hospital services were on the agenda in early stages of the project, the skeleton legislation does not include much that is new for hospitals. It confirms the earlier situation: the responsibilities of services that require a large population base are given to federations of municipalities (e.g. hospital districts) to the extent determined by municipalities. At the beginning of 2009, the total number of municipalities decreased by 67 so the total number is now 348.

Sweden

In Sweden, the National Committee on Public Sector Responsibilities gave its proposals to the Minister of Health and Social Affairs in February 2007 (SOU 2007). The arguments behind the proposals resembled those behind the Norwegian, Finnish and Danish reforms: economic, efficiency and equity. The committee suggested that the number of counties should be reduced from the present 18 plus two regions to six to nine regional authorities by 2015. The proposed larger regional authorities and health care units are assumed to be more cost-effective and to have resources to make long-term strategies, as they would have more capacity (economic, information and medical), for the development of the whole health care system. Hence, geographic equity was expected to improve and regional variations in quality and accessibility to decrease. According to the proposals, the equity aspects should also be promoted by the government's new, more active role in follow-up, evaluation and regulation.

The proposals of the committee have not given rise to substantial changes in health care legislation in Sweden, although many of the experts welcomed them. Yet, a change of attitude towards concentrating at least parts of specialist hospital care to larger regional units can be traced, for example in the very recent proposal of the Committee on National Cancer Strategy for the Future (SOU 2009).

9.3 Vertical integration

Integration or coordination has been pursued in many ways in different health systems, and there are a plethora of terminologies that have variously been described as integrated care, coordinated care, collaborative care, managed care, disease management, case management and so on (Nolte and McKee 2008). The common theme is the ultimate goal of improving outcomes for those with (complex) chronic health problems by overcoming issues of fragmentation through linkage of the services of different providers along the continuum of care. Vertical integration brings together organizations at different levels of hierarchical structure.

Vertical integration of provider responsibilities is rather well developed in Sweden, Finland and Denmark and was considerably less in Norway even before the hospital reform.

Sweden

In Sweden, counties are responsible for the major part of health services, including financing of medicines. There are, however, still large problems associated with the coordination between hospital care, primary care, institutional care and home-based care. Elderly patients and patients with chronic mental illness, in particular, have been shown to suffer from lack of coordination between health services provided by the counties and social services provided by the municipalities. National projects and allocations of extra funds for the development and coordination of psychiatric services have not solved the problems, which are regarded as largely structural. The Committee on Public Sector Responsibilities did not propose changes in the responsibilities between municipalities and regional authorities (county/regional municipalities).

Finland

Finland is the only country where the same authority is responsible for medical and social services (i.e. care of the elderly), but it does not cover use of medicines and private service (e.g. private doctors, examinations, occupational care), which are partly financed by another public source (national health insurance). However, one can argue that a small population base as well as lack of expertise and economic power at municipal level has prevented the efficient vertical integration of production services. Since the mid-1990s, several local reforms have been conducted to integrate the service provision to single organizations. The purpose of these reforms has been to enhance cooperation between primary and secondary health care and social welfare services (Vuorenkoski et al. 2008). The reforms include merging of health centres and regional hospitals into one organization, creating a new regional self-regulating administrative body for all municipal services (including health care, social services, upper secondary schools and vocational services), with its own regional councils, and hospital districts taking responsibility also for primary health - care. In 2008, approximately 10 per cent of the Finnish population lived in areas where most of the primary and secondary health care is provided by the same organization.

This trend was supported by a working group set by the Ministry of Social Affairs and Health on a new Health Care Act (Ministry of Social Affairs and Health 2008). The working group presented two models, which could coexist. In the first model, the organizational responsibility for primary and specialized care would be merged to the same regional organization, called a health district. In the second model, organizational responsibility for primary care would remain the responsibility of municipalities (with a minimum size of 20,000) while specialized care would be the responsibility of a hospital district. The cooperation between these two would, however, be increased by several measures, for example by hospital districts providing some basic specialist level services at municipal level. In addition, it was suggested that the organizational responsibility for ambulance and emergency on-scene services should be centralized to hospital districts.

The proposed reforms in Finland have not touched the highly sensitive and political question of the existence of the two-tier public system. An increasingly higher share of primary care is provided by occupational health care, which is not integrated into the public system. Consequently, the working population has a better access to primary care and this has maintained inequity in the use of services between socioeconomic groups. The income-related inequity in the use of primary care doctors in Finland is one of the highest among OECD countries (van Doorslaer et al. 2004). As the share of the elderly increases, the incentives built into this two-tier system are likely to worsen this picture (Häkkinen 2005).

Denmark

In Denmark, the regions have the responsibility for most health care activities (hospitals, including psychiatric and prenatal centres; GPs; funding of medicines). The reform in 2007 changed only slightly the responsibilities of the two main regional authorities. Municipalities gained overall responsibility for rehabilitation that is not given during hospitalization, which was previously shared with the counties. In addition, municipalities now have primary responsibility for prevention and health promotion, with the goal of integrating these activities with other local responsibilities (such as day care, care of the elderly).

In order to ensure coordination between regional and local activities within the health care system, regions and municipalities will have to enter into bidding partnerships within health coordination committees. They should also make agreements on certain topics such as on procedures for patients discharged from hospital (such as the elderly). Municipalities also finance a part of hospitals by activity-based payments. This is thought to be an incentive for municipalities to make extra efforts to prevent excess use of hospital care.

Norway

The Norwegian reform placed the responsibility of specialist health care with regional health enterprises. Also in Norway there is a growing concern among decision-makers that increased specialization and complicated sets of rules in health and social sectors will lead to a lack of continuity of care and reduce the quality of care (Johnsen 2006). A reform proposed in June 2009 suggests a model of municipal co-payment for hospital services, in line with the present Danish model. Also, a recent committee (NOU 2005, p. 3) discussed appropriate balance between primary health care and specialist health care. One suggestion was to direct the municipalities and the health enterprises to create a cooperation agreement in order to achieve a more seamless delivery of patient treatments. The most recent suggestion on development of integration in Norwegian health care includes consideration of three broad categories of reform: 'linkage', which would operate through existing structures according to recommendations of the earlier committee (NOU 2005, p. 3); 'coordination', which would operate mainly through existing structures but would be a more structured approach involving additional explicit structures and processes (e.g. new delivery, financial and governance arrangements); and 'integration', which would create a single system with responsibility for all services, resources and funding in a single managed structure or through contractual agreements between different organizations. Kaiser Permanente was mentioned as an example of this type of fully integrated system (Oxman et al. 2008).

9.4 Public and private mix

9.4.1 Hospitals

There is a tendency towards the introduction of commercial-style management principles in Nordic hospitals (Pettersen 2004; Pedersen 2005). For example, the Norwegian reform gave the health enterprises a higher freedom than hospitals previously had with regard to investments, flexible planning and health service production, organization and the use of resources across their organizations, and accounting. However, since the state is responsible for their commitments they cannot go bankrupt. Although health enterprises are separate legal entities, the central governments own and control them. For example, central government appoints the regional board members and uses owner control though the articles of association, steering documents (contracts) and through decisions adopted by the enterprise meetings. In addition, major investments are regulated by ministries, and the regional health enterprises are not allowed to borrow money from the private market. The future direction of these enterprises is still unknown. Although it seems certain that public ownership will not be abolished, there is to some extent a growing parallel private market for health care services where some personnel can be recruited from the private sector (Johnsen 2006).

Contracting-out of nonclinical (like catering and laundry services) services is common in the Nordic countries (Pedersen 2005), although it is impossible to give any exact figures on its extent. In Finland, some hospital districts have also transformed laboratory services into publicly owned companies that can provide services to hospital districts, municipalities and to the private sector. In addition, some nonmedical services are outsourced in some hospital districts (e.g. catering and laundry services).

Private hospitals still have only a small role in all Nordic countries. The reason is quite clear. If a for-profit hospital is to survive, there needs to be a good base of health insurance, contract work with the public financier or a political preference for the use of private hospitals. In Denmark, Finland and Norway, the development of the private sector is based on contracts. In Denmark, a more automatic mechanism was created in 2002 with the law on expanded free choice. This means that any citizen has the right to treatment either at a private hospital or abroad after a waiting time of two months for elective surgery at a public hospital, with full public payment. In Finland, the National Sickness Insurance Scheme automatically reimburses procedures and doctors fees given in private hospitals, but the reimbursement level has been so low that this has prevented its popularity.

In Sweden, the question has been more clearly political. In the late 1990s in Stockholm, one hospital with an emergency department was sold (by the non-socialist local government) to private investors and several others in Stockholm and Region Skåne became limited companies to prepare for further privatizations.[3] These changes caused much tension within the Social Democrat Government, and a new act preventing county councils from contracting out emergency hospitals to for-profit owners was passed in 2001. In 2006, new rules for management of publicly financed hospitals came into force. The county councils should manage at least one hospital themselves and responsibility for managing regional hospitals and clinics could not be delegated to others. The centre-right wing coalition that came into power in 2006 has, however, overturned this piece of legislation. The Committee on Public Sector Responsibilities 2007 suggested that the role of regional hospitals should be strengthened in the development of specialist health services.

9.4.2 Primary care

The situation is rapidly changing in Swedish primary care as a consequence of the proposals formulated by the National Committee on Patients' Rights, and a government proposition on Freedom of Choice in Primary Health Care was handed to the Swedish Parliament in December 2008 (Ministry of Social Affairs 2008). According to the proposition, the Swedish Health Care Act is to be changed in order to give the population in each county /region full freedom to choose their GP. The monetary reimbursement, the content of which is to be decided by each county/region, will follow the patient. All public and private providers who fulfil the general requirements set up by the county /region have the right to establish and run their practices and are to be treated on equal terms by the reimbursement system. The reform is to be implemented in the whole country in January 2010.

Further developments toward more freedom of choice for patients, and more equal opportunities for private providers compared with public ones, are under way. The Committee on Patients' Rights is now working on a proposal for a new system that would allow private providers to establish themselves not only in general practice but also in the provision of specialist health services not requiring inpatient care. This proposal is expected to be completed by the end of September 2009.

The municipalities (providers) and hospital districts (producers) in Finland have started to reorganize models of production. In general terms, the aim of these local projects has been to contain costs by cooperation between both different sectors within municipal health services (primary care, specialist care and care of the elderly) and the private sector. Local projects and experiments have taken quite different directions. These projects include the development in one hospital district of a clearer purchaser–provider model, in which smaller municipalities have formed cooperative purchaser organizations for arranging specialized services; a municipality buying its health services from the non-profit third sector; and an instance of the merging of health centres and a district hospital into a single organization providing all health services for inhabitants of the municipalities in the area. In addition, cooperation with the private sector has increased. One example of a new form of public–private partnership is the highly specialized hospital (Coxa) that was founded in Tampere in 2002 to perform endoprosthetic operations. It works as a limited company, and it was founded by Pirkanmaa hospital district (and three other hospital districts), four cities, one Finnish foundation and a German private hospital company. In 2005, the German company sold all its shares to the Finnish National Fund for Research and Development. The Coxa Hospital is responsible for all elective endoprosthetic operations within the Pirkanmaa hospital district area. It also provides these services for patients from other hospital districts as well as for private patients.

Public employers have had great difficulty recruiting primary care physicians in Finland. This has led to an increase in 'rental doctors', who take economically advantageous short-time contracts. In 2008, the private sector provided approximately 60 per cent of all emergency services in primary health centres. In addition, some of the health care centres are now run by private corporations although with public funding. The private corporations often also provide occupational health services.

9.5 Payment structures

In all Nordic countries, most hospital staff are salaried. However, there are significant differences in the payment structures for primary care physicians.

Norway

In Norway, a central goal of introducing the General Practitioner Scheme of 2001 was to facilitate the recruitment of family practitioners to remote areas and communities with lack of health care staff and hence to improve the population's access to primary care services. The scheme is a contractual system based on patient listing and capitation (approximately 70 per cent capitation financed by the municipalities, and 30 per cent per item paid by the National Insurance Scheme). Primary care physicians, having been public employees, were now encouraged to work as private consultants contracted by the municipalities. As the reform was implemented, very few physicians chose to carry on as salaried employees.

The shift to the new model went relatively smoothly, which is partly explained by the economic conditions attached to it. The cost of the reform to the state was high, but the number of primary care physicians increased as did the number of visits to them. In addition to the attractive economic conditions offered to the physicians, the higher degree of freedom in planning a personal workload and individual adjustment of the length of the patient list have been given as explanations to why the reform attained at least some of its goals.

Denmark

Danish primary care physicians were previously practitioners contracted by the counties, which were responsible both for the financing and the organization of health services. In the reform of 2007, the duties of the counties were mainly shifted to five newly established health care regions, which now contract the practitioners. The municipalities are responsible for 'health centres': institutions that do not treat acute diseases but promote health by primary and secondary prevention.

Sweden

In Sweden, primary care services have been delivered under quite varied conditions and by several categories of producer. While the number of individual private family practitioners in Sweden is very small, since 2000, many of the counties have contracted primary care centres run by other producers. In some of the counties, up to 50 per cent of the units are now run privately; for example in Stockholm, more than 40 per cent of the visits to primary care physicians are paid to these centres. Most of the physicians are salaried employees, but the arrangements may vary. In addition, the lack of physicians especially in remote areas has opened up a market for 'rental doctors'. Because of the high cost of these services to the counties, and possibly also because of problems with the continuity and quality of care, many of the counties try to avoid this type of solution, but the lack of physician staff is undermining more long-term solutions (Socialstyrelsen 2006). Some of the counties have tried to recruit physician employees directly from abroad and are more or less succeeding in the battle against physician shortages.

As mentioned above, the situation now in Sweden is changing under the implementation of new legislation on freedom of choice in primary health - care, which will be in force by January 2010. The public and private providers are to be treated equally by the public reimbursement system, the details of which are to be decided upon at the county/regional level. Already today, three counties/regions have independently introduced a freedom of choice reform in primary care. The principles of the reimbursement models have varied between counties and the consequences of the reforms have not yet been evaluated. It has been claimed that success with the models requires generally positive attitudes towards competition and diversity, as well as willingness to reallocate resources according to the factual choices of the population (Anell 2008). Critics have claimed that the introduction of the models has neglected tentative negative consequences on socioeconomic equity of access to health care (Burström 2008).

Finland

In Finland, as in Sweden, primary care services are delivered by several categories of producer. In addition to primary care centres run by the municipalities, there are single-doctor private practices with competence in family medicine. As opposed to other systems occupational health care in Finland often covers the diagnosis and treatment of diseases. This, in fact, has been pointed out as a factor creating inequity in the Finnish system, as the well-developed, easily accessible occupational health services financially supported by the employers are not matched by comparable services to those outside the labour market.

9.6 Discussion

Increasing the diversity of provision can be seen as a means of increasing competition, both based on costs and quality. Creating prerequisites for patient freedom of choice – as a part of a more general patient empowerment movement – has been another motive for increasing diversity into the production of services. It should also be noted that the potential for citizens of EU member states to have access to care in other EU countries adds to the diversity and the complexity of freedom of choice. The Nordic countries seem to be in agreement that the ambition to deliver homogeneous high-quality services to the whole population is the motivating force for tighter government control of services and providers than was the case in the 1990s. More effective monitoring, evaluation and regulation (in a modern sense) are being initiated, as illustrated by the establishment of the Danish Institute for Quality and Accreditation in Healthcare (IKAS) in 2005 (Jonsson et al. 2006).

The main difference between the Nordic countries is that in Finland the municipalities act as purchasers of hospital care whereas in other countries the role has been given to larger units (counties, regions). In the early 2000s, purchasers in each country were directly responsible politically to the population in local elections and also the financing was at least in part based on local taxes. Since then, the situation has been changing in Denmark and Norway. In Norway, the change was radical since direct democratic control was abolished.[4] In Denmark, the new regions responsible for hospital care are financed mainly by block grants, with some activity-based payments from central government.

The role of private hospitals in hospital care is still modest. A few – but much talked about – private hospitals have been established in all the Nordic countries and these are signals that the health care sector is drastically different from that of the late 1980s. The possibility of using the private sector has been regarded as a safeguard for waiting-time guarantees. In Denmark, it has at least temporarily increased the use of private hospitals (Vrangbæk 2008). However, there are no comparative figures and even the exact trend since 2000 on the role of private hospitals is not available. In Norway in 2005, the private hospitals without regional authority agreements treated approximately 3 per cent of inpatient hospital stays and 4 per cent of day cases. In Finland in 2005, private hospitals treated approximately 8 per cent of all patients in somatic hospital inpatient care and produced 6 per cent of inpatient hospital stays, 8 per cent of bed days and 8 per cent of surgical operations. The private hospitals also have a significant role in the care of diseases of the eye and musculoskeletal system. The private sector has a more significant role in the whole health care in Finland than in the other Nordic countries. In 2004, the share of total health expenditure taken by private producers was approximately 23 per cent (4 per cent nonprofit-making organizations and 19 per cent for-profit firms). Their share of personnel was somewhat lower (17 per cent, of which nonprofit-making organizations was 5 per cent and for-profit firms 13 per cent) (STAKES 2007).

It cannot be assumed that the private hospitals in tertiary care will increase substantially in the near future in Norway, Denmark and Finland. The situation may be different in Sweden where the current government has shown a more positive attitude towards the private sector; here a change in ownership of the existing hospitals is also possible. In Finland during 2006 to 2009, foreign investment companies bought the most important Finnish private companies operating in health care, which may increase the potential for private sector investments. The role of the private sector is likely to increase in medical specialties with increasing demand, especially if the public sector is too inflexible to respond to demand. For example, in Finland, the private sector has been expanded quite rapidly in recent years for elective endoprosthetic operations. During 2000–2006, the share of the private sector for hip and knee replacements increased from 8 to 23 per cent. However, over 70 per cent of the 'private' sector operations in 2006 were carried out in three hospitals, of which two are owned by nonprofit foundations and one (Coxa) is owned partly by hospital districts.

Commercial-style management methods (such as contracting out nonclinical services) have gradually been introduced in Nordic hospitals and it is assumed that this trend will continue. Recent reforms in Norway and Denmark have increased the role of central government in hospital care. This opens up possibilities for large-scale structural changes (in scale and scope), new managerial/

organizational forms and public–private partnerships, which are all dependent on centralized decisions.

The situation is rather different in Finland and Sweden, where actual changes are based on voluntary decisions made at local level. In Finland, government activities has been mostly organizational (increase of size of municipalities) without much discussion on contents of care, such as the integration of care providers or closer coordination of services. Local projects and experiments have taken quite different directions, increasing the diversity within the country. In Sweden, the organizational structures (such as the role of political bodies in provision and purchasing) among the country councils are in continuing change. Stenberg (2007) classifies counties as high-frequency changers (counties that changed governance structure for health care after each election) and the still dominant low-frequency changers (counties that do not change organizational model often, but do continual changes). The change of political governance structure has effects on organizing structure of purchasers and providers in Sweden. As in Finland, it is assumed that it will increase diversity within the country.

There is now increasing evidence that Finnish hospitals are more efficient than hospitals in other Nordic countries. Results from a study comparing Finnish and Norwegian hospitals in 1999 indicate that Finnish hospitals were approximately 30 per cent more efficient than Norwegian hospitals, and there were clear difference in favour of Finland even after adjusting the wage differences of hospital staff between the countries (Linna et al. 2006). A more recent study included Finnish and Norwegian hospitals from 1999 to 2004, Swedish hospitals from 2001 to 2004 and Danish hospitals from 2002. After adjusting for wage differences, the Finnish hospitals were, on average, approximately 10 per cent more efficient than Danish or Norwegian hospitals and 25 per cent more efficient than Swedish hospitals (Häkkinen and Linna 2007). Although the Norwegian hospital reform somewhat decreased the gap between the Norwegian and Finnish hospitals, the difference between the countries was still considerable in 2004 (Kittelsen et al. 2007). The reasons for these differences have not yet been fully explored, but one explanation may be that cost control by municipalities (financed mainly by local taxes) is more effective than that of counties or governments. However, so far, there is no comparative information on the differences in quality or outcome between the countries.

The health care reforms carried out in Norway have been subject to extensive monitoring and evaluation. Although it may be too early to draw conclusions on the long-term effects of the reforms, short-term consequences have been analysed and documented more systematically than for most other reforms. According to the recently published evaluation report, the Norwegian hospital reform contributed to somewhat increased productivity and hence better accessibility to hospital services as well as somewhat shorter waiting lists (Norges forskningsråd 2007). The previous variations between the counties diminished, but variations between the five regions persisted. The impact of the reform on the medical quality of services, including patient safety aspects, has not yet been evaluated.

In primary care, the Norwegian system has adapted the Danish model where physicians work as independent practitioners. The lack of physician workforce is still a problem in Sweden and Finland. The differences between countries can be seen also from international comparisons. According to OECD Health Data (2007), the number of visits to a doctor per capita in 2004 was clearly higher in Denmark (7.5) than in Sweden (2.8) or Finland (4.2). In the beginning of the 2000s, income-related inequity in the use of doctor's services was particularly apparent in Finland but also occurred in Sweden more than in Norway and Denmark (van Doorslaer et al. 2004).

The consequences of the Norwegian General Practitioner Scheme for the recruitment of physicians and the accessibility of primary care services have been mostly positive (Norges forskningsråd 2006). The monetary cost to the government has been high, but apparently not beyond what was expected or what the government actually seems to be able – or willing – to pay. The effects on the quality of services, at least in terms of continuity, have been positive. The traditional role as a gatekeeper, however, has been experienced as somewhat problematic by some GPs, as they are at the same time competing for the favour of patients entering their lists. The experience from Norway indicates that with more resources and a new contractual model, the position of primary care could be strengthened also in Finland and Sweden. However, care should be taken that contracts as well as financial incentives are such that they promote coordinating care of people with chronic conditions (Busse and Mays 2008; Oxman et al. 2008).

Notes

1. The merging of two regional health enterprises East and South in 2007 will lead to a restructuring and further reduction in the number of health enterprises in 2009.
2. The Association of Danish Regions has published a homepage with the rebuilding programme of each region: www.Godtsygehusbyggeri.dk
3. There is some evidence that company formation in Skåne has had positive effects (Aidemark and Lindkvist 2004).
4. Originally there were no politicians on the board of the health enterprises. But from 2006 the professional boards were replaced by boards with local politicians because of fears of 'democratic deficit'.

References

Aidemark, L. and Lindkvist, L. (2004) The vision gives the wings: a study of two hospital run as limited companies, *Management Accounting Research* 15: 305–18.
Anell, A. (2008) Vårdval på gång i dagens primärvård. Stora skillnader mellan olika modeller och stort utvecklingsbehov, *Läkartidningen* 105: 2007–10.
Burström, B. (2008) Vårdval: evidens och effekter för 'vård på lika villkor'. *Läkartidningen* 105: 2992–94.
Busse, R. and Mays, N. (2008) Paying for chronic disease, in Nolte E. and McKee M. (eds) *Caring for People with Chronic Conditions: A Health System Perspective*. Buckingham: Open University Press.
Evans, D.C., Nichol, P.W. and Perlin, J.B. (2006) Effect of the implementation of an enterprise-wide Electronic Health Record on productivity in the Veterans Health Administration, *Health Economics, Policy and Law* 1: 163–9.

Feachem, R.G.A., Sekhri, N.K. and White, K.L. (2002) Getting more for their dollars: a comparison of the NHS with California's Kaiser Permanente, *British Medical Journal* 324: 135–43.

Häkkinen, U. (2005) The impact of changes in Finland's health care system, *Health Economics, Supplement 1* S101–18.

Häkkinen, U. and Linna, M. (2007) *Suomessa pohjoismaiden tehokkaimmat sairaalat*. Stockholm: Centre for Health Equity Studies (CHESS), Stockholm University/ Karolinska Institute;CHESS ON LINE 2: 4–5 (http://groups.stakes.fi/NR/rdonlyres/F87820D6–3485–4072-A045-E8C11E60567B/0/CHESS_207a.pdf).

Johnsen, J. (2006) Norway: Health System Review. *Health Systems in Transition*, 8(1): 1–167. Copenhagen: WHO Regional Office for Europe on behalf of the European Observatory on Health Systems and Policies.

Jonsson, P.M., Agardh, E. and Brommels, M. (2006) *Hälso- och sjukvårdens strukturreformer: Lärdomar från Norge, Danmark, Finland och Storbritannien*. Ansvarskommitténs skriftserie [Responsibility Committee Papers]. Stockholm: Statens Offentliga Utredningar.

Kirkman-Liff, B., Huijsman, R. T., van der Grinten, G. and Brink, C. (1997) Hospital adaptation to risk-bearing managerial implications to changes in purchaser–provider contracting, *Health Policy* 39: 207–23.

Kittelsen, S., Magnussen, J. and Anthun K. (2007) *Sykehusproduktivitet etter statlig overtakelse: En nordisk komparativ analyse*. Oslo: Health Economic Research, University of Oslo.

Linna, M., Häkkinen, U. and Magnussen J. (2006) Comparing hospital cost efficiency between Norway and Finland, *Health Policy* 77: 268–78.

Ministry of Social Affairs and Health [Sosiaali- ja terveysministeriö] (2008) *Uusi terveydenhuoltolaki. Terveydenhuoltolakityöryhmän mietintö*. Helsinki: Ministry of Social Affairs and Health.

Nolte, E. and McKee, M. (eds) (2008) *Caring for People with Chronic Conditions: A Health System Perspective*. Buckingham: Open University Press.

Norges forskningsråd (2006) *Evaluering av Fastlegereformen, Sammenfatning og analyse av evalueringens delprosjekter*. Oslo: Norges forskingsråd [Research Council of Norway].

Norges forskningsråd (2007) *Resultatevaluering av sykehusreformen. Tilgjengelighet, prioritering, effektivitet, brukermedvirkning og medbestemmelse*. Oslo: Norges forskningsråd [Research Council of Norway].

NOU (2005) *NOU 2005:3. Fra stykkevis til helt. En sammenhengende helsetjeneste. Statens fortvaltningstjeneste*. Oslo: Ministry of Health and Care Services.

OECD (2007) *OECD Health Data 2007*. Paris: OECD.

Oxman, A.D., Bjørndal, A., Flottorp, S., Lewin, S. and Lindahl, A.K. (2008) *Integrated Health Care for People with Chronic Conditions*. Oslo: Norwegian Knowledge Centre for Health Services.

Pedersen, K.M. (2005) The private–public mix in Scandinavia, in Maynard, A. (ed.) *The Public–Private Mix-for Health: plus ca change, plus c'est la meme chose?* Oxford: Radcliffe, pp. 161–90.

Perlin, J.B. (2006) Transformation of the US Veterans Health Admistration, *Health Economics, Policy and Law* 1: 99–105.

Pettersen, I.J. (2004) From bookkeeping to strategic tools? A discussion of the reforms in the Nordic hospital sector, *Management Accounting Research* 15: 319–35.

Regeringens proposition 2008/09: 74 Vårdval i primärvården. Stockholm: Government Offices.

Siciliani, L. and Hurst J. (2003) *OECD Health Working Paper No. 7: Explaining Waiting Times Variations for Elective Surgery across OECD Countries*. Paris: OECD.

Socialstyrelsen [National Board of Health and Welfare] (2006) *Uppföljning av överenskom-*

melser om en fortsatt satsning för utveckling av primärvård, äldrevård och psykiatri. Stockholm: National Board of Health and Welfare.

SOU (2007) *SOU 2007: 10. Hållbar samhällsorganisation med utvecklingskraft, Ansvarskommitténs slutbetänkande.* Stockholm: Slutbetänkande. Statens Offentliga Utredningar [Government Offices].

SOU (2009) *Utredningen om en nationell cancerstrategi 2009. Nationell cancerstrategi för framtiden.* Stockholm: Statens Offentliga Utredningar [Government Offices].

STAKES (2007) *Yksityinen palvelutuotanto sosiaali- ja terveydenhuollossa 2004. [Private Service Provision in Social and Health Care 2004.]* Helsinki: STAKES, University of Helsinki.

Stenberg, J.G. (2007) *Changes in Political Structures in Swedish Health Care: Models Variations and Implications.* Stockholm: Medical Management Center, Karoliinska Institute.

van Doorslaer, E., Masseria, C., Koolman, X. for the OECD Health Equity Health Group (2004) Income-related inequality in the use of medical care in 21 OECD countries, in *The OECD Health Project: Towards High-performing Health Systems.* Paris: OECD, pp. 109–65.

Vrangbæk, K. (2008) *Rapid Growth in Private Health Care.* Westphalia: Heath Policy Monitor http://www.hpm.org/en/Search_for_Reforms/Search.html.

Vuorenkoski, L., Mladovsky, P. and Mossialos, E. (2008) Finland: Health System Review. *Health Systems in Transition,* 10(4): 1–168.

ten

Changing perceptions of equity and fairness

Johan Calltorp and Meri Larivaara

10.1 Introduction

The equity principle is at the heart of the 'Nordic health model'. During the whole period since the Second World War, it has been one of the strongest common denominators when comparing the systems, both with each other and with the rest of the western systems. The health systems are a key component of the welfare systems and the equity principle underpins the whole Nordic welfare state idea – or maybe more specifically the way welfare is organized the 'Nordic way'. Naturally, there are differences in detail arrangements between the four countries, but by and large the Nordic communality has been quite robust.

This chapter reviews how equity as a policy goal has evolved over the last decades in Denmark, Finland, Norway and Sweden. The concept of equity is considered from two different perspectives: geographical distribution of resources and the principles behind priority setting. The extent to which equity has been accomplished is analysed by focusing on the utilization of health services. Comparisons will be made between the four countries to illuminate the similarities and differences. Finally, the question of whether perceptions of equity in the four countries have changed will be addressed and, if so, in what ways. Through looking at recent developments, attempts will be made to anticipate the future trends.

Before going into empirical data, some conceptual definitions are necessary. What is meant when we talk about equity? First, it is important to distinguish between (in)equality and (in)equity. While 'inequalities' usually refer to mere descriptive differences between various groups, 'inequities' are perceived to mean social differences that are deemed to be unjust. It is important to recognize, however, that these concepts do not have a universal well-defined meaning. They are, therefore, both used and interpreted differently within academic and within policy-making circles.

To understand some of the difficulties in assigning a precise meaning to these concepts, consider the term 'need'. One possible definition of need would be 'capacity to benefit'. Then if you are able to benefit greatly from a service your need of that service is high; conversely if you do not benefit from the service it is difficult to argue that you need it. By using this approach, allocating resources according to need would imply allocating resources according to capacity to benefit. Therefore, an equal (or even just) solution would be to distribute resources according to the ability to benefit. This is what is often termed horizontal equity, for example people with similar problems should receive similar treatment. ('Similar' here is interpreted as similar ability to benefit.) Another way of looking at this, however, is to say that the goal of the health care system is to get as close as feasible to an equal distribution of health. Then need is not defined by ability to benefit but by deviation from the average level of health in the population. People in poorer health will have a higher need than people in good health, regardless of their ability to benefit from services. A distribution of resources aimed at providing equal levels of health is said in this case to pursue a goal of vertical equity.

It is one of the challenges of most health systems that they present preferences for solutions that will simultaneously provide both horizontal and vertical equity. Therefore, we often hear stated as a general policy goal that one should get as much health as possible out of the resources used (which can be interpreted as horizontal equity), while countries also are concerned with social differences in health and aim to reduce these (which can be interpreted as vertical equity, and will not imply maximizing the amount of health obtained from given resources).

In all four Nordic countries, universal access to high-quality health care services is an indisputable goal of the health care system, shared widely across the political parties. Each of the four countries has adopted a public health programme that states reducing health inequalities as one of its central goals (Chapter 12). Furthermore, through various international agreements, Denmark, Finland, Norway and Sweden have committed themselves to providing sufficient and comprehensive health services to their entire populations. Such agreements include the Universal Declaration of Human Rights and the Constitution of the World Health Organization, to name but a few. However, there is evidence that social differences in mortality and morbidity persist in Denmark, Finland, Norway and Sweden, and that these inequalities follow similar patterns over the occupational groups in each country (Lahelma et al. 2002).

Equity in health services can be approached from different dimensions, including access to services, patterns of utilization, health outcomes, financing of health services, distribution of resources and allocation of health services. This chapter focuses on three perspectives: models for distribution of resources, mechanisms for priority setting and utilization of health services. The aim is to examine what kinds of instrument have been recently developed in Denmark, Finland, Norway and Sweden to guarantee equity and then to explore how they work in practice.

Health and health services can be distributed differently according to a citizen's economic position, educational background, occupation, place of living, sex, sexual orientation, native tongue, ethnicity, age and other factors.

This chapter's focus is on socioeconomic, gender and regional equity. Socio-economic and gender inequities have been studied most in the four countries. Regional equity will be discussed mainly from the perspective of resource alloca-tion that, in itself, aims to level regional inequalities.

10.2 Distribution of resources

The Nordic countries are all decentralized in the sense that the responsibility for providing health care (as well as other welfare) services to the populations lies at municipal, county or regional level. This decentralization implies that local governments may have different preferences over which level of services should be provided. Furthermore, local governments may have different levels of tax income, and thus income-based differences in service level are a possibility. Geographic distribution has been an important component in that national funds or supplementary financing to the basic local tax financing have been used to redistribute health resources according to population characteristics and needs, seeking to counteract a situation in which less purchasing and taxation power is linked to older age, less education, lower socioeconomic class and worse health.

Sweden

The allocation of resources among counties in Sweden is influenced by tax equali-zation, by differences in population characteristics and by differences in cost structure. Given the high level of fiscal decentralization in Sweden, state trans-fers account for less than 20 per cent of total county income. Sweden also has a system of need-based state transfers for pharmaceuticals, although this is provided separately from other health care-related transfers.

Denmark

Denmark also has a system of state transfers to its five regions. However, since regions cannot levy taxes themselves, this system effectively provides the main part of each region's income, with a minor part coming from municipal activity-based financing (ABF). These Danish state transfers consist of two parts: a small lump sum and a large needs-based allocation. There are discussions about the adequacy of the present system, with some regions arguing forcefully that cur-rent criteria do not capture regional variations in need adequately, and so some regions gain (lose) funds as a result of an inappropriate formula.

Norway

The Norwegian system for state transfers consists of two parts: 40 per cent of the transfers for somatic patients are based on actual levels of activity, while the remaining 60 per cent as well as funds for other health care services and capital are distributed according to a need-based formula. This formula was revised after the hospital reform in 2002 but was severely criticized and a new formula was implemented in 2009. The allocation of resources is now based on three factors: activity, need and the regional costs of providing services.

Finland

The Finnish system of state transfers – like that of the other Nordic countries – is based on a needs-based capitation formula. Since the municipalities in Finland are free to set their own tax rates, the state subsidies also provide tax equalization. Differences in cost structures are captured by allocating a higher level of resources to rural areas. There is, at time of writing, a process aiming to simplify the capitation-based models in Finland by merging the formula for health and social services with the formulae for other services.

Comparison of countries

There are, therefore, commonalities as well as differences in resource allocation between the four Nordic countries. The common feature is that all countries apply some sort of needs-based capitation formula for the distribution of resources. The types of criteria included in the formula differ, however, substantially. To some extent, this reflects the fact that the state transfers cover different types of service in the four countries, but also the fact that different analytical as well as political perspectives have been present. The formulae in two of the four countries (Norway and Denmark) have generated a lot of political noise. In all probability, this reflects the more centralized fiscal structure of these two countries. Also their approach to adjusting for differences in local cost structures varies. While Denmark has no such explicit adjustment, Finland and Sweden both use the urban/rural distinction to compensate for differences and Sweden also now compensates for differences in wage levels. The last is explicitly rejected in Norway, the argument being that the level of wages is largely determined by managerial actions, thus compensating regions with high wages would effectively enable them to pass the bill to the central authorities.

The overall conclusion is that the Nordic countries actively seek to enable the local authorities to provide their population with equal access to health care services. Providing a geographical resource allocation that is adjusted for variations in need is, however, only the first step. We now move to the questions on how explicit the four countries are in their principles for priority setting.

10.3 Priority setting

Interest in priority setting and in model development within this area has become an important aspect of equity in the Nordic region.

Norway

Priority setting developed first in Norway with the report of the Lønning I Committee, published in 1987 (NOU 1987). This document focused on applied equity and on the appropriate mechanisms to safeguard a health system in a period of fiscal pressure and change. It should be noted that the basic dimensions of this issue were first outlined by Victor Fuchs in 1974 (Fuchs 1998).

Although the Lønning Committee focused attention on financial pressure with its description of how the 'demand curve' was crossing the 'resource curve', it was also closely linked to the planning and resource distribution and redistribution perspective, with its well-known description of the five priority groups. An interesting aspect was, even in 1987, to introduce the technology assessment perspective and the need to implement this knowledge into a priority model. Although influential in policy discussions, the Lønning Report was also criticized for lacking substantive references to the principles of economic evaluation: that is, the discussion of benefits was rarely linked to the corresponding costs. Its practical impact was, therefore, negligible. The Lönning I Report was followed by the Lønning II Report (NOU 1997), now including a discussion of costs as well as benefits and trying to operationalize the concept of a basic benefit package through what was termed 'necessary health services'. The practical result of Lønning II was a broad description of priority principles, though these also were generally found to be too vague to provide meaningful guidance for health care providers. At the time of writing, however, the Norwegian Directorate of Health is completing a number of speciality-specific guidelines that are intended to provide a more practical guide to the principles of priority setting within the Norwegian health care system.

The thinking of the Lønning Committee strongly influenced health policy discussions in the other three Nordic countries. In Sweden, the final report of the 1995 Einhorn Committee had a similar content, as did the report of the Palo Committee in Finland (Working Group on Health Care Prioritization 1995) and similar documents in Denmark. The work of these committees brought forward a specific perspective linking the equity principle to the functioning of the health care system. It also illuminated the mechanisms that are at play to reinforce or counteract equity.

The international literature on prioritization has grown considerably, as have linkages to how relevant tools and measures function in different types of health care system, for example explicit and implicit rationing and the Oregon list experiment (Calltorp 1999).

Sweden

Some 12 years after the publication of the Swedish Priority Committee Report, the concept of priority setting is still a strong area of activity among the county councils. A national centre for priority setting has been organized within a health economic and technology assessment university centre at Linköping University. Other important activities in Sweden include:

- an agreed national model for vertical prioritization, which is a rank order model for medical conditions that can be applied for all medical specialities
- one county council, Västra Götaland, has required medical specialties to describe their medical activity according to this agreed model and has successively linked resource measures to priority groups and experimented with a

horizontal priority model; this includes tests to agree on open criteria for the resource distribution between medical areas (Calltorp 1999)
- the National Board of Health and Welfare has developed national guidelines for different diagnoses – such as coronary care – which incorporate detailed medical advice on prioritization.

Finland

In Finland, the Medical Society Duodecim in 1997 assembled a consultative committee on priority setting. A consensus meeting on priority setting in 2000 was followed by a report that emphasized rationalizing the health care system. While concrete measures for priority setting were not adopted, in March 2005 the principle of access to treatment within a reasonable time period was put into effect, introducing indirect measures for priority setting. The primary objective was to ensure better access to care, which had previously been compromised by long waiting times for certain services in ambulatory and hospital care. As part of the process, the Ministry of Social Affairs and Health, with the help of expert proposals, put together national guidelines defining the limits of access wait for nonurgent specialized care procedures. Guidelines were made for 193 disease or treatment groups covering approximately 80 per cent of nonemergency hospital care. The guidelines define which patients should be guaranteed treatment within a certain time period, but they are not legally binding. Scoring systems are used in some of these guidelines. In March 2007, 87 per cent of the health centres reported using the guidelines. Although developed for ensuring access to care, these guidelines are also a tool for priority setting when put into effect. In comparison with Sweden, the Finnish guidelines define, within each disease or treatment group, the severity of condition that entitles treatment, while in Sweden conditions are grouped into those that require treatment and those that do not.

Comparison of countries

Overall, priority setting is an important perspective on operationalizing equity. It has so far mostly focused on theoretical and policy formulation. There have been a number of interesting attempts to develop tools for implementation, which have tested concrete actions on the service provision level.

10.4 Equity in utilization of health services

In the Nordic countries, improvements in health outcomes have been achieved through a combination of social, educational and health policies and with services that are largely guided by egalitarian principles. Therefore, health experiences and outcomes cannot be attributed to the efforts of health services only. Nevertheless, it is essential to examine equity in utilization of health services, because health services are a place where accomplishment of egalitarian health policies of the Nordic countries is put to test.

All the Nordic countries maintain national hospital registers that have information about hospital inpatient episodes and increasingly about visits to ambulatory specialist care at hospital polyclinics. The registers in Denmark, Finland and Sweden include the personal identification number, making linkages between these and other registers possible. Hospital registers have shown to be reliable according to international standards, although some inaccuracies exist in the data for some diagnoses and procedures (Thorsen et al. 2002; Smedby 2003). Visits to primary care physicians are not recorded in registers in any of the Nordic countries, making it necessary to rely on survey data in the analysis of utilization of primary care. Differences of sampling methods, response rates and wording of the questions complicate international comparisons based on survey data.

We first examine how physician visits and hospital care are distributed between different social groups. Then we take coronary heart disease as an example of a severe disease and look at its treatment in more detail. Finally, we draw attention to what is known about differences in dental care. When looking at the data, it is worth keeping in mind that a consistent socioeconomic gradient in health for the benefit of those better-off has persisted in each Nordic country (Lahelma et al. 2002). Consequently, the lower socioeconomic groups are likely to need more services than the higher socioeconomic groups. As for gender differences, women suffer from more symptoms and illnesses than men, but yet they live longer.

10.4.1 The distribution of physician visits and rates of hospitalization

Comparisons of health care utilization in the four Nordic countries are rare. Haglund (2004) has analysed the data of national surveys (Denmark 2000, Finland 2000, Norway 2002, Sweden 2000 and 2001) to compare the visits to a doctor because of the individual's own illness or injury or, in the Danish case, contact with a doctor, including telephone consultations. The share of population who had visited a doctor at least once during the previous 12 months (Finland and Norway) or previous three months (Denmark and Sweden) decreased with increasing educational level in all countries for both sexes, with the exception of Finnish women. The results are likely to reflect differences in morbidity, so indicating equally accessible services. However, when adjusting the data for health status, the less educated visit a physician less commonly than the more educated in Denmark, Finland and Sweden, while in Norway no evidence for inequality can be found (Haglund 2004 and its Table 2). A comparative Nordic study on children's utilization of physician services found no social inequalities in the use of GP visits in 1996, but use of specialist services was associated with parents' higher socioeconomic status among children with chronic health conditions (Grøholt et al. 2003).

Need-standardized differences in physician use in Nordic countries have also been examined in an OECD study that compared 21 countries in the late 1990s and early 2000s. According to this study, all visits to a physician and visits to a GP were distributed fairly equally in Denmark and Norway, while a significant pro-rich inequity was observed in both cases in Finland. Use of ambulatory specialist services was evenly distributed in Norway, but a pro-rich inequity was discovered in Denmark and Finland. A pro-rich inequity in all visits to physicians was observed in Sweden, but the data did not allow separating visits to GPs from those to specialists. No need-standardized socioeconomic inequities in the number of hospital nights and the probability of hospital admissions were found in Denmark, Finland and Sweden. Data were not available from Norway (van Doorslaer et al. 2004). We now turn to look at each country individually in order to see what national studies reveal about the distribution of health services.

Denmark

In Denmark, national survey data showed that the proportion of the population who visited a GP or a medical specialist over a three-month period increased in all social groups over the period 1987–2005. The least-educated group continued to visit a GP more commonly throughout the study period, while the most educated group visited a medical specialist more commonly. The differences have remained in the same level during the study period, except the difference in visits to a medical specialist. This difference grew between the educational groups over 1987 to 1994 and has remained at approximately the same level ever since. In all age groups, a larger proportion of women than men visited a GP or a medical specialist. Regional differences are small in Denmark, except for the significantly higher number of visits to a medical specialist in the capital area, where the increase has been most remarkable between 1987 and 1994 (Ekholm et al. 2006, pp. 170–5; see also http://susy2.si-folkesundhed .dk/susy.aspx). As for waiting times in Denmark, men with higher education have been reported to experience the shortest waiting times for elective inpatient treatments in the late 1990s, while men with basic education wait longest (Sundhedsministeriet 2000). A survey and register-based study in one Danish county has suggested that hospitalization rates and visits to specialists and GPs are equally distributed over socioeconomic groups when utilization is standardized for age, gender and health status. As for specific types of care, however, the least advantaged consumed a lower than expected share of dentistry, medication and physiotherapy (Gundgaard 2006).

Finland

In Finland, national survey data reveal that need-standardized number of all physician visits has favoured higher socioeconomic groups in the period 1987–2000. The lower socioeconomic groups visited a GP at a primary health care centre more commonly than the higher socioeconomic groups, but the higher socioeconomic groups have more physician visits to occupational health services, specialists at hospital polyclinics and to physicians at private sector. The differences have remained at approximately the same level throughout the study period (Manderbacka et al. 2006). The difference in all physician visits may have increased in the early 2000s, however, as the number of GP visits at primary health care centres has decreased, while the number of physician visits to occupational health care has increased. Hospitalization rates in Finland have been higher for the lower socioeconomic groups, which is in accordance with the higher morbidity in these groups. Yet those with higher socioeconomic status receive more surgical services than those with lower socioeconomic status despite greater need among the latter (Keskimäki 2003). Women visited a physician more frequently than men, at least since the 1960s, and the difference between the genders has grown, particularly between 1996 and 2004. The number of days in hospital treatment is also higher among women than men (Hemminki et al. 2006). The likelihood for a referral to specialist care is significantly larger in cities than in the rest of the country (Keskimäki 1997).

Norway

According to the Norwegian national strategy to reduce social inequalities in health, the use of specialist health services increases with the length of education and size of income. The pattern is reversed for the use of primary health care services, but not if higher morbidity among those with shorter education and lower income is taken into account. The less educated are referred to a specialist less frequently than the more educated, when poorer health among people with low education is taken into account (Norwegian Ministry of Health and Care Services 2006, p. 25). Furthermore, those with university education visit a private specialist more commonly than those with basic education (Finnvold 2002). A single-hospital study near Oslo found no socioeconomic or gender differences in waiting times for inpatient surgical treatments (Arnesen et al. 2002). Those who live in cities use more health services and are more likely to be referred to a specialist than those who live in the countryside (Fylkesnes 1993). It is not possible to sketch trends in Norway on the basis of the published data.

Sweden

As for Sweden, the higher occupational groups more commonly had a personal physician in the 1980s, while the lower occupational groups paid emergency visits more frequently. In the 1990s, those in higher occupational or income groups seemed to have visited a physician more frequently in relation to their need than those in lower groups (Burström and Foree 2001). A recent study of Stockholm County suggests that those with higher education and income visit a specialist and a private physician more commonly, while those with lower education and income are more likely to visit a GP at a primary health care centre (Walander et al. 2004). Several studies have also reported that those in lower occupational, income or education groups, or unemployed persons, refrain from seeking health care when needed more commonly than those in higher occupational, income or education groups, or employed persons (Burström and Foree 2001; Burström 2002; Westin et al. 2004; Åhs and Westerling 2006). At the end of the 1980s, hospital rates were higher among the lower income groups, but the difference had disappeared by the mid-1990s (Burström 2002). The studies from Sweden do not reveal any clear trend, although there might have been a weak tendency in the 1990s towards the higher socioeconomic groups consuming relatively more services than in the 1980s. Women have used more outpatient and inpatient health care services in Sweden, at least since 1980s (Burström and Foree 2001). Women also tend to refrain from seeking health care more commonly than men (Westin et al. 2004). The threshold for referral to specialist care seems to be lower near larger hospitals (Burström and Foree 2001).

Comparison of countries

To summarize, there is no clear evidence that social differences in the use of health services have been changing in the Nordic countries. There may have been some change towards higher socioeconomic groups visiting a specialist more commonly in Denmark in 1987 to 1994 or in Sweden in the 1990s, but the tendencies are too weak to draw any conclusions. The Finnish data suggest that higher income groups benefit first from new surgical procedures, but the socio-economic differences grow smaller over time as the procedures become more common. In general, the lower occupational, income or educational groups use more GP services in each country, while the higher occupational, income or educational groups use more outpatient specialist services. Therefore, some socioeconomic differences prevail in the use of services – especially when taking into account the fact that lower socioeconomic groups have poorer health and higher need of services. Women use more services than men. Regional differences exist in Finland, Norway and Sweden, which each have large, sparsely populated areas in the north, also in the east in Finland. As an area-wise small and evenly populated country, Denmark does not have such regional differences except for the higher use of specialist services in the capital area.

10.4.2 Coronary heart disease as a case study

Coronary heart disease provides an interesting example as it is a significant cause of mortality. Although the lower socioeconomic groups are affected more commonly by coronary heart disease, studies show that they are treated less intensively in terms of both medication and surgical operations in Denmark (Rasmussen, Gislason et al. 2007; Rasmussen, Rasmussen et al. 2007), Finland (Hetemaa et al. 2003; Keskimäki et al. 2004) and Sweden (Socialstyrelsen 2004). In general, women are affected by coronary heart disease at an older age than men. The symptoms of myocardial infarction may also differ between men and women, with the latter having more associated symptoms such as shortness of breath, nausea and palpitation.

In Sweden, data from a quality register for intensive coronary care (Riks-HIA) show that in 1996–97 females received thrombolytic treatment or percutaneous transluminal coronary angioplasty (PTCA) less commonly than men. The same register data show that women also received coronary angiography less often than men. Age-specific gender differences turned out to be relatively small, however, although they still persisted. In order to build a more comprehensive picture of the gender differences, a more detailed analysis of the Riks-HIA data was conducted to compare the use of bypass operations and PTCA between men and women. The study covered 150,000 patients who had been treated in hospital for acute coronary heart disease during 1991–2000. It revealed that bypass operations were more common among men than women in all socioeconomic and age groups, except for the small group of patients younger than 35 years. In general, men were 1.9 times more likely to receive a bypass operation within two years of onset of acute coronary syndrome. After controlling for age and morbidity other than coronary morbidity, the difference persisted between men and women. When taking into account the severity of coronary changes among men and women, the difference was reduced to 1.7 times more operations for men. The difference was not explained by women having more PTCA operations, as the likelihood that a man would receive bypass operation or PTCA was 1.5 times higher than that a woman would receive either (adjusted for severity of the disease) (Socialstyrelsen 2004, pp. 55–62).

Although the gender differences are considerable, there may be medical reasons behind them. Women tend to have fewer indications for operative treatment and they run a greater risk of death shortly after the operation. Although the Swedish study took into account the severity of the disease, the gender differences persisted. This suggests that gender inequities exist when it comes to invasive treatment for coronary heart disease. According to the study, the differences remained at approximately the same level throughout the 1990s (Socialstyrelsen 2004, pp. 61–2). It has been reported that in Finland, too, women receive invasive treatment for coronary heart disease less commonly than men. The number of coronary operations increased 2.5-fold overall between 1988 and 1996. This increase equalized gender differences to some extent but did not abolish them (Hetemaa et al. 2003).

10.4.3 Dental services

The comparative study of OECD countries revealed pro-rich distribution of dental care in each study country – including Denmark, Finland and Sweden – while Norway was not included in the comparisons (van Doorslaer et al. 2004).

Denmark

Danish national health surveys show that dentist visits have become more common in the adult population in the period 1987–2000, but between 2000 and 2005 there was some decline in the proportion of adults who had visited a dentist within a three-month period. Although the differences between educational groups appear to have grown smaller over the years, the data show consistent socioeconomic gradient, with more dentist visits among the more educated (Ekholm et al. 2006, pp. 178–9). Similarly, a recent survey and register-based study revealed lower use of dental services among the lower socioeconomic groups, attributing it to high levels of co-payments (Gundgaard 2006). Women use dental services more than men, but the differences are smaller than in the use of other health services (Ekholm et al. 2006, pp. 178–9).

Finland

National studies in Finland show similar trends to those in Denmark with regard to increasing use of need-standardized dental services in each income group in 1987–2000, and a small decline in middle income groups in 2000–2004. A consistent socioeconomic gradient similar to that in Denmark can be observed throughout the study period. Differences between income groups decreased in the early 1990s but did not diminish after that. The lower income groups visit a dentist at primary health care more commonly, while the higher income groups use the services of private dentists more frequently (Manderbacka et al. 2006, p. 48). Gender differences in the use of dental services are similar in Finland to those in Denmark (Hemminki et al. 2006). Although the differences are parallel in Finland and in Denmark, it is not possible to compare the degree of inequalities on the basis of existing publications.

Norway

Studies from Norway have not examined longitudinal changes in the use of dental services, but a cross-sectional study in Oslo revealed that the more educated visited a dentist more commonly than the less educated (Grøtvedt 2002a,b). A recent survey study found no association between income and the use of dental care. Differences between men and women were small, although women used dental services slightly more (Holst et al. 2005).

Sweden

Sweden also seems to lack longitudinal studies of the use of dental services. The Swedish National Surveys in 2004 and 2005 observed poorer oral health and lower utilization of dental care services among the lower socioeconomic groups. The lowest socioeconomic group was considerably less likely to seek dental treatment even when they needed it. Men were slightly less likely to have visited a dentist within a two-year period (Wamala et al. 2006).

Comparison of countries

To sum up, the lower socioeconomic groups used dental services less in each Nordic country. There are long-term data available from Denmark and Finland which suggest that socioeconomic differences have decreased to some extent since the end of the 1980s. Women visit a dentist more frequently than men, but gender differences are smaller than in the use of other health services.

10.4.4 Structural factors behind the socioeconomic differences in use of health services

In Finland, Norway and Sweden, the adult population needs to contribute co-payments for visits to health services (except for occupational health services in Finland, see below). This may partly explain the differences in the use of health services, although the co-payments are sufficiently low that they create significant barriers of access only for those least well-off. The Danish and

Finnish health care systems have some specific features that may further contribute to some of the socioeconomic differences observed.

The socioeconomic differences in the use of health services in Denmark have been attributed at least partly to the existence of two health service reimbursement schemes, known as Group 1 and Group 2 and the 'free choice'. The Group 2 scheme allows more freedom than the Group 1 in visits to specialist services without referral, but involves co-payments. The 'free choice' scheme allows Danish patients to visit a specialist or a hospital anywhere in the country, but they must pay travel and associated costs. Although the population shares of Group 2 insurance and the 'free choice' scheme are small (approximately 2 per cent), they have been chosen more commonly by those in higher occupational and education groups. In 1990, individuals in Group 2 used specialist services more than those in Group 1, but this was not because of higher morbidity (McCallum 2004). In 1996, the group with the highest level of education used 'free choice' 33 per cent more than the general population (Sundhedsministeriet 2000).

In Finland, inequities exist also in the use of primary health care services. They have been attributed mainly to the coexistence of municipal primary health care and occupational health services. The latter provide outpatient services with shorter waiting times and no user fees. Use of different primary health care services by different socioeconomic groups affects the socioeconomic differences in public sector specialist services as well, as large amount of referrals to public sector specialist care comes from occupational health care system and private health care (see also Häkkinen 2005).

Citizens in all Nordic countries – except for children and certain special groups – have traditionally needed to contribute significant co-payments for dental care. This is likely to explain part of the socioeconomic differences in the use of dental services. For example, Swedish evidence suggests that the lowest socioeconomic groups refrain more commonly from seeking dental care even when in need of it (Wamala et al. 2006).

10.5 New production environment and new tools

Where priority setting models have been shaped by the planning perspective of health services, they have become outdated (or did not get implemented) because new issues and challenges have emerged. (To be fair, the Lønning I Report referenced technology assessment and Lønning II discussed the health production environment). There are a number of important perspectives now affecting equity.

To define true benefits, risks, adverse effects and also individual patient benefit from a specific medical technology. Health technology assessment (HTA) is an established international approach with analytic methods to assess key dimensions, cost–benefit relations and so on. All HTA agencies, however, struggle with the implementation issue. The implementation and use of HTA results in the management of health systems and the medical practice is a particular challenge. Observed practice patterns, outcomes and results are often quite different from scientifically established practice. This is one explanation for large variations in medical practice and in individual patient use of a technological intervention (e.g. for inequities in medical practice).

To develop and maintain an effective and efficient production system of health services. Several international movements address this issue, for example the quality movement (linking methods and experience from other service industries and other production areas of society) moves to ensure that overuse or underuse of resources does not occur. Those movements also have strong Nordic presence.

To develop definitions of service provisions. A third new issue concerns the services to include in publicly funded health provision (the service basket). This issue has emerged as a result of priority setting exercises, but it has also been highlighted by recent major changes in the financing and delivery of services that challenge the old planning model. The issue is linked to technology assessment but also to new mixes of public–private delivery of services. It should be the best example of explicit prioritization or rationing, clearly a key task for politicians, but not a very popular one.

10.6 Handling the challenges: knowledge-informed health management

The issues discussed above are addressed in all the four Nordic countries. After evolving over five to ten years in the academic health research sphere, they have begun to influence operational health management and health policy. They also have been picked up by national authorities. A good example is Nasjonal kunnskapssenter for helsetjenesten in Oslo, a 120 person unit (mostly researchers) independently based but closely linked to Helsedirektoratet. The main task is to deliver the summarized scientific evidence base for activities over the entire spectrum of the health services. STAKES in Finland can be seen as a similar body (although shaped earlier). Sweden still has a more diversified structure on these issues. There are in Sweden, however, good examples of national registries and practice monitoring (60 different medical quality registries), which illuminate key dimensions of performances clearly be linked to the performance (equity) of the system. The National Board of Health produces knowledge-based guidelines incorporating evidence perspectives with detailed advice/directives for different conditions: 'not to do-list' and so on. A similar line of activity is found in all four Nordic countries.

The equity perspective should be safeguarded with additional new measures and tools that reflect the future agenda. However, the 'old' tools such as resource allocation, payment mechanisms and incentives should not be forgotten. An important issue is to maintain the tradition of collecting statistics and monitoring the system. Open and accessible data collection forms one dimension of this. In a far-reaching privatization scheme, it is possible that this openness could become an issue. Any decline of the quality of data through poor functioning of the public system could become another threat. A linked concern is the possibility that, in the public political sphere, a gap between rhetoric and reality could emerge, again making publicly assessable data a key to a more informed discussion.

10.7 Concluding remarks

The equity principle is deeply embedded in the Nordic health services systems. As has been noted in Chapter 1, it may very well be the dimension that is most central in what is somewhat loosely termed the 'Nordic model'. This is a basic value in all the Nordic societies and it is closely linked to other concepts such as 'solidarity'. A main argument for tax financing has, of course, been linked to equity, and the controlling role of politicians in the use of tax money is motivated by this. Therefore, the very construction of these systems is thought to safeguard equity.

A number of instrumental mechanisms have been developed to direct Nordic health systems toward equity goals:

- health care laws specifically outline this goal
- mechanisms for resource allocation have been key elements to link resources and services to needs
- the needs-based service goal has been underscored in law, in distinction to a demand-based system
- techniques to measure health in different population groups have advanced considerably, making it possible to contrast planning goals with the actual outcome for particular groups; it has also become possible to further refine the resource distribution models
- other techniques and tools direct services toward equity goals: reports on the general picture and the situation for specific groups create awareness; ethics committees can focus on ethical analysis of the fundamental dilemmas in health services and concrete links to changes service delivery.

The priority setting models described earlier in this chapter seek to safeguard equity in the new situation that started to emerge more clearly between 1985 and 1995. Norway was the pioneer in this aspect, in 1987, and was soon followed by similar committees and public documents in Sweden, Denmark and Finland. The priority setting commissions discussed the health systems goal of achieving – and safeguarding – equity in a situation with a marked change in production circumstances for the health systems. The era of limitless expansion was over and the issue of how to handle finite resources in relation to steadily increasing demands became the main concern for the priority commissions. Important new dimensions for health politics, policy and management, were introduced through the discussion documents that the priority commissions published. The concept of *limits* was important although it was perhaps mainly understood as limits motivated by the lack of resources – and the priority setting discussion may still have this perspective. There also are important observations of medical systems that in *actual working* have considerable variation in the results obtained from the resources put into it. The original methods and techniques developed with priority groups mainly linked to resource distribution did address some of these issues.

Considerable development work was done subsequently, stimulated by the priority setting exercises of the 1990s. One example is the work with national guidelines in Sweden, incorporating key elements addressing effects and results of defined interventions. This work is also linked to the national quality registries that are at present only partly used as sources for information on the outcome of interventions. Another approach incorporates quality and process development activities. These present a different perspective on the issue of resource constraints, namely that improvement of work processes can have very significant effects.

Both the technology assessment movement and the quality movement are important areas of activity internationally. The Nordic countries are actively involved and often used as good examples of successfully introducing these methods into planned health systems that gave greater scope for results than in the less-planned systems, such as in the United States, where much of the basic development of these methods first occurred.

There is, therefore, a 'developmental path' where the priority setting exercises and models of the 1980s and 1990s move on to what has been named the era of 'assessment and accountability' (Relman 1988). Measuring the outcome of different interventions, both in a test bed and in regular practice, will become increasingly important. Physicians and other decision-makers will be held accountable for the use of resources in relation to new standards. Work on more sophisticated guidelines is under way, and there are interesting prospects for computerized medical records, when physicians will be able to monitor clinical outcomes easily, and also compliance to guidelines both for patient groups and for individuals. Prototypes for this are already under way in the United States integrated systems (for example, the Kaiser Permanente system) and these methods will presumably also have great potential for effective use in Nordic systems.

This development and its meaning for the actors in the health system can best be summarized under the phrase 'knowledge management'. It will build on a number of multidisciplinary competencies now emerging and being linked to the tradition of registration and measurement within health services. This is an area where the Nordic health systems have a long tradition, and it will be important for the development path for the equity dimension within Nordic systems.

Despite the significance of the equity principle for Nordic health service systems, each Nordic country has a systematic socioeconomic gradient in health that benefits those in higher socioeconomic groups. Nevertheless, the gradients are less steep than in many other countries, for example the United Kingdom and Germany. It is difficult to estimate the influence of health services in reducing health inequalities between different socioeconomic groups, as more general mechanisms in the welfare systems are also likely to play a role. Yet it has been suggested recently that the influence of health services has been increasing, owing to the early detection and treatment of certain cancers and significantly improved treatment results for major diseases (Leppo 2007). Up to half of the decrease in deaths from coronary disease has been contributed by the actions of health services in recent research in the United States (Ford et al. 2007). Therefore, it seems that health services can have an increasing role in health promotion and in narrowing health inequalities (see also Nolte and McKee 2004).

There is no general pattern in the Nordic countries that implies a development of increasing – nor decreasing – socioeconomic difference in the use of health services. This is true especially for primary care. However, there are observations of socioeconomic gradients in more highly specialized services, such as coronary care. Where this is observed, there are well-established links to higher social class and better access to services to explain better outcome. The Finnish experience suggests that inequalities decrease when new treatment forms become more common. The socioeconomic differences can result from many factors, such as attitudes towards health, care-seeking patterns and doctor–patient interaction, but certain structures in health care systems seem to produce and maintain inequalities in Denmark and particularly in Finland. There are still insufficient published data on other equity dimensions such as regional differences, gender and ethnicity.

In summary, the Nordic countries have put equity at the forefront of their health systems. It is part of a value base that underpins the whole society and this goal is reflected in the construction of these health systems. A number of mechanisms have also been developed to address the issue in concrete terms: the resource planning instruments and the population perspective. The priority setting models marked a phase of awareness and concern for equity when resource constraints started to be visible. At the same time these models – and especially the discussion around them – pointed to new issues and circumstances that needed to be addressed to safeguard equity. Effectiveness and efficiency regarding outcome and a perspective of organizational and process improvement are new important perspectives and tools. The political pendulum has also introduced new ideas such as 'new public management' (Chapter 1). Concrete action within the political sphere in the Nordic countries has now introduced more free choice for patients, some competition between providers and also some degree of private financing. As free choice and the share of private financing increase, socioeconomic differences are likely to increase, because the most vulnerable groups in society may not be capable of utilizing these options to the same extent as the general population.

The lesson learned so far is that equity is not safeguarded solely by relying on planning models and resource distribution formulae. Even before market and competition elements were really introduced into the Nordic systems, the limitations of this approach could be seen.

One important characteristic of the health system is the way new tools (summarized under the term 'knowledge management') can be added to the old ones. It is not likely that there will be a replacement or total shift, more likely the system will learn to use the new tools to enhance functions in the earlier ones.

References

Åhs, A.M.H. and Westerling, R. (2006) Health care utilization among persons who are unemployed or outside the labour force. *Health Policy* 78: 178–93.

Arnesen, K.E., Erikssen J. and Stavem K. (2002) Gender and socioeconomic status as determinants of waiting time for inpatient surgery in a system with implicit queue management, *Health Policy* 62: 329–41.

Burström, B. (2002) Increasing inequalities in health care utilisation across income groups in Sweden during the 1990s? *Health Policy* 62: 117–29.

Burstörm, B. and Foree, L.N. (2001) *Vård på lika villkor? En litteraturgenomgång av studier av vårdutnyttjande I olika grupper.* Stockholm: Socialmedicin.

Calltorp, J. (1999) Priority setting in health policy in Sweden and a comparison with Norway. *Health Policy* 50: 1–22.

Ekholm, O., Kjøller, D.M., Hesse, U., Erisken, L., Illemann, C.A. and Grønbæk, M. (2006) *Sundhed og sygelighed I Danmark 2005 and udviklingen siden 1987.* Copenhagen: Statens Institut for Folkesundhed.

Finnvold, J.E. (2002) *Bestemmer behovene broken av legespesialistene? Sosialt utsyn 2002: Helse og omsorgstjenstene.* Oslo: Statistisk Sentralbyrå.

Ford, E.S., Ajani, U.A., Croft, J.B. et al. (2007) Explaining the decrease in US deaths from coronary disease, 1980–2000, *New England Journal of Medicine* 356: 2388–98.

Fuchs, V.R. (1998) *Who Shall Live? Health, Economics, and Social Choice*, expanded edn. London: World Scientific Publishing.

Fylkesnes, K. (1993) Determimants of health care utilization: visits and referrals, *Scandinavian Journal of Social Medicine* 21: 40–50.

Grøholt, E.-K., Stigum, H., Nordhagen, R. and Köhler, L. (2003) Health service utilization in the Nordic countries in 1996. Influence of socio-economic factors among children with and without chronic health conditions, *European Journal of Public Health* 13: 30–7.

Grøtvedt, L. (2002a) *Helseprofil for Oslo:Voksene. Nasjonalt folkehelseinstitutt.* Oslo: Program for storbyrettet forskning.

Grøtvedt, L. (2002b) *Helseprofil for Oslo: Eldre. Nasjonalt folkehelseinstitutt.* Oslo: Program for storbyrettet forskning.

Gundgaard, J. (2006) Income-related inequality in utilization of health services in Denmark: evidence from Funen County, *Scandinavian Journal of Public Health* 34: 462–71.

Haglund, B. (2004) Social differences in utilization of ambulatory care, in *Health Statistics in the Nordic Countries 2002.* Copenhagen: NOMESCO, pp. 222–37.

Häkkinen, U. (2005) The impact of changes in Finland's health care system, *Health Economics* 14(Suppl): S101–18.

Hemminki, E., Luoto, R. and Gissler, M. (2006) Sukupuolierot terveyspalveluiden kohdentumisessa, in Teperi J., Vuorenkoski, L., Manderbacka, K., Ollila, E and Keskimäki, I. (eds) *Riittävät palvelut jokaiselle: Näkökulmia yhdenvertaisuuteen sosiaali- ja terveydenhuollossa.* Helsinki: STAKES, University of Helsinki, pp. 56–63.

Hetemaa, T., Keskimäki, I., Manderbacka, K., Leyland A.H. and Koskinen S. (2003) How did the recent increase in the supply of coronary operations in Finland affect socio-economic and gender equity in their use? *Journal of Epidemiology and Community Health* 57: 178–85.

Holst, D., Grytten, J. and Skau, I. (2005) Den voksne befolknings bruk av tannhelsetjenester i Norge i 2004, *Den Norske Tannlegeforenings Tidende* 115: 212–16.

Keskimäki, I. (1997) *Social Equity in the Use of Hospital Inpatient Care in Finland.* Helsinki: STAKES, University of Helsinki.

Keskimäki, I. (2003) How did Finland's economic recession in the early 1990s affect socio-economic equity in the use of hospital care? *Social Science and Medicine* 56: 1517–30.

Keskimäki, I., Aalto, A., Häkkinen, U. et al. (2004) *Raportteja 286: Sepelvaltimotauti ja eriarvoisuus. Kyselytutkimus sepelvaltimotautia sairastavien oireilusta, hoidosta ja elämäntavoista.* Helsinki: STAKES, University of Helsinki.

Lahelma, E., Kivelä, K., Roos, E. et al. (2002) Analysing changes of health inequalities in the Nordic welfare states, *Social Science and Medicine* 55: 609–25.

Leppo, K. (2007) Kansanterveys, terveyserot ja yhteiskuntapolitiikka. Jäähyväisluento

24.10.2007. [Public health, health inequalities, and social policy. Farewell lecture 24.10.2007]. *Sosiaalilääketieteellinen aikakauslehti [Journal of Social Medicine]*, 44: 228–38.

McCallum, A. (2004) Socio-economic differences in use of specialist services in Nordic countries, in *Health Statistics in the Nordic Countries 2002*. Copenhagen: NOMESCO, pp. 204–22.

Manderbacka, K., Gissler, M., Husman, K. et al. (2006) Väestöryhmien välinen eriarvoisuus terveyspalvelujen käytössä, in Teperi J., Vuorenkoski, L., Manderbacka, K., Ollila, E and Keskimäki, I. (eds) *Riittävät palvelut jokaiselle. Näkökulmia yhdenvertaisuuteen sosiaali- ja terveydenhuollossa*. Helsinki: STAKES, University of Helsinki, pp. 42–55.

Nolte, E. and McKee M. (2004) *Does Health Care Save Lives? Avoidable Mortality Revisited*. London: Nuffield Trust.

Norwegian Ministry of Health and Care Services (2006) *Report No. 20 (2006–2007) to the Storting: National Strategy to Reduce Social Inequalities in Health*. Oslo: Norwegian Ministry of Health and Care Services.

NOU (1987) *NOU 1987: 23. Retningslinjer for prioritering innen norsk helsetjeneste*. Oslo: Ministry of Health and Care Services.

NOU (1997) *NOU 1997:18. Prioriteringer på ny*. Oslo: Ministry of Health and Care Services.

Rasmussen, J.N., Gislason, G.H., Rasmussen, S. et al. (2007) Use of statins and beta-blockers after acute myocardial infarction according to income and education, *Journal of Epidemiology and Community Health* 61: 1091–7.

Rasmussen, J.N., Rasmussen, S., Gislason, G.H. et al. (2007) Persistent socio-economic differences in revascularisation after acute myocardial infarction despite a universal health care system: a Danish study, *Cardiovascular Drugs Therapy* 21: 449–57.

Relman, A.S. (1988) Assessment and accountability. *New England Journal of Medicine* 319: 1220–2.

Smedby, B. (2003) Validity and comparability of Nordic day surgery statistics, in *Health Statistics in the Nordic Countries 2001*. Copenhagen: NOMESCO, pp. 211–64.

Socialstyrelsen [National Board of Health and Welfare] (2004) *Jämställd vård? Könsperspektiv på hälso- och sjukvården*. Stockholm: National Board of Health and Welfare; www.socialstyrelsen.se, accessed May 2008.

Sundhedsministeriet [Ministry of Health] (2000) *Sundhedsanalyser 2000:2. Social ulighed i sundhed. Forskelle I helbred, livsstil og brug af sundhedsvæsenet. 2. delrapport fra Middellevetidsudvalget*. Copenhagen: Nyt Nordisk Forlag Arnold Busck.

Thorsen, G., Nikiforov, O., Lynge Sandegaard, J., Segadal, L., Serdén, L. and Virtanen, M. (2002) Validity and comparability of Nordic hospital statistics on surgical procedures, in *Health Statistics in the Nordic Countries 2000*. Copenhagen: NOMESCO, pp. 213–72.

van Doorslaer, E., Masseria, C., Koolman, X. for the OECD Health Equity Health Group (2004) Income-related inequality in the use of medical care in 21 OECD countries, in *The OECD Health Project: Towards High-performing Health Systems*. Paris: OECD, pp. 109–65.

Walander, A., Ålander, S. and Burstörm, B. (2004) *Sociala skillnader I vårdutnyttjande. Yrkesverksamma åldrar. Värd pä lika villkor Rapport 1/2004*. Stockholm: Smahällsmedicin.

Wamala, S., Merlo, J. and Boström, G. (2006) Inequity in access to dental care services explains current socioeconomic disparities in oral health: the Swedish National Surveys of Public Health 2004–2005, *Journal of Epidemiology and Community Health* 60: 1027–33.

Westin, M., Åhs, A., Bränd Persson, K. and Westerling, R. (2004) A large proportion of Swedish citizens refrain from seeking medical care: lack of confidence in the medical services a plausible explanation, *Health Policy* 68: 333–44.

Working Group on Health Care Prioritization (1995) *From Values to Choices*. Helsinki: STAKES.

chapter eleven

Reforming primary health care

Allan Krasnik and Bård Paulsen

11.1 Introduction

The role of primary health care has been a major health policy issue since the Second World War. Community medicine with a focus on primary care, community health centres and population health was seen as an interesting and promising trend by many public health experts, health service researchers and primary health care professionals during the 1960s (Kark 1974). The Alma Ata Declaration in 1978 was an important inspiration for many health policy-makers around the world, leading to national official goals to promote primary health care as the key mechanism for promoting population health through the delivery of basic health services and gatekeeping roles for specialized care. During the 1970s and 1980s, the WHO under the leadership of the Danish General-Director Halfdan Mahler gave strong support to this development – with a special focus on low-income countries with serious population health problems, limited resources for health care and few specialized services. However, in most countries, health budgets and policy initiatives were still mainly directed towards specialized hospital care, not least in the wealthy industrialized countries, leading the rapid biotechnological development that mainly supported the specialized care of individual patients.

The Nordic countries were not an exception to this rule in spite of the differences in the structure and the development of primary health care in the five Nordic countries. Whereas hospital care in all the Nordic countries has been based on the same general principles of tax-funded public hospital services, the role and organization of primary health care has varied substantially according to historical trends, geography and human resources, but also according to social and cultural factors affecting public administration and services in general. However, in all the Nordic countries, health policy discussions and health care reforms during recent years have given attention to the potential of primary care, the problems related to lack of integration and continuity of care, the growing needs for rehabilitation of patients with chronic disorders, and prevention and health promotion for the general population.

The concept of primary health care is not very distinct. The Alma Ata statement emphasized a broad, multidisciplinary and population-oriented perspective on primary care (Cueto 2004). However, many articles discuss primary care as a kind of extended general practice (Moore and Showstack 2003; Meads 2006). Types of service considered as parts of primary health care may vary considerably, even between closely related systems such as those in the Nordic countries, as will be shown in the discussion in this chapter. The term primary care is usually associated with a local community perspective (Haggarty et al. 2007). It may, however, be organized and financed at municipal, county or state level. When discussing primary care, we must allow for both the ambiguity of the concept itself and the diversity between countries.

As a starting point, Barbara Starfield's (1998) much cited definition highlights several important common elements:

> Primary care is that level of a health system that provides entry into the system for all needs and problems, provides person-focused (not disease-oriented) care over time, provides care for all but very uncommon or unusual conditions, and coordinates or integrates care provided elsewhere by others.
> (Starfield 1998, pp. 8–9)

Important in Starfield's definition are:

- accessibility: low threshold, combined with a wide and inclusive perspective on people's needs and problems
- continuity of care over time
- a gateway to the overall health care system
- an agent for coordination of care provided in other parts of the health care system.

In the Nordic countries, these elements, alongside tax-based funding, are constitutive in the various primary health care systems, even though the organizational and political/administrative solutions differ very much between countries. The variations in primary health care and related health care reforms across the five Nordic countries, despite many social and cultural similarities and being Beveridge-type health systems, provide fine opportunities for comparative analyses. This chapter provides a short overview of the reform trends related to primary health care in Denmark, Norway, Finland and Sweden during recent decades and discusses some of the key policy issues that have dominated reform trends. These include:

- problems of access, staffing and quality
- balancing public–private provision of primary care
- introducing new organizational models
- interactions of primary health care, social services and hospital care, with a special focus on initiatives related to coordination and continuity.

This presentation excludes private practising specialists as part of primary health care as their roles and functions parallel the specialized hospital services.

Lastly, the chapter examines the future prospects for a possible 'Nordic model' for primary care in the light of general characteristics and trends regarding accessibility, continuity, gatekeeping and coordination.

11.2 Reforming primary health care in Denmark

Historically, private practising GPs were distributed very early across the whole country and were more numerous in Denmark than in most other countries for centuries (Vallgårda and Krasnik 2007). This was partly because of the relative wealth of the country, but also because private non-profit health insurance organizations were established – first by craft guilds and then, during the last part of the nineteenth century, also by groups of local citizens and farmers. These organizations ensured a reasonable income for the private practising GPs even outside the urbanized areas as well as health care for members on the basis of an annual fee. The state increasingly gave financial support and in 1933 compulsory membership was established for people with low incomes. More and more people joined and public funding gradually increased. In 1973, the health insurance system was taken over by the counties because 90 per cent of the population were members and the expenses were mainly covered by tax-financed public money. However, the general structure and payment systems were maintained. The GPs were still private practitioners and their reimbursement was based on a mixture of fee for service and capitation. An exception to this rule occurred in the City of Copenhagen where GPs were employed by the Municipality of Copenhagen (which had county as well as municipal roles) and reimbursed almost entirely through capitation. However, in 1987 the system was changed also in Copenhagen, and since then the organization and financing of general practice has been the same in the whole country.

From 1973, the counties and municipalities were the major political–administrative health agents in primary health care: the counties mainly through their role in the financing of the national health insurance system and the municipalities through their responsibilities as employers of certain groups of health professionals.

As a consequence, the Danish health care system has been separated into three major elements: (1) the private health care providers (GPs, most of the dentists, physiotherapists and private practising specialists), (2) the public (and the few private) hospitals, and (3) the municipal primary health services (public health nurses, home nurses and child dentistry). This division of care has been a major challenge for achieving a coordinated, integrated health care system that ensures a clear division of tasks and continuity of care for the patients.

The state has played a very limited role, mainly as a partner in the annual budget negotiations between the state and the counties and the municipalities, the last being introduced in 1980 and having a strong impact on resource allocations to health care. The state, however, has tried to cope with the division of health care since 1994 by mandating coordinated health plans every four years between counties and municipalities. The health plans included a description of the health status of the population and the available services as well as an indication of the nature and extent of cooperation between municipalities in the region and the county – and with other counties. The coordination process varied from county to county but is often based on meetings, seminars and joint committee work focusing on specific subjects such as the elderly or mental health. However, the effect of this has been quite limited (Seeman 2003; Strandberg-Larsen et al. 2007) and it mainly serves as a symbolic act to demonstrate willingness to collaborate more than a tool for actual coordination.

The GPs have been seen as key actors in the health care system on the basis of their role as continuous health care providers for the individual and the family and as gatekeepers to specialized services (Christiansen 1999). The free-standing individual position as the 'advocate' of the patient, the frequent contacts with the patients (about six contacts per year for the general population) and the rather even distribution of GPs over the country have been described as major characteristics ensuring easy and equal access to qualified services in the country. Also financing by a mixed fee for service and capitation has been seen as a positive factor, combining the advantages and reducing the disadvantages of both systems (Mooney 2002). However, the free-standing position, the many single practices and the more and more dominating role of fee for service might have an adverse impact on the quality of care by creating problems of continuity of care, resistance to change and large variations in the patterns of care.

The 2007 structural reform and new initiatives regarding health centres, quality indicators and special fees are trying to deal with these problems.

The major structural reform of the Danish political–administrative system in 2007 mainly changed the platform for hospitals in Denmark. However, primary health care was also affected directly and indirectly by the changes. Whereas the GPs have been transferred from the counties to the regions without changing their general position, functions or financing, the larger municipalities have been given new and stronger roles in prevention and rehabilitation in order to reduce blurred borders between the regional and local responsibilities and to strengthen activities focusing on prevention and rehabilitation of chronic diseases. New requirements regarding health plans have also been introduced. Regional consultative committees are established with representation from the region, the municipalities and private practice, and the plans must include agreements on discharge from the hospital for weak and elderly patients, social services for people with mental disorders and, not least, agreements on prevention and rehabilitation.

In order to support prevention and rehabilitation by municipalities with limited traditions and competence in these areas, the government has initiated a programme of health centres. Special funding for a limited time and limited number of centres has been established, and 19 proposals for new centres have been funded around the country. Teams of professionals with different tasks are employed, and the very different profiles and functions of these centres will be evaluated over the coming years in order to provide guidelines for future health centres. Many GPs, however, have been quite negative towards these initiatives, fearing political–administrative dominance and interference with their professional freedom. The GPs are, therefore, not represented in the health centre teams, but they are in some cases close collaborators and referring agents. Therefore, the problems of continuity of care are still not solved and the centres might even add to the fragmentation of the system by introducing a new element within the health care organization.

The role of the GPs as coordinators of care might be strengthened in the future by the introduction of a new fee for service. The GP will get a special annual fee for coordinating the care of each patient with a chronic disease. This requires that the GP identifies the patients included and agrees to carry out certain tasks defined in the programme for the specific patients involved. The first phase of this new agreement includes patients with diabetes. Using specific fees in order to stimulate new activities among GPs has always been an element in the general agreements between the Organization of General Practitioners (PLO) and the counties. Examples of this include a fee for preventive visits with the GP, including examinations and advising, and a fee for collaboration with social welfare authorities regarding social/medical problems of patients.

Strengthening collaboration between primary health care and hospitals has been a clear objective, but difficult in practice. Special practice coordinators representing GPs in the catchment area have been appointed by hospitals in order to facilitate collaboration, and joint emergency services based on collaboration between GPs and hospitals have been established.

A national quality indicator programme has been initiated based on general and national standards and monitoring procedures; however, this only includes primary health care activities to a very limited extent at present. Whereas waiting times have been a major issue in relation to hospital care, it has not been as important in primary health care. Limitations regarding waiting times for planned visits in general practice are in place, but new proposals have been put forward for maximal waiting time for other services in primary health care. A national initiative regarding the quality of public services has been established by the government. This will probably lead to the development of further standards for services including primary health care as well as new monitoring systems based on consumer surveys and other quality indicators.

Freedom of choice of GP has always been a right for citizens, but this has been gradually extended regarding distance and frequency of changes. The 2007 reform introduced new patient rights regarding choice of municipal rehabilitation programmes, which implies that patients can decide to opt for a programme in another municipality. As with the free choice of hospitals, this complicates coordination between different services as the number of potential partners will increase.

The public–private mix has been an issue in several ways (Krasnik 2004). The GPs as private practising professionals working almost entirely on the basis of tax-based remuneration have been a key feature of Danish primary health care for many years, and there is little support for publicly employed GPs. In contrast, municipal primary health care is based on publicly employed health staff, including some physicians responsible for public health activities focusing on special groups (e.g. children, the elderly, socially disadvantaged), but they do not provide individual care. Out-sourcing of home care has been a theme, but so far only limited in extent. However, the possibility for patients to choose private alternatives for some services, financed by the municipality, might strengthen the role of private providers. This has been the case for some time for child dentistry, where private dentists are entitled to provide publicly financed preventive dental care for children below 18 years of age.

During the last decades, status and income have improved for GPs, and recruitment of doctors to primary care has been relatively easy. This has partly been facilitated by the introduction of general medicine (family medicine) as a specialty, the establishment of university departments in general practice and new chairs and research units financed jointly by the counties and the Association of General Practitioners. However, the general lack of trained medical doctors in the country has recently started to cause problems for recruitment to general practice especially in rural areas and districts with many social problems, such as a high number of immigrants. This will certainly threaten the further development of primary health care; patients will have to travel further to see a doctor and some of the tasks which are today seen as part of the role of the medical doctor will have to be taken over by other professional groups. The same trend is seen in municipal primary health care, where recruitment of fully trained nurses is getting more difficult.

11.3 Reforming primary health care in Norway

Primary health care in Norway is a municipal responsibility. The legislative basis for modern Norwegian primary care is the Law of Municipal Health Care, which took effect in 1984. The law gave Norwegian municipalities both responsibility and funding for planning and organizing what today is termed municipal health services: general practice, physiotherapists, public health nurses, home nursing and home helpers. New political/administrative structures were established. To ease collaboration and integration between the various health care services, many municipalities chose to organize health care centres, responsible for well-defined geographical areas. Four years after the reform, nursing homes were included. Caregiving to old people or others who need it is a dominant and growing part of the activity in the 431 Norwegian municipalities, and this is very important for understanding current trends in Norwegian primary health care.

Geographical inequalities between central communities and more remote ones in access to health services has traditionally been an important issue in health politics in Norway. Recruiting GPs to sparsely populated communities has been difficult. Physiotherapists were found almost exclusively in towns of some size. As a remedy, a municipality could choose to offer a GP or a physiotherapist a fixed salary, to reduce risk and cost when establishing a practice. However, this was insufficient to solve the problems. A salaried position is easy to take and equally easy to leave. And so many smaller communities experienced a very unstable situation, with GPs just passing through on their way to a more attractive private practice in a bigger city.

In 2001, a list patient system was introduced. The reimbursement system was changed, leaving the doctors with approximately 30 per cent per capita and 70 per cent fee for service. When introducing the list patient system in 2001, the fixed salary option was abolished (except for GPs already hired on such terms), and general practice was thereby privatized. The patient-payment share was kept at approximately the same level as before the reform. The list patient system gave every inhabitant a right to a place on a GP's list. During the process of patient listing, however, GPs in the bigger cities experienced a lack of patients because of the traditional excess of doctors there. Many newcomers to the GP profession were forced to establish their practice outside the most central municipalities. In the years after the reform, the list patient system seemed to contribute to a more even geographical distribution of GPs in Norway (Finnvold et al. 2005). Even so, inhabitants in many remote communities continue to experience unsatisfactory access to primary care (Lian 2003).

By the nursing home reform in 1988, municipalities acquired overall responsibility for nursing and home-help services for elderly people and others who need it. An important consequence was the introduction of a sharp division of responsibility between specialist medical care to be given in hospitals, and nursing services to be given by the municipalities. In the years that followed, heavy pressure was put on municipalities to take responsibility for old long-term patients waiting in hospital for municipal care. During the next decade, the volume of caregiving service within the municipalities grew, including care for mentally disabled persons and mental health care. Using the consumption of person-labour per year as a measure, municipal care today more than outnumbers the hospital sector (Sosial- og helsedirektoratet 2006).

For economic and planning purposes, many bigger Norwegian municipalities have introduced a functional split between the assessment of needs (purchaser) and the provider of services within the municipal organization. In some municipalities, an internal quasi-market within the municipal organization was created; in other, municipalities created a real market with competing public, private voluntary organizations or private commercial ones. Since the mid-1990s, private for-profit enterprises have provided both nursing homes and home-based services for the elderly in many Norwegian municipalities. The introduction and growth of private service is heavily debated and is an important political question in the municipal elections. Privatization on the provider side, however, has not been followed by privatization on the consumer side.

Traditionally, the Norwegian health authorities have well-developed statistics concerning the resources used and the number of clients served, but not concerning quality of the services rendered. In 2003, the Ministry of Health introduced a regulation on quality standards in municipal care. At the same time, the municipalities were obliged to establish routines to ensure their fulfilment, and make data on quality of care available to their inhabitants. On the national level, however, no systems were established for standardizing, reporting, processing and publishing these data, which would have enabled a comparison to be made of patient satisfaction between the municipalities. The IPLOS system, an elaborated user register, was implemented in 2006, giving detailed information on the functional status of the municipal clients, their needs and the help given; this was in preparation for systematic reporting nationwide. A system called SEDA was established for monitoring general practice, based on data from 80 representative GP journals from doctors situated in various part of the country. This system is, however, not aimed at comparisons between municipalities.

11.3.1 *Integrating primary health care*

Lack of integration between the various parts of the health care system became increasingly a central issue in Norwegian health policies. The problems addressed and the measures taken may be discussed at a patient level, as a question concerning coordination within the municipal primary health care organization and as a question concerning the relationship between primary health care and hospitals.

On the patient level, 'the individual plan' is intended to be an important integrative mechanism. Psychiatric patients, patients with learning difficulties, the elderly and people living with chronic and disabling illnesses often have to face the problem of lack of coordination between the various parts of the health care system, on which they are dependent. Since 2004, people who need coordinated services from different sources for a longer period or continuously are entitled to an 'individual plan'. The individual plan is a formal document specifying the applicant's needs, measures to be taken and persons responsible. Personnel in both primary health care and in hospitals are obliged to initiate an individual plan when those entitled to it seek their help.

On the organizational level, the municipalities are facing new challenges. In the years after the 1984 reform, when primary health care obtained its legislative, financial and organizational foothold in the municipalities, a district- or area-oriented model of organization was implemented in most cities and bigger municipalities in order to facilitate collaboration and integration. Health centres were built, in some municipalities including social services as well. When introducing the patient list system in 2001, however, people were free to choose a doctor wherever they pleased, not limited by municipal district or area organization. In many Norwegian municipalities, the introduction of the list patient system challenged a strategy of integration by colocalization and a shared-area responsibility between GPs and other parts of the primary heath care organization.

A growing number of people with physical disabilities, both young and old, being cared for in their own homes are dependent on efficient collaboration between nurses and doctors for medical service. However, a study undertaken by the central state medical supervising authorities during 2006 revealed that the collaborative patterns between GPs and home-care personnel were inefficient in large part: these patients were not able to go to their GP's office very often; they had to wait a long time for their doctor's visit and very often had to turn to the emergency ward for help (Sosial- og Helsedirektoratet 2006). Similarly, a study of municipal services in primary health care for patients with mental health problems revealed that GPs were often very reluctant to engage in collaborative structures concerning their patients (Ådnanes and Bjørngaard 2006).

For residents in nursing homes, medical service is given by a visiting doctor, contractually hired for some hours a week. This practice was not changed by the list patient reform. Studies showed that the amount of medical service in nursing homes varied greatly between municipalities, some places probably being reduced to what was considered unacceptable levels (Sosial- og helsedirektoratet 2005). The findings triggered a debate in the Norwegian Parliament, where several representatives argued that a system of central state regulations on the level of medical service within nursing homes was needed to secure an acceptable standard in the care of the elderly. The proposal of state-regulated minimum standards was rejected. Instead, a system of annual reports of GP hours in nursing homes was introduced. Although not using explicit norms, state surveillance and comparative statistics are intended to force the municipalities to raise the standard of medical service in nursing homes.

At the turn of this century, the Norwegian health sector went through major reforms at both hospital and primary care levels. On the hospital side, ownership was transferred from counties to central state health authorities. Important aims were to reduce the many conflicts between local county authorities and central state, to create more efficient structures for planning and leadership, and to achieve more efficient production of hospital services. Today, the Norwegian health sector has only two political/administrative layers: municipalities and the central state. However, the process of parallel growth, reform and developmental work, within both hospitals and the municipal health service, was triggered in each sector by its own culture and organizational rationality, leaving many important questions of coordination between them unresolved. As the county–state axis vanished, the hospital–primary health care axis received more attention and became more negotiable. In 2006, an agreement was made between the Ministry of Health and the Association of Norwegian Municipalities stating joint obligations to improve the patterns of collaboration between the five regional state-owned enterprises of specialist health care and primary health care. Important topics included the patterns of collaboration related to admittance and discharge from hospitals, especially for the elderly needing medical attention and nursing after discharge.

The term integrated care is based on the assumption that an episode of care should be experienced by the patient as a smooth and foreseeable process, with necessary help given at the right time and in the right amount (Haggerty et al. 2003). An example of the practical measures instituted is the organization of intermediate wards, economically a joint venture between hospitals and municipalities and organized like a nursing home with extended medical and nursing service; these take care of fragile elderly patients temporarily after hospital treatment. The purpose of the stay at the intermediate ward is to prepare the patients for returning to their own homes. Other practical measures are the development of district medical centres, giving outpatient medical service in centres in remote districts, various projects aimed at developing electronic communication systems between hospitals and primary health, and a consultant system giving doctors working in primary health care better access to specialists in hospitals.

11.4 Reforming primary health care in Finland

The organization and function of primary health care in Finland is strongly affected by the decentralized political–administrative system, with 448 municipalities. The long historical tradition of local governing and its role in primary health care was further strengthened by the 1972 Primary Health Care Act, which defined the obligation of municipalities to provide general health care for their citizens. This obligation was described in broad terms and allowed for large variations in the actual performance of these functions. The concept of health centres, however, was a key element and a platform for services – either as centres owned by the municipalities individually or as ones owned jointly with others. As an alternative, municipalities were allowed to purchase primary health care from private providers, but this has been limited in take-up at present. The very different geographical and demographic characteristics of the municipalities, including large variation in the size of the population, gave rise to different solutions for primary health care provision across the country. Only 25 per cent of the municipalities had more than 10,000 inhabitants and 20 per cent had fewer than 2000. The state had little power or tools to influence developments, and this was further reduced by the State Subsidy Reform in 1993, which gave more independence to municipalities regarding changes in the organization of care (Häkkinen and Lehto 2005).

Health centres are not always 'within walls'. Many spread over different locations especially in larger, urban areas. The personnel are publicly employed and include various professionals such as GPs, nurses, midwives, dentists, physiotherapists and medical specialists in different combinations. The centres can also include one or more inpatient departments, typically with 30–60 beds and mostly providing care for elderly, chronically ill patients, but in some instances even short-term curative functions. Some centres have taken over smaller hospitals as part of their function.

Problems with continuity of care have been an issue since the establishment of the centres, as no direct link between the doctor and the patient was estab-lished in the form of patient lists for individual doctors. This was dealt during the 1980s by some municipalities through the development of a 'personal doc-tor system' within the health centres or with a number of private physicians responsible for a population of 1600–3100 patients as part of a special project (Vohlonen et al. 1989). Some of the biggest municipalities have divided their populations into several local integrated social and health service stations, which are responsible for the local listed citizens' primary social and health services. The units have their 'own' listed patients/clients, and every citizen should know his/her 'own' physician, if appointed, or at least should know the particular social and health station where he/she should go if necessary. Waiting time for a visit with a doctor has been an issue as well, and the 'personal doctor system' seemed to reduce waiting time substantially.

In order to enhance the team approach and general continuity of care, a system of 'population responsibility' has been introduced in most centres. This implies joint team work between doctors and nurses, with a responsibility for a defined population within a certain geographical area, thereby aiming for a community focus. This was an important initiative within larger health centres, whereas the many small centres covering limited population groups could, in principle, already build on such a team-oriented community approach in their practice.

The fact that municipalities are responsible for both primary care and hospital care and the placing of bed units within the health centres seems to offer fine incentives for coordinating the different levels of care and collaborating across health centres. In 2002, the Ministry of Social Affairs and Health financed

32 local development projects in order to strengthen the effectiveness of social welfare and health care and enhance collaboration between local authorities. An evaluation of the whole programme in 2005 (Virtanen and Tontilla 2005) showed that no uniform interpretation could be achieved regarding the sub-regional collaboration and its significance. In particular, it was found that geographical factors such as long distances between the centres did affect views regarding local cooperation and its benefits. Individual projects produced local innovations and collaboration between authorities, but new cross-administrative service models did not play a significant role.

During the 1990s, there was a clear government policy to reduce institutional care and strengthen social and medical support outside institutions. This was partly motivated by the high incidence of hospitalizations compared with other countries. However, there are indications – for instance from mental care – that the necessary means for supporting outpatient care and social services were not provided and the objectives were, therefore, not met (Järvelin et al. 1992).

The Social Welfare and Health Care Target and Operating Plans require that a four-year social and welfare and health care plan be developed when a new government is in place in order to ensure the collaboration between government, municipalities and other actors in the field. The Public Authorities' Collaboration in Rehabilitation Act says that the municipalities must establish a leading group, called the local coordination group of rehabilitation services, for the collaboration of the state's local authorities with the local representatives of the Social Insurance Institution. The task of the group is to arrange the necessary services for people in need of various forms of rehabilitation. The same law established the regional coordination boards for the rehabilitation services as well. A nationwide body of rehabilitation was established to coordinate the rehabilitation processes at the macro-level (Niskanen 2002).

Case managers are also used as a tool for better coordination of care. The case manager's task is to supervise and help the clients/patients through the care processes or 'care bureaucracy' so that a single individual patient/client actually gets the required services in every phase. The case managers can also receive complaints from the patient/client and/or give information about the different options in social or health service. The rehabilitation case manager works in the hospital and is responsible for the management of the patient's rehabilitative care. The rehabilitation case manager arranges, for example, postoperative rehabilitation for a patient with heart or lung disease, and also visits the patient's home to make sure that the services are actually carried out.

The lack of strong instruments for the government to implement general changes and the very decentralized nature of the system means that local projects have been an important agent for change. As indicated above, these projects have focused on local collaboration between municipalities and health centres, but purchasing services from others, and even the merging of health centres and district hospitals, have also been elements in such projects. Seamless patient flows have also been a target in a number of projects developing joint information technology in order to achieve better continuity of care.

The free choice of provider by the individual patient is an issue in Finland; however, opportunities are limited because of the sparse population in some areas, the long distances and the small units responsible for primary care. This problem is further intensified by the growing lack of health personnel – especially in health centres in the rural areas of the country.

The main challenges for primary health care in Finland were summarized at a seminar arranged in June 2006 by the Ministry of Social Affairs and Health as part of the National Health Care Project (Ministry of Social Affairs and Health 2007). The following measures were suggested:

1. *Defining the basis tasks of health centres.* The role of the different agents should be defined and the various development projects need to be merged into broad-based, holistic and long-term activities for the development of health centres. Clarifying basic tasks should include legislative reforms.
2. *Strengthening patient-directed orientation.* Health centres need to create new models for various kinds of need and for different population groups in order to diminish differences in health. The status of the patient should be reinforced by increasing freedom of choice and by facilitating access to services across municipal borders.
3. *Developing competence and capacity.* Training and continuing education should be improved, administration and leadership strengthened and monitoring of services enforced.
4. *Creating a network of health centres.* New networks of health centres should be supported by regional development units; regional primary health care representatives should be elected and a national forum established to coordinate the steering of regional data processing and comparisons.
5. *Utilizing information technology-facilitating research and development.* An online database for good practices and development projects should be established as well as a support system for research on primary care.
6. *Developing the organization and operations.* The implementation of care chains must be intensified. Service structures must be developed as single municipalities have limited possibilities to reform their primary health care operations.

11.5 Reforming primary health care in Sweden

The description and discussion here of primary health care in Sweden are based on two main sources: the European Observatory on Health Systems and Policies' report on Sweden (Glenngård et al. 2005) and Anders Anell's (2005) discussion of important dilemmas in Swedish primary health care.

In Sweden, 21 county councils (including three larger/merged counties) are responsible for health services. In 1982, parliament adopted the Health and Medical Services Act, stating that political and financial responsibility for health services was decentralized from central state to county council level. A fundamental value was equity: good health and health care on equal terms to the entire population. Both primary health care and health service at specialist level were included in the county responsibility. In 1985, the Dagmar Reform followed, changing the reimbursement system to extend the county councils' responsibility and control of private physicians. A nationally administered fee-for-service system was replaced with per-capita grants to the counties, strengthening their planning capacity regarding private providers of health services.

Another important change in Swedish health policy was the ÄDEL Reform, implemented in 1992. With this reform, responsibility for providing long-term care to elderly and disabled people was separated from the county councils' general health service responsibility and made a municipal responsibility. An important aim of this reform was to achieve a better integration between services for the elderly, by gathering relevant services at the municipal level. With this reform, a clear line was drawn between hospitals and municipalities regarding the problem of discharges from hospitals of old people needing care after discharge. Prior to the reform, many of these patients experienced unnecessarily long (and unnecessarily expensive) hospital stays, waiting for appropriate care. As a part of the reform, hospitals were entitled to charge (on a per diem basis) municipalities that did not fulfil their obligations to take their patients home once medical treatment was finished in hospital. The ÄDEL Reform established a clear distinction between medical treatment and long-term care, grouped caregiving services at the municipal level, and created financial incentives to make hospital treatment of elderly people more cost-efficient. Over the period 1993 to 2003, the average length of stay in hospitals decreased by 1.9 days. In addition to the impact on the bed-blocker problem, the reform increased both housing facilities for the elderly and qualified nursing personnel in the municipalities (Andersson and Karlberg 2000).

Three years after the implementation of the ÄDEL Reform, the stated municipal obligations were extended to include psychiatric patients. The municipalities were obliged to take care of psychiatric patients after they had been fully treated in hospitals, including housing, occupational services and rehabilitation services.

A further health policy change at the core of Swedish primary health care was the family doctor reform, legislated through the Family Doctor Act and the Act on Freedom to Establish Private Practice. These laws were short lived, as they were introduced by the 1991–1994 non-socialist government but did not survive the return of the Social Democrats to power. However, they gave way to important changes in many counties, as implementation was underway when the laws were withdrawn.

With these laws, a list patient system was introduced for general practice in Sweden. All inhabitants were asked to choose a family doctor (a GP). This choice also included doctors who did not currently have a contract with the county in which they worked. These acts altered the basic framework for the organization of primary health care, in which the district-oriented primary health centre had been the established model. The health centres were designed to stimulate collaboration between doctors and nurses within a geographically defined area (Spri 1983). When the family doctor system was implemented, however, patients were invited to choose their family doctor unrestricted by geographical borders. At the same time, the reimbursement system for doctors was changed, replacing fixed salary with a combination of fee for service and a per capita payment. This reform thus weakened doctors' ties to defined geographical areas, and public primary care physicians found themselves in competition for patients with each other and with private GPs. Conversely, this new arrangement facilitated better continuity of care, since the patient became the responsibility of only one physician instead of a series of different clinic doctors, and it also encouraged higher compliance rates from patients with physician instructions. Both of these changes were seen as particularly important in dealing with growing numbers of elderly and/or chronically ill patients. Although these laws were short lived, some counties decided to continue implementation of this new arrangement and of the family doctor system. Today, both the geographically defined health centre system and the family doctor system can be found in different counties in Sweden. In recent years, there has been increased interest from counties in a new version of patient choice of GP, termed 'vardval', which has extended the reach of patient choice of primary care physician into additional county councils.

Swedish health care has been traditionally viewed as predominantly hospital based, with a large proportion of physicians working in hospital. In most county councils, GPs have no gatekeeper function, and direct access to specialist health - care is traditionally taken for granted. Glenngård and co-workers (2005, p. 110) describe health care services overall as still somewhat fragmented, with insufficient coordination between different levels of care. A growing number of elderly, often chronically ill, patients in need of an integrated, well-coordinated chain of medical services, nursing and social support have sometimes faced considerable challenges in having their needs met. As the economic pressure on specialist health service increases, more people will be cared for at primary health level, in their own homes or in municipally organized accommodations.

Anell (2005) discusses the dilemmas surrounding the future development of primary health care organization in Sweden, following the challenges mentioned above. Two important health political values seem to be at stake: consumers' free choice and the need for an integrated primary health service where doctors play their roles as a part of a team (Anell 2005, p. 67). As discussed above, the family doctor system, where consumer choice is a basis for organization, tends to loosen the ties between the GP and the geographic catchment area he or she had been responsible for, which implies looser ties to the nurses, physiotherapists and other health personnel. Anell discusses various compromise solutions for this dilemma. One of the possibilities mentioned is to allow consumers themselves to decide, by choosing between the alternatives, offered as concrete options: team-organized or individually working GPs. Another is to organize larger integrated health centres with a diversified team, also including key medical specialists, serving an area big enough to give the inhabitants the possibility to choose between doctors, and with the capacity to offer 24 hour acute service.

A major change in primary health care organization will need support from both those dependent on health care services and the personnel providing the services. Personnel experience seems to point in different directions. A study undertaken during 1995, shortly after the family doctor reform was discontinued, concluded that family doctors experienced greater demands and lower levels of competence development than colleagues who worked within the catchment area and team-organized model. At the same time, district nurses, traditionally working in close collaboration with GPs in the catchment area organization, experienced deteriorating working conditions (Wilhelmsson et al. 1998). However, a qualitative study from Stockholm in 1999 concludes that doctors seemed to be in favour of the family doctor model and a strengthening of GPs' position in the health care system by a well-defined gatekeeper function (Quaye 2001). During recent years, gatekeeping has been implemented in some counties, and the principle of gatekeeping has gained support in parts of the political system. Anell (2005, p. 66), in his discussion, cautions against trying to strengthen primary health care through political decisions that may have little political support from the patients themselves.

11.6 Discussion

Primary health care is an important element of health services in the Nordic countries but generally attracts less political attention and resources than does specialized hospital care. However, reforms toward further decentralization during the last decades in all four countries, and the ongoing changes in demographic and disease patterns towards more elderly and more chronic diseases, have created a growing interest in coordinated, qualified primary care, including preventive and rehabilitative services.

This leads to the key questions. Is there a common Nordic model for primary health care? Where does primary health care differ between the Nordic countries? What are the important questions to be answered, and what are the options?

Table 11.1 provides a starting point for this discussion. The table provides a summary of the common organizational traits and differences in primary health care among the four Nordic countries. Despite common characteristics of the mainly tax-based health care systems with major public providers, GPs working independently of hospitals (not providing services to inpatients) and an emphasis on regional and local agencies, there are some important historical variations in the organization of primary health care. Yet, the reform processes seem to include many common features, which tend over time to diminish the cross-country variations.

The general Nordic model of tax-based funding including primary health care has not been changed and is still a basic feature in all Nordic countries. However, some elements of co-payment do exist for dental services, physiotherapy, drugs and in nursing homes; in Norway and Sweden co-payments also exist for GP visits. Co-payment for seeing a doctor, in order to reduce unnecessary visits, has sometimes been an issue for debate in Denmark but is still rejected by the majority of politicians.

The position of the providers, however, is more blurred and shows large variations between the countries, with different combinations of private practice/public employment and private versus public (tax-based) financing. Further privatization and outsourcing have also, to some extent, been seen as means to achieve better efficiency in primary health care, but these have only had a rather limited role in most settings and primary care is predominantly still based on financing by public funds. In Denmark, all GPs have traditionally been private practising but financed from counties (now regions). In the other countries, a mixture of publicly employed doctors and private practitioners has been the main feature, creating a rather complex picture and with a tendency towards an increased number of private practising doctors. A general trend towards an

Table 11.1 Important features of the current organization of primary health care in Nordic countries

	Denmark	Norway	Finland	Sweden
Political/administrative responsibility	GPs and other private practitioners at the regional level, other services on the municipal level	Municipal responsibility	Municipal responsibility	Primary health service at county level; long-term care at municipal level
Consumer choice	Free choice of GP within a list patient system; restricted number of GP changes per year	Free choice of GP within a list patient system; restricted number of GP changes per year	Mixed: area or list patient organized	Mixed: area or list patient organized
Financing	Mainly tax based	Mainly tax based	Mainly tax based	Mainly tax based
Public or private providers	GPs in private practices; otherwise mainly publicly employed primary care providers	GPs in private practices; both public and privately provided long-term care	Mixed: both private GP practices and publicly employed doctors	Mixed: both private GP practices and publicly employed doctors
Gatekeeping function in the overall health care system	Patient access to specialists, physiotherapists, hospitals and some other services regulated by GP referrals	Patient access to specialists, physiotherapists and some other services regulated by GP referrals	GP gatekeeping function in the public sector, but patients have direct access to specialists and hospitals in the private sector	GP gatekeeping function in some counties, while patients have a free access to specialist care in others
Integrating health: initiatives for coordination	Individual patient plans; practice coordinators; regional health plans jointly with municipalities	Individual patient plans; state actions to strengthen collaboration between GPs and long-term care; municipal payment for long hospital stays; practice coordinators; intermediate care	Joint team work; developmental projects for collaboration, national health care plans; local and regional coordination groups/boards	Joint team work; municipal payment for long hospital stays
Centralization/ decentralization: changing the balance between local autonomy and central state authority	A mix of decentralization from regions to municipalities and centralization through merging of municipalities and state interference through standards and monitoring	Stable decentralized political/ administrative structures; increased state influence through standards and monitoring	Stable political structure with strong local autonomy and little state interference	Gradual decentralization from state to counties and from counties to municipalities

increasing role for fee for service, sometimes in combination with capitation fees, is sometimes used effectively by health authorities to stimulate certain desired activities, for example prevention. Most of the other professionals in primary health care are employed directly by the municipalities on a fixed salary basis. Some outsourcing of services, such as nursing homes and home-based services, by the municipalities to private providers is taking place in all four countries but is still a subject of debate and political controversy. An example is the introduction of commercial enterprises in primary health care (such as large companies with a profile within the cleaning business providing nursing home care in Sweden) or health trusts that might at some stage take responsibility for larger sections of health care (as in Finland). This kind of outsourcing (based on public funding), or privately funded health enterprises establishing themselves on a free market basis, is very different from the traditional individual private practitioners in primary care and is likely to introduce major changes in the organization and financing of health care in the Nordic countries if national and local policies are willing to support such developments.

In all four countries, municipalities play an important role, most clearly in Finland where many small municipalities have a high degree of independence with little state interference. Danish and Norwegian municipalities have also had a strong position in primary health care over many years, and this position has been strengthened recently for specific aspects of health care. In Sweden, the regional level has been more important, but a gradual process of decentralization towards the municipalities has taken place over several decades. Even if a decentralized political/administrative structure concerning primary health care seems to be the preferred model, tendencies of increased state influence may be observed.

Saltman and co-workers (2007) discuss the question of increased inequalities as a consequence of decentralization. Decentralization may be a rational strategy to increase allocation efficiency. However, an important dilemma is that local autonomy, distributing welfare benefits by local standards, rationality and community knowledge, may create inequalities between municipalities (Saltman et al. 2007, p 16). Inequalities in health care between municipalities are not politically important as long as they are not visible. Until a few years ago, statistical monitoring of activity in primary health care was not well developed apart from annual statistics on person-year and number of clients. Today, transparency increases as elaborate administrative systems are introduced into primary health care; electronic systems for communication are under development, and a higher degree of standardization of electronic patient journals is being implemented. As a result, the possibility of deriving more elaborated and more comprehensive comparative statistics on municipal performance in the primary health care will increase, effectively monitoring differences and inequalities between municipalities. The inherent dilemma between two important values in Nordic primary health care – local autonomy and national equality – will probably be both more visible and more politically controversial. Political debates on observed inequalities in primary health service will result in a call for national standards. If so, many decisions concerning primary health care that have been traditionally municipal ones may be taken out of individual municipality remit and replaced by (formalized or informal) national standards. In this way, the local political system may steadily lose some of its autonomy and authority, even if the formal political/administrative structures are unchanged.

The aim of the ongoing reform processes in Nordic primary care is to strengthen the health service systems' abilities to meet patient needs. In Starfield's (1998) terms, this means that it should offer an accessible, low-threshold health service characterized by continuity in patient–helper relationship, serve as the patient's gateway to the overall health care system and, at the same time, act as an agent for coordination of care provided in other parts of the health care system. To what degree do the Nordic primary health care systems meet these demands?

11.6.1 Accessibility

Tax-based funding is considered an important prerequisite for fulfilling the aim of equal access to health services irrespectively of who the patient is and where they live. Another means to secure access to health service is the patient list system, implemented on a nationwide basis in Denmark and Norway, and partially in Sweden and Finland. A study by van Doorslaer and Masseria (2004) of GP usage in 11 OECD countries concludes that income-related variations in GP use are small (data from 2000–2001). Non-standardized user rates showed higher usage in the poorer parts of the population in all the countries studied. When controlling for variations of needs, this inequality decreases and becomes insignificant in most countries, including Denmark, Norway and Sweden. An exception from this overall pattern is Finland, where a very small but significant pro-rich deviation is observed. According to van Doorslaer and Masseria, this may be an effect of the extended use of company doctors in Finland. A traditional and probably more important dimension in the discussion of equal access to health services in the Nordic countries is geographical distribution. In Sweden, Norway and Finland, some of the populations live in less-populated areas with long distances between centres and this is associated with a persisting problem in recruiting GPs (Lian 2003). Even in Denmark, there are now signs of similar problems in rural districts in spite of the limited size of these areas.

11.6.2 Continuity, coordination, gatekeeping and consumer choice

Continuity of care is an important part of Starfield's (1998) model of primary health care. The question of continuity, however, is multidimensional and complex. Leona Bachrach (1981) discusses several important dimensions in the thinking about continuity of care. Continuity of care means that care is patient centred, well coordinated regarding collaboration and information concerning the patient, flexible in the understanding of the patient's needs, continuous regarding personal relations between patients and caregivers and accessible when needed. All dimensions mentioned represent important values in primary health care. The complexity of the continuity concept may, however, at the same time create important dilemmas.

Consumer choice is a growing feature in Nordic health care, and in primary health care this is associated with the concept of family doctors, with patients receiving care from the same doctor over time. Patient choice regarding municipal primary care has previously been quite limited in the Nordic countries, but some choice has been introduced, for instance for home care and child dental care. The trend towards individual choice is at the same time threatening the ambition to achieve more integrated care. For example, the patient listing associated with the family doctor system may to some extent weaken primary health care teams oriented towards geographically target areas. Hjelmgren and Anell (2007) have studied population preferences regarding primary care models in Sweden. In their study, they found that 'older individuals and individuals in poor health preferred the option to register with a GP whereas working individuals and individuals living at a greater distance from hospital preferred the option to register with a primary care team' (Hjelmgren and Anell 2007, p. 315). Different dimensions within the concept of continuity had different values for different groups, according to their life situation. A trial of a combination of the family doctor system and the team-based organization in the four largest cities in Finland during 1983 to 1987 showed a substantial 'leakage' of patient visits to GPs outside the individual's residential area (Vohlonen et al. 1989), illustrating how continuity may conflict with other values.

Traditionally, both Norway and Denmark have relied on GPs to have a gatekeeping function to regulate use of specialized health service and to act as coordinators in the overall health care system. The role as gatekeeper, however, does not automatically follow the family doctor system – clearly seen in Sweden, which still allows direct access to other health services without referral from the GP. Clearly, from a patient point of view, gatekeeping may be considered a means to restrict the use of other services. A European study of patient satisfaction with their GPs showed a higher degree of satisfaction in countries where other health services were directly accessible than in countries where referrals from GPs were needed (Kroneman et al. 2006). However, the Danish case clearly illustrates that the population is ready to accept the GP as the gatekeeper even when given the choice of selecting a 'health coverage category' that implies direct access and public remuneration of specialist services (but some co-payment). Only 1–2 per cent of the Danish population has selected this second option. Even if the GP as the gatekeeper to other services is in an ideal postion for taking the role of coordinator, that role is hampered by lack of interaction with other professionals and lack of information and feedback. This is caused by organizational barriers, lack of general incentives and lack of common information technology systems across health care systems.

Ensuring continuity of care – especially for patients with chronic conditions – is one of the main challenges in primary health care. This is further complicated by the distribution of responsibilities between different agencies and political–administrative levels, as particularly seen in Denmark and Sweden. Many initiatives in Nordic countries seek to cope with this problem on the patient as well as the organizational level. Individual plans are used on a mandatory basis in Norway when patients need coordinated care and in Denmark for rehabilitation after hospital discharge. Case managers are seen as a solution in some cases: in Denmark a special fee for GPs was introduced in 2007 in order to encourage them to develop individual plans for diabetes patients.

In order to improve coordination, joint committees between political–administrative levels and institutions have been set up and joint or coordinated health planning mandated (as in Denmark and Finland). Defining population responsibility for several professionals has also been used as a strategy, sometimes in combination with the establishment of new health centres with general primary health care services (as in Finland and Sweden) or health centres with special functions (such as the centres in Denmark with a focus on prevention and rehabilitation). In Denmark and Finland, national strategies, including financial incentives, have been used in order to stimulate local development projects in the municipalities. This might lead to better integration of care but also carries a risk of adding another unit to those already in place, as in Denmark where GPs are mainly not involved in the new health centres.

11.7 Concluding remarks

This review of primary health care reforms in the Nordic countries shows that in this sector the 'Nordic model' is neither homogeneous nor stable. The term primary care means different clusters of services in the different countries, organized in different ways and the objects of various reform processes. Yet some basic principles are common, including mainly tax-financed services, general entitlement, decentralized responsibility for care and important roles for GPs and for municipal health authorities. The reform initiatives in most cases are not very dramatic for primary health care and appear to relate to similar kinds of problem: patient choice, local governance, integration and continuity of care, equity and quality. The problem of coordinated care within a system of distributed health - care providers with different roles and differing financing and organizational frameworks is still a major issue in spite of many attempts to improve coordination. Patient choice seems to be given greater priority in Nordic reforms but is, at the same time, threatening attempts to improve continuity. Privatization or other financial reforms in relation to primary care has been limited, except for the development towards private practising rather than publicly employed physicians. Contrary to hospital care, strict quality issues have not played a strong role in primary care reforms so far and there is still only scarce evidence on the quality of primary health care services. However, new general initiatives such as plans for a Danish national quality reform for public services and national requests for standards and better monitoring in all the Nordic countries are most likely to sharpen the focus on ensuring a high quality of primary care services in the future.

References

Ådnanes M. and Bjørngaard, J.H. (2006) *Fastlegen og det psykiske helsearbeidets tiltak for voksne med psykiske lidelser*. Trondheim: SINTEF Helse.

Andersson, G. and Karlberg I. (2000) Integrated care for the elderly, *International Journal of Integrated Care* 1: e01.

Anell, A. (2005) *Primärvård i Förendring*. Lund: Studentlitteratur.

Bachrach, L. (1981) Continuity of care for chronic mental patients: a conceptual analysis. *American Journal of Phsychiatry* 138: 1449–56.

Christiansen, T. (ed.) (1999) *International vurdering af organisation og finansiering af det danske. Sundhedsvæsen.* Odense: University of Odense Press.

Cueto, M. (2004) The origins of primary health care and selective primary health care, *American Journal of Public Health* 94: 1864–74.

Finnvold J.E., Svalund, J. and Paulsen, B. (2005) *Etter innføring av fastlegeordning: bruker-vurderinger av allmennlegetjenesten.* Oslo: Statistisk sentralbyrå.

Glenngård, A.H., Hjalte, F., Svensson, M., Anell, A. and Bankauskaite, V. (eds) (2005) *Health Systems in Transition: Sweden.* Copenhagen: WHO Regional Office for Europe on behalf of the European Observatory on Health Systems and Policies.

Haggerty, J., Reid, R.J., Freeman, G.K., Starfield, B., Adair, C.E. and McKendry, R. (2003) Continuity of care: a multidisciplinary review, *British Medical Journal* 327: 1219–21.

Haggerty, J., Burge, F., Lévesque, J. et al. (2007) Operational definitions of attributes of primary health care: concensus among Canadian experts, *Annals of Family Medicine* 5: 336–44.

Häkkinen, U. and Lehto, J. (2005) Reform, change, and continuity in Finnish health care. *Journal of Health Politics, Policy and Law* 30: 79–96.

Hjelmgren, J. and Anell, A. (2007) Population preferences and choice of primary care models: a discrete choice experiment in Sweden, *Health Policy* 83: 314–22.

Järvelin, J., Rico, A. and Cetani, T. (eds) (1992) *Health Care Systems in Transition: Finland.* Copenhagen: WHO Regional Office for Europe for the European Observatory on Health Care Systems.

Kark, S.L. (1974) *Epidemiology and Community Medicine.* New York: Appleton-Century-Crofts.

Krasnik, A. (2004) The strong public tradition in Danish health care, in Maarse, H. (ed) *Privatisation in European Health Care.* Maarseen: Elsevier.

Kroneman, M.W., Maarse, H. and van der Zee, J. (2006) Direct access in primary care and patient satisfaction: a European study, *Health Policy* 76: 72–9.

Lian, O. (2003) *Pasienterfaringer i primærlegetjenesten før og etter fastlegereformen.* [ISM skrift-serie] Tromsø: University of Tromsø.

Meads, G. (2006) *Primary Care in the Twenty-first Century: An International Perspective.* Oxford: Radcliffe.

Ministry of Social Affairs and Health (2007) Seminar 11 May 2007. Helsinki: Ministry of Social Affairs and Health; http:/www.stm.fi/Ressource.phx/publishing/documents/8615/summary_en.htx.

Mooney, G. (2002) The Danish health care system: it ain't broke, so don't fix it, *Health Policy* 29: 161–71.

Moore, G. and Showstack J. (2003) Primary care medicine in crisis: toward a reconstruction and renewal, *Annals of Internal Medicine* 138: 244–8.

Niskanen, J.J. (2002) Finish care integrated? *International Journal of Integrated Care* 2: e16.

Quaye, R. (2001) Internal market systems in Sweden, *European Journal of Public Health*, 11: 380–5.

Saltman, R.B., Bankauskaite, V., Vrangbæk, K. (2007) *Decentralization in Health Care.* Maidenhead: McGraw Hill/Open University Press for the WHO European Observatory.

Seeman, J. (2003) *Sundhedsplanlægning i et interorganisatorisk perspektiv.* Copenhagen: Forskningscenter for organisation og ledelse.

Sosial- og helsedirektoratet (2005) *Report IS-1293: Normering av legetjenester i sykehjem.* Oslo: Sosial- og helsedirektoratet.

Sosial- og helsedirektoratet (2006) *Report IS-1420: Legetjenester til personer med kommunale omsorgstjenester utenfor institusjon.* Oslo: Sosial- og helsedirektoratet.

Spri (1983) *Primärvårdens organisation.* Stockholm: Spri.

Starfield, B. (1998) *Primary Care: Balancing Health Needs, Services, and Technology.* New York: Oxford University Press.

Strandberg-Larsen, M., Nielsen, M.B. and Krasnik, A. (2007) Are joint health plans effective for coordination of health services? *International Journal of Integrated Care* 7: e35.

Vallgårda, S. and Krasnik A. (eds) (2007) *Sundhedsvæsen og sundhedspolitik.* Copenhagen: Munksgaard.

van Dorslaer E. and Masseria, C. (2004) *OECD Health Working Papers No. 14: Income-related Inequality in the Use of Medical Care in 21 OECD Countries.* Paris: OECD.

Virtanen, P. and Tontilla, J. (2005) *Making the Service System More Effective: Assessment of Sub-regional Development Projects and Development Trials Regarding the Health Service System.* Helsinki: Ministry of Social Affairs and Health.

Vohlonen, I., Pekurinen, M. and Saltman, B. (1989) Re-organizing primary medical care in Finland: the personal doctor program, *Health Policy* 13: 65–79.

Wilhelmsson, S., Faresjö, T., Foldevi, M. and Åkerlind, I. (1998) The personal doctor reform in Sweden: perceived changes in working conditions, *Family Practice* 15: 192–7.

chapter twelve

Addressing the dual goals of improving health and reducing health inequalities

Signild Vallgårda and Juhani Lehto

12.1 Introduction

Like many other countries, Denmark, Finland, Norway and Sweden have adopted public health programmes in the period since the mid-1990s with the dual goals of improving the health of the population and reducing health inequalities. While improvement of the health of the population has been a political issue at least since the second half of the eighteenth century, the explicit focus on health inequalities is a recent phenomenon in the political arena in the Nordic countries, first becoming apparent in the 1980s and 1990s.

This chapter examines how population health and health inequalities are defined as political problems, with special focus on (1) where responsibility for health is placed, with the individual citizen or the state; (2) whether public health policies correspond to the ideas of a Nordic welfare state; and (3) the importance of the political orientation of the government in charge for the policies suggested. Policy documents from four Nordic countries provide the basis of the analysis but whether or how the policies are implemented is not considered.

12.2 Analytical framework

Problematization, or defining a phenomenon as a political problem, is a crucial step in any political process. It frames an issue as relevant and accessible to political action; it involves defining the nature of the problem, pointing to reasons for dealing with it and identifying its causes as well as its possible solutions. In the words of Michel Foucault (1994), '[t]his transformation of a group of obstacles and difficulties into problems to which diverse solutions will attempt to produce a response, this is what constitutes the point of problematization'. In this chapter, political problematization is analysed in public health policies in general and policies of social inequalities in health in particular. Health programmes are examined to identify how public health problems are defined, how the policies are legitimized, which causes are identified and which initiatives are suggested. In political science, the concepts of agenda setting and framing are used to describe central elements of this problematization process.

12.2.1 Welfare policy models

The Nordic welfare states are often characterized as adhering to a common and particular Nordic or social democratic idea (Esping-Andersen 1990), with emphasis on ensuring social security for all citizens through universal benefits and with all citizens entitled to health, social and education services. Welfare policies may be characterized as either universal or residual. The latter focuses on the poorest part of the population, giving professional discretion or means testing a central role in deciding who should receive services and benefits. Universalism is characterized by providing services and benefits to all citizens regardless of income. Universal policies can be subdivided according to entitlement and of allocation of services and benefits (Rothstein 2001; Kildal and Kuhnle 2005). Child benefits and old age pensions are examples of universal allocations, where identical benefits are given to all citizens in the relevant age group. In health care, all citizens are entitled to health care, but it is up to professional discretion to decide who should actually get which services. In this respect, the four Nordic countries are similar: they adhere to basically the same welfare model, although they organize health care in different ways, as shown in other chapters of the book. The Nordic welfare states are often characterized as universal. The degree of universalism and residualism in actual policies does, however, depend on the area concerned. If, as Esping-Andersen (1990) and others maintain, a common Nordic welfare model exists, one would expect that the public health policies would be similar and not influenced by the colour of the national governments in power.

Another reason for expecting similar policies in the four countries and an equally central role of the state is what the Swedish historian Lars Trägårdh (1997) labels as 'statist individualism'. He claims that citizens of the Nordic countries, in contrast to many other Europeans, tend to view the state as benevolent and as a shelter against dependency on the family. If this is the case, the state is likely to be given a central role in caring for citizens' health and also before they fall ill, that is with a role in disease prevention and health promotion.

12.2.2 Responsibilities

Is the health of the population and thus of the individuals a responsibility of the state or of the individual citizens? The answer to this question, of course, depends on political values or ideology. One would expect market liberals to place most of the responsibility on individuals, who are considered to have both the ability and the right to decide for themselves how to live and which risks to take. The state is left with the task of providing relevant and sufficient information and to enable the individuals to make informed decisions.

Social democrats or socialists, with a perception of human beings shaped by social and physical environments outside the scope of individual influence, would give the state a greater role in ensuring conditions that are not harmful to the citizens' health. Similarly, one would also expect conservatives to give the state authority to prevent people from leading an unhealthy life (Heywood 2003; Vallgårda and Krasnik 2007). On this generalized background, one would expect that public health policies of a given country could potentially change with the ideology of the political majority.

12.3 Public health programmes as policy source

The material used in this study comes from recent public health white papers and programmes developed by the Finnish (Ministry of Social Affairs and Health 2001), Norwegian (Norwegian Ministry of Health 2003), Swedish (Regeringen 2002a, 2008) and Danish (Regeringen 2002c) Governments. It also includes the Norwegian plans for reduction of health inequalities (Directorate for Health and Social Affairs 2005; Ministry for Health and Care Services 2007). The programmes are studied as expressions of how the respective governments construct and present their overall objectives, concerns and intentions on public health policy.

The white papers of the four countries differ in at least in two respects. First, they differ in terms of the preparatory work invested in the papers. The most effort was invested in the social democratic Swedish Government (Regringen) white paper from 2002 (Regeringen 2002a), much less in the white paper from 2008 (Regeringen 2008) launched by the liberal government that came into power in 2006. Also in Norway, both the liberal government's programme in 2003 (Norwegian Ministry of Health 2003) and the social democratic programme specifically addressing social inequalities in health (Ministry for Health and Care Services 2007) were preceded by green papers. Much less preparatory work was done to elaborate the Danish programme of 2002 (Regeringen 2002b) issued by a liberal-conservative government. The Finnish white paper (Ministry of Social Affairs and Health 2001) was issued by a coalition of social democrats with greens and right-wing parties and prepared by a smaller group of experts and civil servants.

The health policy documents also vary in size and style. The Norwegian and social democratic Swedish white papers are much more comprehensive and refer explicitly to research. The target groups are the respective parliaments. They were also presented to politicians at other levels, to civil servants and to other public health professionals who were supposed to become involved with the implementation of the recommendations. Finally, they were communicated to the general public (via the mass media). The Danish programmes (Regeringen 1999, 2002b) also seem to aim at a broad target group. Their size, text and layout indicate an ambition to make them readable outside the central political–bureaucratic establishment. The Finnish document (Ministry of Social Affairs and Health 2001) is framed as a purely administrative document, but the content seems to address a larger audience. In spite of these differences, it is reasonable to assume that the white papers give a sufficient and fair account of the ideas the governments wish to present.

There are language issues. In the Scandinavian languages and Finnish a distinction is made between the health of the population (folkehelse, folkhälsa, folkesundhed, kansanterveys) and the activities undertaken to improve it, meanings which are often both included in the English concept public health. Four countries imply four languages, which in addition are described using a fifth language, English. The words ulighed, ulikhet, ojämlikhet and (väestöryhmien) erot are translated here as the word inequality, assuming that they are roughly understood in the same way. The Scandinavian languages do not distinguish between inequality and inequity, and for reasons of simplicity we have chosen to use only the concept inequality, which is also often used in the United Kingdom (UK Department of Health 2003). This concept has also been used when the Nordic programmes have been translated into English (Ministry of Social Affairs and Health 2001; Regeringen 2002c; Swedish National Institute of Public Health 2004; Directorate for Health and Social Affairs 2005).

12.4 Old or new concerns?

Public health policies formulated in terms of the dual goals mentioned above – improving the health of the population and reducing social inequalities in health – are fairly recent. The health of the population in general and the health of the poor in particular have, however, been on the political agenda in the Nordic countries more or less prominently since the eighteenth century. For different reasons and with different means, governments have taken it as their task to improve the health of their populations by influencing behaviours and, above all, the environment. Interventions have concerned food quality; sanitation; alcohol; water supply; housing; working conditions; protection against contagious diseases by isolation and vaccinations and through health care, education and employment, doctors and midwives and building of hospitals (Johannisson 1991; Qvarsell 1991; Vallgårda 2000, 2004; Moseng 2001; Schiøtz 2003; Harjula 2007). These measures, of which several are now labelled welfare state interventions, were thus introduced long before the concept was coined.

General public health programmes have been published from the 1980s and onwards (SOU 1984; Ministry of Social Affairs and Health 1987; Regeringen 1989, 1991, 1994, 1999; Sosialdepartementet 1993; NOU 1998). But the countries have been rather asynchronous when it comes to introducing health inequality as an issue on the political agenda. Equality in access to health - care, education and so on has been on the agenda in all the Nordic countries for a long time, while the equality problem, phrased as 'social inequalities in health', has only fairly recently become a political issue. The representatives of the Ministries of Health of all four countries were in agreement with the WHO policy launched in 1984, *Health for All by the Year 2000*, where the reduction of health inequalities in and between countries was one of the central goals.

This, however, did not have an immediate effect on the policies presented in Denmark and Norway, wheras in Sweden, the policies towards health inequalities have been on the agenda since 1984 (Vallgårda 2007a, 2008). However, the programme for 2008 virtually excluded this issue. In Denmark, inequality was addressed on a national political level only as late as in 1998, and in Norway it was mentioned at the beginning of the 1990s but not elaborated on until after 2000. In Finland, the equality agenda was very strong in the late 1960s and early 1970s (Puro 1973) and even before the Second World War (Kuusi 1932). It could be said that, then, public health policy was still 'a part of (equality oriented) social policy'. It was also transferred to the emerging public health policy in the late 1960s. This ethos, however, lost much of its strength in late 1970s until the end of the 1990s (Tervonen Goncalves and Lehto 2004). The Finnish strategy of 1987 (Ministry of Social Affairs and Health 1987) did mention that the disadvantaged should have priority and that equal access to health services should be ensured, but otherwise social inequality in health was practically absent. Later there was a separation of health and social policy, which then led to the reemergence of the equality agenda within a new narrower health policy after 2000.

To sum up, timing has differed, but by the start of the twenty-first century the dual goals were addressed in all four countries, although the latest Swedish programme does not explicitly state goals.

12.5 How are policies and activities legitimized?

A policy must be considered justified and legitimized in order to be accepted by politicians, doctors, nurses and others responsible for carrying it out, as well as by the public at large. A central part of making a given issue into a political problem (i.e. putting it on the political agenda) is, therefore, to state the reasons for dealing with it. When it comes to the overall objectives and justification of the policies, there are few differences between the four Nordic public health programmes. They focus on creating better lives for citizens and strengthen the economy of the public sector and that of society as a whole. As stated in the Danish programme, 'Targeted efforts are therefore required based on human, health and economic considerations' (Regeringen 2002c). The Finnish programme has the principal argument that 'Attaining the maximum possible health is also a basic human right' (Ministry of Social Affairs and Health 2001), which is the only Nordic government to state this explicitly. It argues that, according to a democratic principle, when people expect better health they are entitled to get it.

Economic arguments are important in all white papers. Bad health is costly and good health is expected to further economic progress. The Norwegian programme finds that 'with prevention we need to repair less', assuming that health care spending could be reduced and states that '(h)ealth is an investment in the good life' (Norwegian Ministry of Health 2003). The Finnish government states: 'Investment in health is an investment in the future. A healthy population is an important precondition for economic growth and competitiveness'

(Ministry of Social Affairs and Health 2001). The social democratic Swedish Government expected that with improved health Sweden would 'achieve sustainable growth, good social welfare and ecological sustainability in Sweden' (Government of Sweden 2002). Sweden's public health policy was, therefore, closely related to welfare state politics, both as a measure of its success – 'the population's state of health is an important indicator of welfare trends' – and as central goal – 'human health is one of the most important issues facing a welfare state' (Government of Sweden 2002). The welfare state has played a central role in Swedish political self-perception (Vallgårda 2003). The present liberal Swedish Government stresses the importance of health for inclusion and employment and the injurious consequences to health of exclusion and unemployment. The reasons given for dealing with the health of the population are similar pointing at a common political ethos.

12.5.1 Why are health inequalities a problem?

Similarities are also evident when it comes to the reasons for reducing health inequalities. In all the Nordic countries, the governments maintain that health inequalities are incompatible with their political values, except for the liberal Swedish Government, which does not explicitly address the issue. The Danish Government states that it 'believes that social equity in health is one of the fundamental values of a welfare society' (Regeringen 2002b), and the Norwegian and former Swedish Governments stress that in a democratic society health inequalities are not acceptable. They put forward the idea that an unequal society is harmful to the health of all its citizens, not only the worst off. The idea fits well with the universal goals of welfare policies as a means to improve the conditions of all citizens. The Danish Government presents another reason in stating that 'the public sector has special responsibility towards the weakest groups in society . . . This is one of the core tasks of the welfare state' (Regeringen 2002b), thereby subscribing to a conservative ideal or a residual welfare policy model. The Finnish programme does not explicitly give reasons for reducing health inequalities. However, the reasons stated for addressing inequalities are based on the ethos of a universal, equality oriented and inclusive welfare policy (Ministry of Social Affairs and Health 2001). The reasons for addressing health inequalities differ among the Nordic governments: the Danish Government and the new Swedish Government distinguish themselves by focusing on residual not general inequalities.

12.6 Which health problems are identified as key issues?

Crucial in any problematization process is the concrete definition or construction of the problem which is to be addressed. Life expectancy, quality of life, functional capacity and health inequalities are problems addressed in all health programmes. The specific diseases mentioned also are very similar: cardiovascular disease, cancer, diabetes, allergy, musculoskeletal disorders and mental illnesses are mentioned by all programmes, but with different weight.

Whereas the social democratic Swedish programme focuses explicitly on risk factors for bad health, it also defines which diseases, among those mentioned above, were the most important to reduce: mental health and musculoskeletal disorders (i.e. non-lethal health problems) (Regeringen 2002a). These health conditions were prioritized because they seemed to be increasing and because they result in illness-related absenteeism at work, a problem that has attracted at lot of attention in Sweden since the mid-1990s. The liberal programme from 2008, referring to effects on disability adjusted life years (DALYs), mentions cancer, cardiovascular and neuropsychiatric disorders. The equally liberal Danish programme lists eight so-called people's or population diseases (folkesygdomme) and cites the economic burden on the public sector and the suffering of the citizens in giving them priority (Regeringen 2002c). In Norway, four criteria for prioritizing health problems are presented: the number of people affected, costs to society, knowledge of causes and availability of effective and acceptable measures (Norwegian Ministry of Health 2003). As in Sweden, the societal costs mentioned are illness-related absenteeism and disability pensions. The Finnish programme focuses on specific health problems of the different age groups. This results in prioritizing of substance abuse problems among young people; violence, accidents and suicide among young adult males; chronic diseases including impaired mental health within an ageing work population; and functional impairments among the elderly (Ministry of Social Affairs and Health 2001). Early retirement is also emphasized as a health-related problem to be solved in Finland.

In spite of different political regimes, by and large the identified health problems are the same, although mental health is given a higher priority in Finland and Sweden and reducing mortality is considered more important in Denmark. Arguments for prioritizing the health problems are similar: costs, suffering and the numbers of those suffering. Costs related to disease such as sickness benefits and disability pensions are not explicitly mentioned in Denmark, while they are prominent in the Norwegian and Swedish programmes. The issue later (especially from 2007) entered the Danish political agenda.

Comparisons often play an important role in the process of defining problems in policy-making, and Nordic public health policies are no exception to this. The Norwegian and Swedish programmes both present positive overall pictures of the health situation in their respective countries. For example, in the 2002 Swedish programme, it is stated: 'Internationally speaking, Sweden has one of the highest average life expectancies in the world' (Swedish National Institute of Public Health 2004). This self-image may be one reason for the higher priority given to non-lethal diseases in Sweden. When comparing life expectancies with other countries, the Danes are less contented: 'Denmark is still in the bottom half of the European Union (EU) countries' (Regeringen 2002c). The Danish programme was, therefore, developed on the basis of dissatisfaction with the general health situation. In Denmark, much attention has been devoted to the mean life expectancy and consequently to the diseases causing high mortality. Finland uses as the main comparative argument the historical development: significant progress with regard to most indicators, but problems, particularly in terms of inequality between socioeconomic groups and new health problems.

Table 12.1 has been included to provide some of the statistical background

Table 12.1 Comparisons of life expectancies: development in mean life expectancy in the Nordic countries 1970–2000

	Men (years)			Women (years)		
	1970	2000	Change	1970	2000	Change
Denmark	70.7	74.5	3.8	75.0	79.0	4.0
Finland	66.5	74.2	7.7	75.9	81.2	5.3
Norway	71.2	76.0	4.8	77.5	81.5	4.0
Sweden	72.2	77.4	5.2	77.1	81.9	4.8

Source: OECD health databases.

that was known to civil servants and politicians when the programmes were prepared. As can be seen from the table, the level and development in mean life expectancy differ substantially. Norway and Sweden have had similar developments, starting from a relatively high level and increasing in a similar pace and consequently remaining at the top both in a Nordic and in a global context. In 1970, Denmark had almost as high a life expectancy as the two other Scandinavian countries but has lagged behind since and is now at the lower end in a European comparison. This has caused some concern in Denmark since the beginning of the 1990s. The Finnish development is the most remarkable, as male life expectancy has increased by almost eight years in a 30-year period.

12.6.1 Describing social inequalities

Social inequalities in health are usually described in one of two ways: as a dichotomy such as the health problem of the most disadvantaged or excluded minorities compared with the rest of the population, or as a gradient, such as increasing health problems with decreasing income or education. In the dichotomy description the problems are confined to an excluded group, while the gradient approach considers the problems as concerning the whole population (Vallgårda 2008). The Danish Government presents the problem solely as that of the disadvantaged groups, defined both by their social and by their health characteristics. The Norwegians in the last programme have two definitions, both the problem of exclusion and the gradient. The former Swedish Government likewise uses both descriptions, but both governments tend to give most weight to the gradient definition. The liberal Swedish Government in 2009 focuses on exclusion and thus has a dichotomous understanding of differences. The Finnish Government defines the problems both as the poor health of 'groups in the weakest position' and as differences between socioeconomic, educational and vocational groups, indicating an understanding of the issue both as a dichotomy and as a gradient. The Finnish, Norwegian and former Swedish Governments all mention health inequalities between the sexes and between geographical areas. In the latest Swedish programme from 2008, these play only a minor role, while five national minorities (who have an acknowledged language such as Finnish, Sámi or Yiddish) are mentioned as groups to focus on. When inequalities are described as a gradient and other social categories are included, the focus of the policies towards health inequalities becomes broader and tends to include the whole population, making universal measures obvious. By comparison, considering health inequalities to be the poor health of a marginalized minority, as the Danes and the liberal Swedish Government do, makes a residual approach more appropriate. In this policy field, the problem definition differs substantially, with Denmark, and now Sweden, presenting the most divergent position.

12.6.2 Comparisons of health inequalities

Comparing social inequalities in health is more difficult than comparing mean life expectancy. The main reason is that categorizations and the content of the categories differ. Another problem is that the regulation of labour markets may influence the results. Inequalities among the employed were more distinct in Sweden than in Denmark. The smaller relative differences in Denmark could partly reflect the fact that dismissing employees on long-term sick leave is easier in Denmark than in Sweden (Lissau et al. 2001). A third issue is whether relative or absolute differences should be considered (Vågerö and Erikson 1997; Diderichsen 2006; Lynch et al. 2006). According to Ringbäck-Weitoft (2001), when looking at relative differences, Sweden has greater inequalities than Denmark, while the result is reversed if the differences are considered in absolute terms. Boström and Rosén (2003) reach the same result (Table 12.2). The probability of dying is higher in Denmark, making the risk of death for Swedish manual employees almost as low as that of non-manual Danish employees. Finland stands out with the greatest inequalities irrespective of measure and has the highest mortality level among male blue-collar workers, while the Danish white-collar employees have higher mortality levels than their Nordic counterparts. We do not know if these figures were actually available to the politicians

Table 12.2 Comparisons of health inequalities: deaths in men aged 30–59 years by socioeconomic group 1990–1994

Country	Socioeconomic group	Deaths per 100,000 person-years	Relative difference	Absolute difference
Denmark	Blue collar	570	1.5	180
	White collar	390		
Finland	Blue collar	690	1.9	330
	White collar	360		
Norway	Blue collar	430	1.5	150
	White collar	280		
Sweden	Blue collar	410	1.6	160
	White collar	250		

Source: Boström and Rosén (2003).

and the civil servants, but there was a clear understanding among them that health inequalities were increasing.

12.7 Causes and responsibilities

Given that the health problems identified are fairly similar, one might expect that this would also be the case for their explanations. Indeed, there are similarities. All programmes mention diet, physical inactivity, alcohol and smoking as important causes of ill health. There are, however, also substantial differences between the programmes. The Danish programme focuses almost exclusively on so-called lifestyles, that is, on risk factors associated with certain forms of behaviour, although it also mentions physical environment and work environment.

In the Norwegian and Swedish programmes, in contrast, living conditions and social relations play a central role. Stress, unemployment, poor social networks and lack of social support are mentioned as important causes of ill health. The Norwegian programme describes both strengthening and debilitating factors. Positive, or strengthening, factors are 'our relations to our nearest and dearest and our social networks, the extent to which our life seems meaningful, is predictable and manageable'. Negative factors mentioned are 'things we eat and drink, and factors in our social or physical environment' (Norwegian Ministry of Health 2003). Psychosocial factors are stressed in the Norwegian programme as being both strengthening and debilitating. The present Swedish Government also mentions all these factors but emphasizes the importance of individual behaviour.

The Finnish Government has a fairly broad scope of explanations: 'everyday conditions, and human interaction, ways of life and choices ... biological, psychological, chemical, physical and social factors in people's normal environments – their homes, housing areas, traffic, schools, workplaces and leisure activities' (Ministry of Social Affairs and Health 2001). In this respect it resembles the Norwegian and Swedish programmes.

While the green papers preceding the earlier Swedish programme considered social capital an important factor for health, this was replaced in the programme of 2002 by the importance of political participation: 'Participation and influence are key issues for a democratic society and have also been shown to affect public health' (Swedish National Institute of Public Health 2004). In addition, characteristics considered typical of the welfare state – 'economic and social security, equality in living conditions, gender equality and justice' (Swedish National Institute of Public Health 2004) – were mentioned as factors influencing the health of the population. The important factors influencing public health policies were thus identical with central elements of social democratic ideals about democracy and welfare state. Likewise the new Swedish programme stresses participation, above all employment, as important to health. Increased employment is central in the policies of the liberal government. Both governments thus combine their general political goals with the health goals.

12.7.1 Who is responsible?

The identification of causes of good and bad health is closely connected with the constructions of responsibility. If unhealthy behaviour is construed as the major cause of disease, and if citizens are seen as capable of making free choices over lifestyles, then the individual is considered to bear the primary responsibility for his or her health condition. If living conditions are considered to be a major cause of ill health, the state and consequently politicians are given more responsibility. In the Finnish programme, emphasis is on both individual and collective responsibility. Some factors can be influenced by individuals, others only by politicians. The programme mentions biological, psychological, physical, chemical and psychosocial stresses; social characteristics of the everyday environment; competition; lack of social support and care; and lack of knowledge, abilities and education. All of these must be seen as mainly collective responsibilities. However, it also emphasizes unhealthy behaviour, which could also be an individual responsibility. The Finnish Government seems to stress autonomy but says less about individual responsibility: 'Ultimately people decide what their lives will be like through the choices they make. The desire for autonomy is a key human characteristic: people are given information, opportunities and challenges, but they make their own decisions.'

In the Norwegian and Swedish programmes, living conditions and social relations are also constructed as important factors, and behaviour is to some extent construed as determined by these, with responsibility for the individual's health to a larger degree seen as belonging to the politicians or society.[1] The Norwegian programme explicitly states that 'the health of the population results not least from developments and political choices outside the single citizen's influence' (Norwegian Ministry of Health 2003), but it also stresses that there is 'a connection between the responsibility and possibility of influencing the health situation between the individual and the society' (Norwegian Ministry of Health 2003). The former Swedish programme characterizes public health as 'society's responsibility' (Swedish National Institute of Public Health 2004) thus stressing the responsibility of politicians even more. The present liberal Swedish Government marks a change by stating that it builds on 'people's need for integrity and freedom of choice' and that 'great improvements in the health of the population can be achieved if the individuals can take and take an increased responsibility for their health' (Regeringen 2008).

Like the liberal Swedish Government, the Danish programme emphasizes the responsibility and autonomy of the individual: 'Individuals are responsible for their own lives. Everyone has the right to live their lives as they wish: to make their own choices'; 'Respecting individual autonomy is decisive. The public sector should not control our lives' (Regeringen 2002c). Although it does mention the government's responsibility, this plays a less significant role than in the Finnish, Norwegian and both Swedish programmes.

In comparison with the Finnish, Norwegian and the Swedish programmes, the Danish programme stands out by devoting far less attention to social relations and living conditions and, therefore, more to individual behaviour, as well as granting politicians a smaller role in improving the health of the population. The latest Swedish programme is somewhat contradictory since it in some respects builds on the former programme and mentions social conditions as crucial, yet simultaneously stresses the responsibilities of the individuals.

12.7.2 Causes of social inequalities in health

Not surprisingly, the explanations of social inequalities follow the general discourse of the programmes. In Denmark, the personal behaviour of the marginalized is seen as the main cause of their poor health, while in Finland, Norway and Sweden other causes such as poverty and, above all, working conditions are mentioned as causing the differences. The 2006 Swedish Government writes about exclusion. These countries also mention behavioural factors such as smoking, diet and physical inactivity as causing higher prevalence of poor health in the lower social classes, but at the same time stress that behaviours are influenced by social conditions. The Norwegian and the former Swedish programmes phrase the notions in exactly the same way: 'Since they follow very clear social patterns, the principle cause of the disparities is not an individual's choice of lifestyle' (Norwegian Ministry of Health 2003; Swedish National Institute of Public Health 2004). While the Danish explanations are open to the interpretation that health inequalities are primarily the responsibility of the individual, that interpretation is rejected by the two other Scandinavian countries.

12.8 Which means are suggested to solve the problems?

The means suggested to improve the health of the population are largely in accordance with the explanations given. The initiatives suggested in the Danish programme primarily reflect a liberal view and respect for the autonomy of the individual. Citizens should be helped to make their own informed decisions: 'One key aspect is giving individuals the necessary knowledge and tools to carry out their own efforts to promote health and care for themselves' and initiatives should mainly be 'based on voluntary participation and respect for individuals' (Regeringen 2002c). According to the Danish programme, the government should be much more active when it comes to people who are labelled 'vulnerable adults', and health professionals should perform tracing and outreach activities. The 'disadvantaged' should be induced to change their behaviour. Freedom is granted only so long as people act responsibly in the eyes of the authorities. The pronounced focus on behaviour and the responsibility of the individual citizen are continuously the hallmarks of Danish public health policy in addition to a focus on vulnerable groups as the means to reduce social inequalities in health. This can be seen from two recent policy papers from the government (Regeringen 2007a, 2007b) and a statement from the dominant party in the governing coalition (Venstre 2007). The liberal Swedish Government expresses similar ideas, saying that people should have their own choice while also wishing 'to promote the interests, responsibility and possibilities of the individual to take care of its own health' (Regeringen 2008). This is to be achieved both through impartial information and by efforts to change people's ambitions by 'motivational interviewing' and so on. The government wants people to choose freely but that freedom should be used to choose healthy behaviours; otherwise the government wishes to help people to change their motives and choices.

Similar ideas are expressed in the Finnish programme: 'Respecting autonomy and supporting the preconditions for it are crucial in all health recommendations. On the other hand, people should always have a strong personal sense of responsibility for the consequences of the decisions they take about their lives'. However, the same programme also supports state interventions and demands action by industries, media and non-governmental organizations. It is also quite specific in advocating European state interventions: 'In legal regulation of many health risks, national sovereignity has already shifted to the EU. This is why there must be a stronger international dimension in new health policy initiatives and impact' (Ministry of Social Affairs and Health 2001).

The social democratic Swedish Government aimed, as does to a lesser extent the present liberal government, at addressing a broad spectrum of social environmental factors such as participation, economic and social security, safe childhood, improved work-related health, healthy and safe environment and products, and individual behaviour such as safe sex, increased physical activity, good eating habits and safe food, and decreased tobacco and alcohol consumption.

The Norwegian paper is the most specific concerning suggestions about both living conditions, physical planning and better facilities for cycling, and behaviour, such as physical activity in general and at the workplace or smoking prohibitions. The government also wishes to 'strengthen the individual's experience of coping ability, social support and participation, the feeling of being useful, capability of being responsible for themselves and using their own resources' (Norwegian Ministry of Health 2003).

All programmes refer to 'partnerships' between individuals, communities, the non-governmental organizations, and the private and public sectors in carrying out public health measures. However, whereas the Finnish, Norwegian and Swedish programmes state that the public sector has a central partnership role, the Danish places more emphasis on individuals and non-public actors and states that, 'partnership is cooperation between equal partners to solve collective tasks' (Regeringen 2002c). It is not discussed what specifically makes partners (e.g. employees and employers) equal. The Norwegian programme argues for 'an active partnership which places responsibility, creates commitment and is an incentive to action' (Norwegian Ministry of Health 2003), emphasizing that responsibility should be taken at all levels.

The Finnish programme focuses on arenas such as working places, schools or the media. It maintains that it tries to balance between individual responsibility and state intervention and ends up in expecting more from the 'communities'.

The Norwegian programme and former Swedish programme do not pay much attention to securing the freedom of the individual citizens, but they do refer to individual responsibility. The Norwegian and the present Swedish programmes are most elaborate with regard to focusing on the state's role in strengthening and shaping the citizens, while the former Swedish programme is the most far reaching in that it allows public health policy to encompass virtually all political areas that may, in one way or another, influence health. This mirrors the wider range of factors included in Swedish identification of health causes, which grants higher importance to the state. In the Danish programme, focus is on changing individual behaviour and little is said about the tasks of the state. Therefore, although the Danish Government is the least content with the health situation in the country, it suggests fewer political measures to improve it.

12.8.1 How to reduce health inequalities?

Three strategies can be identified in the efforts to reduce health inequalities. Two focus on the worst off (i.e. a residual approach), one by trying to influence the behaviour of the disadvantaged (the Danish programme and to some extent the Swedish) and the other by trying to tackle exclusion (mainly the Norwegian, the present Swedish and the Finnish), as stated in the Finnish programme: 'Exclusion for reasons of age or cultural differences must be avoided, not least because of the obvious effects it has on health' (Ministry of Social Affairs and Health 2001). The third strategy is to use universal measures to address the social conditions of the whole populations in order to level out the gradient. This policy is mainly advocated in the Norwegian programme and the earlier Swedish programme of 2002.

The problem definitions or agenda settings are therefore quite different when it comes to solutions or interventions, and the four governments (or rather five, since the two Swedish government are so dissimilar) stand out with different approaches, although Norway and Sweden show some similarities both in addressing living conditions and by having a more universalist approach. The Danish focus on the disadvantaged is an expression of a residual welfare state approach, while the new Swedish approach hardly addresses the health issue as an inequality problem.

12.9 Concluding remarks

12.9.1 Who is responsible?

The way public health issues and social inequalities in health are problematized differs substantially among the Nordic countries, and in Sweden between different governments, social democratic and liberal. This occurs for the identification of causes and solutions and also for allocating responsibilities and in the understanding of social health inequalities. The political agendas differ, not least when it comes to placing responsibilities, where Denmark stands out as the country leaving least to the politicians and most to the individuals and the Norwegians most clearly stating that public health is a political responsibility.

12.9.2 Stable national approaches or changing agendas?

Are the national differences identified a result of longer traditions or path dependence in the policy-making and agenda setting, or are they expressions of a specific political climate and change with the political ideology of the government? The focus on the behaviour of citizens as the central cause of health problems and the central target for interventions has been predominant in Denmark at least since the first public health programme of 1989 (Regeringen 1989; Vallgårda 2003), while the Swedish policy statements from the 1980s and onwards have included living conditions and social relations, not least working conditions, as important causal factors and foci of interventions (SOU 1984; Folkhälsogruppen 1989; Vallgårda 2003). The paths followed in public health policies seem to have been in existence for several decades and the solutions point at certain nationally specific ways of understanding and solving health problems.

It would be tempting to claim that the differences of the four programmes reflect the different ideological composition of the government at the time of adopting the programmes. During the last two decades, Sweden has had social democratic governments, and in shorter periods liberal governments; Norway has had both liberal and social democratic governments launching programmes, and so has Denmark. Finland has had a rainbow coalition of social democrats with greens, right wing parties as well as the left union from the left side of the social democrats. The differences between the programmes of governments of different political colours in the same country are small. In spite of some changes in the public health programmes during the last decades, there seems to be rather consistent national approaches that do not change radically with the political ideology of the government (Vallgårda 2007b, 2008). However, the latest Swedish programme does not fit this conclusion. This government is following a new path and its new ideology implies a major change in the content of the policy.

12.9.3 A Nordic model?

We have to conclude that the countries do not adhere to a common model that could support the concept of a common Nordic welfare state model, though there are similarities. The policies are all based on an epidemiological and economic perspective in selecting diseases that are to be addressed. The same main causes of death, early retirement and sickness absence are identified. They all construe citizens as individuals capable and competent of making choices and the state as a legitimate guardian of the health of the population. They give similar reasons for dealing with the health of the population and identify similar health conditions and public health problems.

But there are, at the same time, important differences in the ways public health is problematized that seriously challenge the idea of a Nordic model in this policy field. More so than in other policy areas, Danish public health policy tends to stress individual responsibility and individually chosen behaviour as the main cause of poor health and the focus of interventions, whereas the other countries emphasize the importance of living conditions (i.e. factors outside the reach of the individual influence) and so place more responsibility on the state. The recent Swedish programme has elements of both. The problematization when it comes to causes and responsibilities is, therefore, quite different. The difference is even more obvious when it comes to the problematization of social inequalities in health, where in Denmark it is defined as the poor health of a marginalized minority caused by their behaviour and remedied by interventions by the health and social sector. In the other countries, the understanding of inequalities is as a gradient mainly caused by living conditions, and thus the responsibility of the state to change, pointing at a universal welfare state approach. In the last Norwegian programme, it is explicitly stated: 'General welfare initiatives are less stigmatising and may prevent people from ending up in the vulnerable situations in the first place. Furthermore, social health differences have impact on all social classes not only the most disadvantaged. We therefore have to continue the Nordic tradition of universal arrangements, combined with targeted interventions for the worst off' (Ministry for Health and Care Services 2007). The most recent Swedish programme is not explicit on the question of health inequalities and their causes.

The Norwegian programme and the former Swedish programme seem to be more clearly 'welfare statist', linking the promotion of public health closely with universalist social policies and constructing a benevolent interventionist public sector. The Danish programme is clearly much more cautious in these respects. It constructs a residual public health policy that relies much more on enlightened individuals and leaves only concern for vulnerable and excluded people for the state. Following a residualist orientation in this respect, the 2006 Swedish Government tends to follow the Danish. The Finnish programme seems to accept both orientations. This can be understood as an attempt to construct a 'third way' between traditional social democratic or welfare statist and traditional libertarian or residualist options.

Policy programmes are also 'only' programmes. Differences between them do not necessarily imply that the policy practices differ as much. Many initiatives labelled public health initiatives in Sweden and Norway are performed in Denmark under other headings such as environment or working conditions or school policy. Although it has importance for what is done whether health is included as an aim or not, the content of the interventions can be fairly similar in spite of different labelling. From the study of the public health programmes, the conclusions must, however, be that no Nordic model exists in the field of expressed public health policies, and that the policies, especially concerning social inequalities in health, subscribe to different welfare state models where the Danish is more residual and the former Swedish and Norwegian programmes have a universalist ethos.

Note

1. Society (samhälle, samfund, Yhteiskunta) in the Nordic languages can mean both the state and (civil) society and nation (Kettunen 2000), indicating another relation between the state and the citizens than in south European and Anglo-Saxon countries.

References

Boström, G. and Rosén, M. (2003) Measuring social inequalities in health: politics or science? *Scandinavian Journal of Public Health* 31: 211–15.

Diderichsen, F. (2006) Ulighed i sundhed: et skæringspunkt mellem etik, epidemiologi og politik, in Vallgårda, S. and Koch, L. (eds) *Forskel og lighed i sundhed og sygdom.* Copenhagen: Munksgaard, pp. 29–42.

Directorate for Health and Social Affairs [Det kongelige helse- og omsorgsdepartment] (2005) *The Challenge of the Gradient.* Oslo: Directorate for Health and Social Affairs.

Esping-Andersen, G. (1990) *The Three Worlds of Welfare Capitalism.* Cambridge: Polity Press.

Folkhälsogruppen (1989) *Folkhälsa: Riktlinjer för folkhälsoarbetet och folkhälsogruppens uppgifter.* [Pamphlet] Stockholm: Folkhälsogruppen [Public Health Group].

Foucault, M. (1994) Polemics, politics, and problematizations: an interview with Michel Foucault, in Rabinow, P. (ed.) *Ethics, Subjectivity and Truth.* New York: The New Press, 111–19.

Government of Sweden (2002) *Public Health Objective Bill* [2002/03:35]. Stockholm: Government of Sweden.

Harjula, M. (2007) *Terveyden jäljillä: suomalainen terveyspolitiikka 1900-luvulla.* Tampere: Tampere University Press.

Heywood, A. (2003) *Political Ideologies: An Introduction,* 3rd edn. Basingstoke: Palgrave Macmillan.

Johannisson, K. (1991) Folkhälsa: Det svenska projektet från 1900 till 2: a världskriget, *Lychnos:* 139–95.

Kettunen, P. (2000) Yhteiskunta: Society in Finnish, in *Finnish Yearbook of Political Thought 2000.* Jyväskylä: Sophi Academic Press, pp. 159–97.

Kildal, N. and Kuhnle, S. (eds) (2005) *Normative Foundations of the Welfare State.* London: Routledge.

Kuusi, E. (1932) *Sosiaalipolitiikka.* Porvoo: WSOY.

Lissau, I., Rasmussen, N.K., Hesse, N.M. and Hesse, U. (2001) Social differences in illness and health-related exclusion from the labour market in Denmark from 1987 to 1994, *Scandinavian Journal of Public Health* 29(Suppl 55): 19–30.

Lynch, J., Smith, G.D., Harper, S. and Bainbridge, K. (2006) Explaining the social gradient in coronary heart disease: comparing relative and absolute risk approaches, *Journal of Epidemiology and Community Health* 60: 436–41.

Ministry for Health and Care Services [Det kongelige helse- og omsorgsdepartment] (2007) *Nasjonal strategi for å utjevne sosiale helseforskjeller.* Oslo: Ministry for Health and Care Services.

Ministry of Social Affairs and Health (1987) *Health for All by the Year 2000: The Finnish National Strategy.* Helsinki: Ministry of Social Affairs and Health.

Ministry of Social Affairs and Health (2001) *Publication 6: Government Resolution on the Health 2015 Public Health Programme.* Helsinki: Ministry of Social Affairs and Health.

Moseng, O.G. (2001) *Det offentlige helsevesen i Norge,* Vol. 1: *Ansvaret for undersåttenes helse 1603–1850.* Oslo: Oslo University Press.

Norwegian Ministry of Health [Det kongelige helsedepartement] (2003) *Resept for et sunnere Norge. Folkehelsepolitikken. Stortingsmelding nr. 16 (2002–2003).* Oslo: Det kongelige helsedepartement.

NOU (1998) *NOU 1998: 18. Der er bruk for alle.* Oslo: Sosial- og helsedirektoratet.

Puro, K. (1973) *Terveyspolitiikan perusteet.* Helsinki: Tammi.

Qvarsell, R. (1991) *Vårdens idéhistoria.* Stockholm: Carlssons.

Regeringen (1989) *Regeringens forebyggelsesprogram: Programdel.* Copenhagen: Government of Denmark.

Regeringen (1991) *Regeringens proposition 1990/91: 175. Om vissa folkhälsofrågor.* Stockholm: Government of Sweden.

Regeringen (1994) *Regeringens skrivelse 1993/94: 247. Investera i hälsa – Prioritera för hälsa.* Stockholm: Government of Sweden.

Regeringen (1999) *Regeringens folkesundhedsprogram 1999–2008: Et handlingsorienteret program for sundere rammer i hverdagen.* Copenhagen: Government of Denmark.

Regeringen (2002a) *Regeringens proposition 2002/03: 35: Mål for folkhälsan.* Stockholm: Government of Sweden.

Regeringen (2002b) *Sund hele livet: de nationale mål og strategier for folkesundheden 2002–2010.* Copenhagen: Government of Denmark.

Regeringen (2002c) *Healthy Throughout Life: The Targets and Strategies for Public Health Policy of the Government of Denmark, 2002–2010.* Copenhagen: Government of Denmark.

Regeringen (2007a) *Bedre velfærd og større arbejdsglæde: Regeringens strategi for høj kvalitet i den offentlige service.* Copenhagen: Government of Denmark.

Regeringen (2007b) *Mulighedernes samfund: Regeringsgrundlag.* Copenhagen: Government of Denmark.

Regeringen (2008) *Regeringens proposition 2007/08: 110 En förnyad folkhälsopolitik.* Copenhagen: Government of Denmark.

Ringbäck-Weitoft, G. (2001) Social differences, vulnerability and ill-health: health in Sweden. The National Public Health Report 2001, *Scandinavian Journal of Public Health* 58(Suppl): 199–218.

Rothstein, B. (2001) The future of the universal welfare state, in Kuhnle, S. (ed.) *Survival of the European Welfare State.* London, Routledge, pp. 217–33.

Schiøtz, A. (2003) *Det offentlige helsevesen i Norge 1603–2005,* Vol. 2: *Folkets helse – landets styrke 1850–2003.* Oslo: Oslo University Press.

Sosialdepartementet (1993) *Stortingsmelding nr. 37 1992–93. Utfordringer i helsefremmende og forebyggende arbeid.* Oslo: Sosialdepartementet.

SOU (1984) *SOU 1984: 39. Hälso- och sjukvård inför 90-talet. HS90. Huvudrapport.* Stockholm: Socialstyrelsen [National Board of Health and Welfare].

Swedish National Institute of Public Health Govt.Bill 2002/03: 35 (2004) Chapter 3: The Swedish public health policy and the National Institute of Public Health, *Scandinavian Journal of Public Health* 32(Suppl 64): 60–4.

Tervonen Goncalves, L. and Lehto, J. (2004) Transfer of Health for All policy: what, how and in which direction? A two-case study, *Health Research Policy and Systems* 21: 2–8.

Trägårdh, L. (1997) Statist individualism: on culturality of the nordic welfare state, in Sørensen, Ø. and Stråth, B. (eds) *The Cultural Construction of Norden.* Oslo: Scandinavian University Press, pp. 253–85.

UK Department of Health (2003) *Tackling Health Inequalities: A Programme for Action.* London: Department of Health.

Vågerö, D. and Erikson, R. (1997) Socioeconomic inequalities in morbidity and mortality in western Europe, *Lancet* 350: 516.

Vallgårda, S. (2000) Om at styre menneskers liv: Danske myndigheders tiltag for at reducere sygelighed og dødelighed 1750–2000, *Tidsskrift for sygeplejeforskning* 16: 9–27.

Vallgårda, S. (2003) *Folkesundhed som politik: Danmark og Sverige 1930 til i dag.* Århus: Århus University Press.

Vallgårda, S. (2004) Power over life: the establishment of hospitals in Denmark in the late eighteenth century, in Andresen, A., Grønlie, T. and Skålevåg, S.A. (eds) *Hospitals, Patients and Medicine 1800–2000.* Bergen: Stein Rokkan Centre for Social Studies, pp. 11–20.

Vallgårda, S. (2007a) Health inequalities: political problematisations in Denmark and Sweden, *Critical Public Health* 17: 45–56.

Vallgårda, S. (2007b) Public health policies: a Scandinavian model? *Scandinavian Journal of Public Health* 35: 205–11.

Vallgårda, S. (2008) Social inequality in health: dichotomy or gradient? A comparative study of problematisations in national public health programs, *Health Policy* 85: 71–82.

Vallgårda, S. and Krasnik, A. (2007) *Health Services and Health Policy*. Copenhagen: Gyldendal Akademisk.

Venstre (2007) *Tre år ekstra om ti år. National forebyggelsesplan med klare mål for danskernes sundhed*. Copenhagen: Venstre.

chapter thirteen

Changing demands for institutional management

Lars Erik Kjekshus

13.1 Introduction

Efficiency, accountability, transparency and enhanced management are common goals for the governance reforms in the Nordic countries. However, it is unlikely that the overarching governance reforms will have such impacts unless changes in the institutional level are instituted. However, how the institutions will respond and adapt to such central governance reforms is uncertain. The objective of this chapter is to give a description of the internal organizational development in the hospitals in the Nordic countries in recent years (1999–2008) and discuss how these changes are related to the governance reforms in the Nordic countries. The Nordic countries have experienced different structural reforms and governance developments and presumably this has provoked differences in management and how work is organized.

The chapter will start with a presentation of an analytical approach that will enable central questions to be raised regarding the internal organizational development. How would institutional management be expected to respond to changes in governance structure? The second part of the chapter gives a presentation of central areas of internal organizational development in the hospitals of the Nordic countries and a discussion of these developments across providers and across countries. Are the changes in management models according to the expectations? The third part of the chapter discusses to what extent these organizational developments actually can be seen as a direct response to changes in governance as such. The chapter finishes by outlining possible future directions for organizational and institutional developments in the Nordic countries.

13.2 Analytical approach

Like many other European countries, the Nordic health systems experience increased demand for effective steering capabilities and management control (McKee and Healy 2002). Each Nordic country has undertaken different changes in government and governance structures. The governance reforms and how the Nordic countries have developed in recent years has been described and discussed in depth in the previous chapters.

These new governance structures can be divided into three main areas of governance (see Figure 13.1 on p. 278):

- *type of ownership relations and/or decentralization of decision-making power and responsibility for service delivery*: changes in the role of politicians and changes in the regulatory interaction between central (state) and decentralized levels (Chapter 5), contracts, purchaser–provider split, network governance versus government, interaction with the primary care (Chapters 11 and 12), political influence on hospital boards, the share of private versus public providers
- *financing*: de-/recentralization of taxation, changes in payment mechanisms to introduce more explicit use of economic incentives, new combinations of global versus activity-based financing (ABF) in order to improve budget discipline and performance (Chapters 5 and 8)
- *regulation*: quality assessment (Chapter 6), degree of quasi-market and market-driven purchasing (Chapter 9), patient choice of hospitals (Chapter 6).

At a general level, the aim of health system governance reforms is to influence the performance of the health system by reorganizing steering, management and organizational features. Specific objectives relate to organizational accountability, patient responsiveness, high-quality services, cost-efficiency and universal and fast access for all citizens (evidenced by short waiting lists). However, the objectives of the reforms are unlikely to be fulfilled unless the hospitals respond to the new governance structure by changing how their work is organized. This chapter will discuss variation in organizing hospital organizations.

There are multiple ways to describe the main features of organizations. This chapter will use an analytical model developed by Morten Egeberg (1989) in his studies of Norwegian public organizations. Egeberg distinguishes between *physical arrangements*, *organizational demography* and the *formal normative organizational structure* of the organization. This approach describes the basic characteristics of the organization and focuses on the organization as a tool for coordinated actions. The independent variables in focus are, in principle, open to redesign and under the control of the central management. They influence decision-making because they define, specify and reduce the amount of available choices in the organization (Egeberg 1989).

The physical arrangements of the hospital would be the architectural design as well as size and location. Location features include whether the hospital is in an area with many other hospitals (high hospital density) or the hospital is rather physically isolated. Hospital mergers would often affect the physical arrangement of the hospital as such.

The organizational demography includes the composition of the workforce and the characteristics of the employees, including gender, tenure and education, and the structure and competencies of management.

The formal organizational structures represent a normative description of core characteristics. The organizational structure can be grouped into four main areas of organizational elements:

- *leadership structure*: unity of command (one responsible leader at the department level of the hospitals instead of a leadership divided between two or three persons, such as troika leadership), scope of authority, jurisdiction and leadership development programmes
- *informatics and digitalization*: digitalization of traditional 'paper-heavy' routines, digital diagnostic services including X-ray and scanning facilities
- *budget routines*: internal pricing, ABF at department level, distribution of diagnosis-related group (DRG) budgets
- *patient logistics*: typical patient pathways, mechanisms for coordination and interaction between different parts of the hospital, 'ring-fencing' of elective surgery, organization of observation units and quality assessment systems.

Other independent variables such as climate, topography, culture, historical institutional arrangements are emphasized less because these variables are seen as relatively constant. They are important but not under the control of the management; they are handled as conditions that each hospital has to be aware of and must adjust their activities for. The focus in this chapter is on changes in organizational demography, physical arrangements and organizational structure in response to new governance initiatives.

By applying this framework, the chapter initially leaves out more detailed discussions of informal or cultural organizational features (Meyer and Rowan 1977; Powell and DiMaggio 1991). While such features are undoubtedly important for organizational performance, they are also very difficult to capture in a comparative light. The discussion of results briefly returns to such perspectives. It is suggested that more detailed studies of informal organizational elements could be an interesting follow-up to the present chapter. Summing up, the core argument of the chapter is that changes in governance make some organizational changes more likely than others, and that it is relevant to study changes in (formal) organizational features as they set the parameters for organizational activities (formal and informal) and thus for organizational performance.

13.3 Institutional response to change in governance

Previous chapters have shown profound changes in the Nordic health care system in terms of relationships between professions, politicians and administrators. Ownership structures have changed and decisions have either been decentralized or recentralized. Financing and payment mechanisms have changed along with more general adjustments of the regulatory structures. There has been an emphasis on explicit economic incentives in all four countries, in addition to more traditional steering mechanisms. Some parts of the region have seen experiments with quasi-market structures. But how do such changes in external governance structures affect the organization and management of health care organizations in the four countries? What is the relationship between change in governance structure and institutional management?

Healthcare organizations are often characterized as relatively resistant to change and are assumed to be difficult to change intentionally through management initiatives. This is partly because of the strong and relatively independent health professions working in hospital organizations and partly because of the size and complexity of organizational features and work processes. McKee and Healy (2002, p. 11) argue that 'external factors may be the most likely and appropriate way to change some aspects of hospitals and hospitals system'. Studies have shown that hospitals exposed to external pressure, such as a hospital merger, are more likely to initiate organizational redesign (Bogue et al. 1995; Kjekshus 2004). However, studies have also shown that changes in the external environment do not necessarily affect the organizational structure immediately and in the ways that were expected (Jakab et al. 2002). The upshot must be that external changes produce pressures that increase the likelihood of changes in particular directions, and make other organizational arrangements less likely. It is important to keep this in mind as we analyse the observed changes.

There are several reasons for being cautious in making exact predictions of the organizational effects of various governance changes. First, organizational change could be initiated by a plethora of different reasons related to both internal and external factors. The same organizational response could, therefore, result from several explanatory conditions. Second, most organizations face multiple pressures for change. The pressures interact but do not necessarily push the organization in the same direction. Third, introducing a new impulse, for example in terms of governance change, may have a different organizational impact in different organizational configurations. Fourth, the organizational interpretation of appropriate responses may differ, and the 'correct' response may not be evident. Several different institutional choices could be effective responses to different organizational contexts. In sum, the link between impulse and organizational response may be affected by many different factors, and we are unlikely to see the exact same response in all cases, although some general trends may be discernable.

These difficulties are acknowledged when mapping the relationship between change in governance and institutional response, although the argument here is that not all organizational responses are equally likely. It is reasonable to presume that some organizational features would be more expected than others. In the following, an analytical model of the relationship is presented. The model is a simplification and only thought of as a sketchy presentation of a possible relationship to be discussed in greater depth based on an instrumental perspective of organizations as presented by Egeberg (1989) (Figure 13.1).

The model indicates two relationships and illustrates how new governance could indirectly affect hospital performance in relationship 2. First, new governance must affect how the service is organized and delivered in relationship 1. Then, how the service is organized and delivered would affect the performance in relationship 2. The relationship between organizing and hospital performance is, if possible, even more complicated and difficult to figure out (Kjekshus

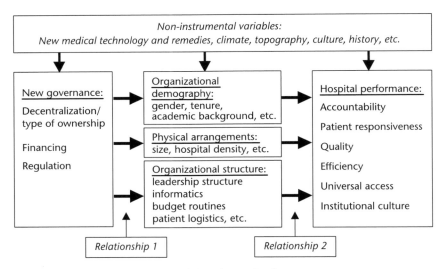

Figure 13.1   An analytical model of the relationship between new governance structures, organizational structures and hospital performance.

2004). However, relationship 2 is not the focus in this chapter and will only briefly be commented on.

In the following, hypotheses about relationship 1 will be addressed before the presentation of the actual organizational development in the Nordic countries is presented. The hypotheses will be the starting point for a discussion on the relationship between change in governance structures and organizational development in the aftermath. It should be noted that the term 'hypotheses' does not refer to formal testable statements but rather to 'working assumptions' for the explorative investigation.

13.3.1 Hypotheses for institutional response to change in type of ownership relations and/or decentralization of decision-making power and responsibility for service deliver

Decentralization and recentralization have been important reform themes in the Nordic countries. Decentralization would imply more responsibility and increased amount of assignments at the lower levels of the system. The following hypothesis could be put forward: a response to decentralized governance structure would involve more personnel with economical and administrative competencies in the hospitals, the introduction of unity of command,[1] professional hospital boards and unit-based budget responsibility in order to meet the new demand for enhanced steering capabilities.

However, some of the Nordic reforms also have elements of recentralizing of decisions, such as questions regarding distribution of highly specialized medical services and acute care. One typical feature of several of the Nordic health care reforms is the wish to neutralize politics in the decision-making processes (Stigen and Opedal 2005). The day-to-day operations should be performed without intervention from politicians. The intention of the reforms is that politicians should be occupied with ideological and strategical questions and leave the implementation and details to professional managers. In Norway, the ownership of the hospitals was transferred from the county level to the state. It could be assumed that the recentralizing would increase the hierarchical lines of authority in the health care organizations and create a more distinct separation of the role of provider and purchaser. However, studies have shown that it has been difficult to formally recentralize politics in an area where the decisions have high priorities in the local communities and where the decisions are controversial (Tjerbo 2007). The politics are still present but find new channels. A potential hypothesis regarding recentralized governance structure is that the disappearance of a formal governmental level will enforce increased network governance and an institutional management capable of handling both the administrative and the political challenges. This would increase the need for more personnel with competencies in media and reputation evaluations and the need to construct a superficial organizational design in response to ambiguous and changing political signals.

13.3.2 Hypotheses for institutional response to change in financing

All the Nordic countries have experienced changes in the financing and payment mechanisms for health care. The effect of the traditional payment mechanisms based on global budgeting was increased waiting time. The introduction of ABF gave incentives for higher productivity in the health care organizations. Organizations with an especially high productivity would no longer be punished with insufficient funding. We would expect to find organizational responses in terms of changes such as patient logistics, changes in accounting and budget routines and changes in management competencies with the aim of increasing the productivity at the hospital.

A response to ABF would be a stronger focus on patient logistics and organizational features that would enhance the productivity of certain medical treatments. Such organizational features could include specialized 'ring-fencing' units, where elective operations are shielded from emergency care. The elective operations are inspired by assembly lines. The operating theatre is set up for a specific procedure with a minimum of equipment and personnel. This enables a fast track for certain types of patient. Another organizational feature directed to improve the flow of patients is observation units. This reduces unnecessary in-bed admissions by enabling observation of patients in a special unit in the emergency department before final decisions are made on admission. Most patients with unclear diagnoses, such as unspecific abdominal pain, improve after a few hours and are no longer in need for in-hospital stay. Other organizational feature we would expect as a response to ABF would be new accounting routines and increased personnel with economical competencies, in order to increase economic control, predictability, transparency and accountability.

13.3.3 Hypotheses for institutional response to change in regulation and market orientation

An important aim in many of the reforms in the Nordic countries has been to enforce a more patient-focused ward with better coordination between primary and secondary care. The introduction of more market orientation in health care systems could enforce more patient-focused care. Healthcare organizations would need to attract patients and try out patient-centred wards as a contrast to the traditional professional bureaucracies.

Reforms that aim to strengthen the interaction between primary and secondary care could give incentives to implement new organizational features to enhance interaction and coordination. Positioning a primary care coordinator at the hospital could be one such response. This would be a person designated to work in coordination with the primary caregivers to ensure fast and smooth communications (Kjekshus 2005). A different organizational response could be to build hospital hotels, to merge GP wards and the emergency department at the hospital, or to provide in-between services such as an ambulant medical team and district medical centres.

A response to a more market-oriented health care system and reforms that enhance the interaction between primary and secondary care would be a patient-centred organizational design to attract patients and organizational features enabling enhanced interaction between primary and secondary care.

13.4 New governance in the Nordic countries

Between 1990 and 2008, all the Nordic countries experienced changes in how their health care system was governed (Chapter 5). Norway experienced a major structural change in 2002 when the responsibility for hospitals shifted from the counties to the state and the hospitals became public enterprises. Use of ABF was implemented in 1997. Free choice of hospitals, unity of command and the GP reform were also implemented during this period. Denmark experienced their major governance reform in 2007, where the responsibility for the hospitals was moved from 15 counties to five health regions. However, as discussed in detail in Chapter 5, Denmark has had several reforms since 1990. It has introduced ABF, free choice of hospitals and a stronger emphasis on economic incentives. Denmark, in contrast to the large-scale and state-driven reforms in Norway, has also had several local reform initiatives leading up to the major structural reform of 2007. Many reform initiatives have focused on internal organization rather than on changing the overall structure of the hospitals.

The Swedish health care system is primarily regional based (18 county councils) and less centralized compared with Denmark and especially Norway. Sweden, compared with Norway and Denmark, has been the tortoise when it comes to implementing large-scale governance reforms. However, although Sweden has mainly relied on regional reforms, some of these have been relative radical in a Nordic context. The many regional reform initiatives led to the expectation that changing demands for institutional management are likely to be as evident in Sweden as in the other Nordic countries, although perhaps with more diversity because of the differences in regional governance systems.

Finland has differed in development from the other Nordic countries. The Finnish health care system is decentralized to the municipal level. During the 1990s, there was increasing deregulation and emphasis on municipal autonomy. The Finnish health care system was facing severe challenges in how to maintain the health care services during and after the economic recession in the 1990s. The Finnish health sector was a pioneer in introducing ABF and the DRG system and has been able to show only a modest growth in health care expenditure and still have a population that is relatively satisfied with the services (more than 80 per cent of Finnish respondents were satisfied compared with EU average of 41.3 per cent (Järvelin 2002)). The country is divided into 20 hospital districts, each responsible for providing specialized medical care and the coordination of the public specialized care services within its area. Each municipality must be a member of a hospital district (Järvelin 2002).

In the following sections, the main institutional responses that have been observed in the Nordic countries will be sketched out and then discussed in light of the hypotheses presented above.

13.5 Responses to changes in governance structure

The number of observations from the four Nordic countries varies in terms of perspective, scope and scale. Our sources for these presentations are comments from country experts together with existing literature describing observations in the different countries. Denmark and Norway to some extent have more systematic registrations of new management structures within the health - care organization. This means that some of the findings, especially from Finland and Sweden, are not fully documented and are based on general statements from country experts. There are significant methodological concerns in applying the same concepts and analytical categories for collecting data in the four countries. For example, is 'ring fencing' or 'observation units' understood in the same manner in the different national contexts? Further validation of the understanding of concepts should be undertaken, but for the present purposes we rely on the relative homogeneity across the countries and the comparative insights of the country experts to provide relatively consistent interpretations. Table 13.1 gives a brief summary of the empirical findings.

The first impression of the summary of findings in Table 13.1 is the variation among countries. Finland and Sweden are characterized by more modest developments and fewer large-scale changes. Norway has had the largest increase in health expenditure (over 80 per cent in yearly expenditure from 2000 to 2006) (SSB 2007).

Table 13.1 Summarized responses regarding internal organizational development among Nordic physical care hospitals 2000–2008

	Denmark	Norway	Finland	Sweden
Organizational demography				
Has the relative number of nurses increased?	2	2	n/a	2
Has the relative number of physicians increased?	2	3	n/a	2
Has the relative number of personnel with administrative and economical competencies increased?	2	2	n/a	1
Has the relative number of personnel with administrative and economical competencies increased at the top level of the hospitals?	2	3	n/a	3
Has the relative number of public relation personnel increased?	2*	2	n/a	2*
Physical arrangements				
Have several hospitals merged during the period?	2	3	2	0
Have there been several hospitals closures?	1	1	1	0
Have the hospitals expanded?	2	1	2	0
Has the total amount of beds expanded?	−1	2	1	1
Have new hospitals been built?	0	3	0	0
Have several hospitals invested in electronically patient records?	3	3	3	3
Have several hospitals invested in new informational technology systems and support?	3	3	3	3
Organizational structure				
Have several hospitals implemented a divisional organizational structure or similar?	2	3	1	3
Have several hospitals implemented ring-fencing surgery or medicine?	3	2	2	3
Have several hospitals implemented observation units in the acute care unit?	n/a	2	2**	1
Have several hospitals engaged in projects to enhance efficiency (e.g. LEAN, logistics)?	3	2	3	0
Have several hospitals engaged in projects to enhance quality (e.g. TQM, ISO certification)	3	2	3	2
Have several hospitals engaged in projects to enhance cooperation with primary care?	2*	1	1	2
Have several hospitals signed formal agreements on cooperation with primary care?	2*	0	n/a	2
Have several hospitals implemented activity-based budgeting on a department level?	2*	3	3**	2
Have several hospitals implemented internal pricing?	n/a	3	3	3

Leadership structure

Have several hospitals implemented unity of command?	3*	3	n/a	2
Have several hospitals implemented decentralized authority to the department level (e.g. authority to hire physicians, making readjustment in investments)?	3*	2	2	0
Do several hospitals gather public relations information and perform strategic analysis of the surrounding (e.g. SWOT analysis)?	n/a	2	n/a	2
Do several hospitals offer management training to their top management?	2*	3	2	2
Are there several hospitals that have leaders with bonus arrangements?	n/a	0	3	0
Has the top management turnover increased?	n/a	2	0	n/a

TQM, total quality management; SWAT, strengths, weaknesses, opportunities and threats; −1, reduction; 0, no observable difference; 1, small increase; 2, medium increase; 3, large increase.
* Baseline.
** University hospitals.

13.5.1 Changes in organizational demography

Changes in organizational demography were particularly expected as an institutional response to changes that involved decentralization, increased private providers and changing financial systems.

Table 13.1 shows a general trend of health care expansion, although that in Norway greatly exceeds that in the other Nordic countries. An interesting and surprising finding is the relatively low growth in administrative and economic personnel compared with other types of personnel. The hypothesis was that recent reforms in the Nordic countries would trigger an increase in such groups; instead it seems that other groups, nurses and especially physicians, have seen a higher growth. The only exception seems to be Finland. The Finnish hospitals have been under increasing pressure to improving coordination of the delivery of health care services and to handle growing deficits. The administrative and economic competencies have increased, although accurate records are not available to show the relative proportion compared with the increase in clinical personnel.

In the other Nordic countries, the administrative and economic competencies at the department level of hospitals are also strengthened. However, the relatively fastest growing group is the physicians and the number of administrative personnel has not increased as much that for physicians. In Norway, there was a 2 per cent increase in administrative personnel from 2002 to 2005 compared with 13 per cent for physicians (Iversen et al. 2006). Among the top executives in the Norwegian hospitals in 2007, 35 per cent had a medical background, 25 per cent a nursing background and only 22 per cent had social science or economics as their main educational background (Kjekshus and Westlie 2008). This blend of top executives was stable and was the same in 2003 and 2005.

An institutional response more consistent with the hypothesis is the increase of media advisors and public relations personnel, especially in Sweden and Norway. In 2003, only 37 per cent of the Norwegian hospitals had a public relations manager as a formal position among their top executives. In 2007, 88 per cent of the Norwegian hospital enterprises had a public relations manager among their top executives and the total number of public relations executives in the hospital enterprise is increasing. In 2005, 49 per cent of the hospitals reported that they perform regular opinion evaluation. In 2007, this trend had increase to 67 per cent of the hospital enterprises.

13.5.2 Changes in physical arrangements

New hospitals have been built in all the Nordic countries in the past decades. There is a trend among the hospital architects to acknowledge the demand for change and flexibility in the physical arrangement. Hospitals are, therefore, designed to be easy to change. The buildings are created with different modules, and walls that are easy to redesign. Often the buildings are designed to be able to expand either in height or width.

Another general trend in all the Nordic countries is that hospitals are merging (Borum and Pedersen 2008). This is also a global trend and could be explained by the need for larger units in order to implement more advanced diagnostic apparatus and more advanced medical procedures. The general trend can also be explained by a popular opinion that larger production units are more efficient and can deliver better quality than smaller units, although recent research questions this opinion (Kjekshus and Hagen 2007). However, the trend of merging hospitals does not necessarily affect the physical arrangements. The ambition is often to reallocate the functions of the hospitals being merged but the reality is that closures and reallocations are difficult to achieve because of local political protest and other conflicting interest (Tjerbo 2007). The trend of hospital mergers is most evident in Denmark and Norway. In Norway, hospital mergers had already started in the early 1990s (Kjekshus and Hagen 2007). However, mergers increased dramatically following the hospital ownership reform in 2002. A common strategy of all the five regional health enterprises in Norway was to merge approximately 70 hospitals into 25 larger enterprise units. Sweden had their wave of hospital mergers in the period 1995 to 2000. This trend could be related to the economic recession Sweden experienced in 1993, and the resulting pressure for increases in hospital efficiency. Since 2000, the trend of mergers has slowed although a large merger and a new hospital is being planned in Stockholm (Calltorp 2008). All the Nordic countries apart from Sweden report a small number of hospital closures.

In Sweden and Denmark, we also observe a trend of vertical integration, both formally and informally. The focus has been on organization of the interaction between levels of cure and care, and initiatives for closer coordination have been introduced. An example of a vertical integration is when the GP on duty call is physically based in the hospital emergency department. In 2007, 37 per cent of the Norwegian hospitals had such vertical integration. A general and strong trend in new physical arrangements in hospitals in all the Nordic countries is towards the implementation of new information technology systems and electronically based systems such as digital patient records and digital radiography records, as shown in Table 13.1.

It seems that the largest changes in new physical arrangements of the hospitals are happening in Norway. Norway is the only country reporting several new hospitals, although Denmark is currently (2009) planning several new facilities. Sweden has had the least amount of change in the physical arrangement of the hospital landscape in the period between 2000 and 2008.

13.5.3 *Changes in internal organizational structure*

All the Nordic countries indicate that the organizational structure in hospitals is changing in a number of areas, including interaction with primary care, patient logistics, systems of quality standards and internal payment mechanisms. The exact distribution of these new organizational features in Sweden and Finland is not known. The data from Denmark and Norway are more comprehensive. In Norway, the INTORG studies have examined organizational development over time (Kjekshus and Harsvik 2007; Kjekshus and Westlie 2008). Figure 13.2 shows central organizational developments in Norwegian hospitals from 1999 to 2007.

Experiments with patient-centred wards, clinics and divisions to replace traditional department structures are taking place in all the Nordic countries except Finland, which to a larger extent still has the traditional department

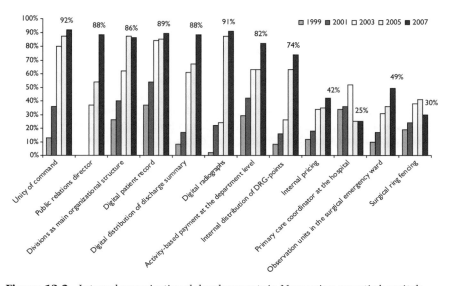

Figure 13.2   Internal organizational developments in Norwegian somatic hospitals 1999–2007. DRG, diagnosis-related group.

Source: Kjekshus and Westlie (2008).

structure (Table 13.1). In terms of organizing patient logistics, several new organizational designs are emerging, such as observatory units in the emergency department, surgical ring fencing and GP on duty call being physically based in the the hospital emergency department (Figure 13.2). Especially in Denmark, several hospitals have implemented ring-fenced surgery. In Norway, it seems that the trend is declining. Several hospitals in Sweden have surgical ring fencing, for example Hesleholm in Skåne. However, there is an ongoing debate on the effect of ring fencing (Kjekshus and Hagen 2005). There is a general trend to focus on logistics and new programmes in redesign, such as LEAN and six sigma, as well as new quality-enhancing programmes such as 'total quality management' (Vrangbæk 1999). In Denmark, there is a general obligation for all hospitals to be accredited as part of the national quality assessment programme. The same trend is increasing in Norway. The largest health enterprise (Helse SØR-ØST) made this mandatory in 2008 for all their hospitals. In Sweden, this trend is not as evident. New trends in logistics in particular have been met with discontent and scepticism among the health professionals (Calltorp 2008).

New electronically based routines have been observed for laboratory text requests, for example, and for communication between primary care and specialist services. There has been an increasing focus on transparency in all the Nordic countries (Levay and Waks 2006) and hospitals report regularly on several quality indicators in all four countries. Changes in budget and accounting routines are observed in all the Nordic countries, particularly the Norwegian and Finnish hospitals. The budgets are more detailed and routines such as internal pricing and ABF at department level have been implemented. Norway and Finland were also first to introduce ABF, whereas Sweden and Denmark have been more reluctant to introduce this type of financial incentives.

13.5.4 Changes in leadership structure

The most common new organizational and leadership structures are within the authority structure and accounting routines in all the Nordic countries. Most hospitals in Norway report increasingly decentralized authority structures. New leadership structure such as unitary command has been implemented in all Norwegian and Danish hospitals. The quest for unity of command is also evident in Sweden and Finland but to a lesser extent.

The trend of decentralizing decision structures is particularly evident in Norwegian hospitals. Decisions regarding issues such as the hiring of physicians and nurses, on-duty call systems, individually differentiated salaries and the coordination of incoming patients are increasingly delegated to the department level of the hospital enterprises. However, decisions regarding extraordinary expenses and making statements to the press are centralized to the top management of the hospital enterprises.

In Sweden, the trend of decentralizations has been evident since the beginning of the 1990s and, therefore, it would not be correct to report an increase in the late period 2000–2008. Finland has a similar trend of decentralizations as in Norway although this is not documented to the same extent. From Denmark, we have a baseline observation showing that decentralization is very common among Danish hospitals. Here, the hospital structure is dominated by centre organizations and divisions. The troika leadership model is still the dominating leadership structure. However, although the trend is centralized coordination, decentralized economical responsibility is also seen.

In all the Nordic countries, training programmes for top management are increasingly common. From Norway, accurate data show increasing turnover of top management, especially after the hospital reform. Similar documentation is not available for the other Nordic countries but the impression is that the same trend is observed in Sweden but not in Finland. Finland is the only country that is introducing bonus arrangements for top management.

The modelling of the hospitals is changing from medical specialities to divisions with unit-based budget responsibility and improved institutional accounting practices. This represents a new way of rethinking hospitals, strongly influenced by the private sector and industry (Bentsen 1997; Timm 1997; Levay and Waks 2006).

13.6 Towards a new Nordic management model

The general empirical evidence on organizational development of the health care systems of the Nordic countries does show variations, although the variations can be larger within countries than between countries. Based on the ongoing debates and case studies from the Nordic countries, some general trends in management responses to new governance can be identified. Hospitals are introducing digital services on a large scale, such as electronic medical records and digital radiography systems (PACS); decentralized budget responsibilities and more advanced accounting systems. They are experimenting with new organizational designs such as ring-fencing day surgery and observation units in the emergency department. These organizational features are as expected and are predicted responses to the changes in governance in the Nordic countries, such as the introduction of ABF. However, while we believe the Nordic health care systems have become more market oriented, with the introduction of patient rights to choose hospitals, we also observe areas with a more unexpected development. There is weak evidence for hospitals organizing to attract more patients. The interaction between primary and secondary health - care services seems to be unsolved although there are some attempts to strengthen administrative coordination. The organizational demography is also developing differently to expectations. Although we do observe a strengthening of the administrative and economic competencies in the Nordic hospitals, we also observe a relative higher increase in physicians than in other personnel groups. This is especially evident in Norway.

13.6.1 *From hospital to health care organization*

An international trend has been that the 'hospital' concept is changing (Scott et al. 2000). This was particularly evident in Norway after the ownership reform.

Where the organizational border of a traditional hospital starts and stops is difficult to define. The traditional old hospital system with the three basic main components of medicine, surgery and administration within a limited geographically area and within the same physical building is eroded. These days, the old hospital is only one among several other health care centres such as specialized patient centres (heart and lung centres), district medical centres and district psychiatric wards. In 1990, there were approximately 80 somatic hospitals in Norway. Today the number is approximately 26 and consists of several merged hospitals plus different types of centre and specialized unit and 'one and a half' services (in cooperation with the primary care services). The merging of the old hospitals was initiated in order to redistribute the medical function and the on-duty system between the hospitals. Several health care enterprises have merged specialities across hospitals, with one medical director in charge of the speciality in several hospitals, as illustrated in Figure 13.3.

The old hospital buildings are still there and patients continue to refer to the buildings as hospitals, but the health care organization no longer uses the term hospital but labels them instead as health care divisions. For example, Healthcare Division 'Gjøvik', Healthcare Division 'Lillehammer' and Healthcare Division 'Hamar' used to be separate hospitals but are now part of the health care enterprise 'Hospital Innlandet'. The health care organization 'Hospital Innlandet' itself has no physical location but consist of 41 units all over Hedmark and Oppland County (Økelsrud 2007). Similar trends can be seen in Denmark, where the structural reform of 2007 further accelerated hospital mergers and experiments with new organizational designs.

13.6.2 Strengthening or weakening the Nordic democratic management model

Several analysts of the Nordic health care system have advocated a new management leadership style in order to meet the challenges in the new governance

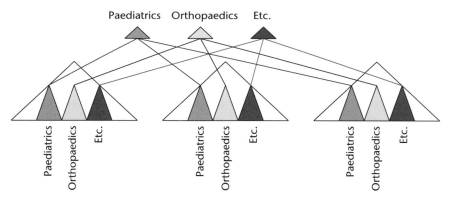

Figure 13.3   Merged hospitals organized in medical divisions with one medical director for each specialty. Etc., indicates other specialties.

structure. A key point has been to enable management to understand medical decision-making better, as well as handling administration, economics and politics. In the National Health Service in the United Kingdom, this type of leadership has been defined as clinical governance. A description of the Nordic management model that has been used by several scholars is as a democratic management model. Decision behaviour and processes are built on democratic traditions where the legitimacy of the processes is based on participation of a broad set of interest groups, including different patient representatives, representatives from the different unions and representatives from hospital stakeholders such as local politicians and primary care representatives.

Vrangbæk and Torjesen (2005) performed a comparative study of hospital leaders' attitude towards leadership issues, economical issues and recent reforms in Denmark and Norway. The study shows an interesting difference between Denmark and Norway. Norwegian leaders tend to be more focused on the formal governance structures than are the Danish hospital leaders. It may be that Vrangbæk and Torjesen are observing the beginning of a new trend where the Nordic management model is moving towards a more hierarchical and formal management model. Norway has chosen a more radical reform path than Denmark in terms of introducing state-owned enterprises and unity of command. Yet, it is possible that the Danish structural reform of 2007 may lead to similar changes in leadership focus. The general findings presented in this chapter indicate a modification of the Nordic democratic management model. The trend is a stronger emphasis on unity of command and a stronger emphasis on centralized decision efficiency and hierarchical management model.

13.7 New organizational structures as a response to changing governance

Healthcare organizations in the Nordic countries are changing. This chapter has attempted to point out some tentative links between changes in governance and organizational changes. Yet, several questions were already apparent about how direct such effects would be and how strongly we can argue for linkages between the ongoing changes in governance and the changes we observe in the Nordic health care organizations. This is a consequence of contextual conditions as well as the complexity of what would be the appropriate response. However, it was also argued that some organizational features would be more likely than others. Even if these assumptions are fulfilled, there are still several unsolved difficulties in the relationships between deciding to implement and de facto having the organizational feature.

Organizational changes have occurred; however, the question is how profound are these changes and to what extent do old structures cease to exist when new ones are introduced? An illustration of this point could be shown in a comparison with the work of geriatricians. It has been argued that the most important work of geriatricians is to unfold the total use of medications to the ageing patient and get rid of medication the patient no longer need – the cessation of medical treatment. In worst cases it could be that the patient is taking a pill that was prescribed to reduce adverse effect of another pill that initially was prescribed to treat a disease the patient no longer had. A parallel description could be drawn of hospitals. Philip Selznick (1957) has shown how organizations institutionalize over time; they are infused with norms and values. The initial arguments and source for the norms and values are forgotten over time and they become taken for granted. Similar observations can be made regarding organizational structures and design. Structures are implemented as layers upon layers of change (Sahlin-Andersson 2003).

In several areas of organizational change we observe that it takes longer for the health care organizations to lose old structures than it does to implement new ones. In Norway, hospitals have an officially implemented unity of command. However, to what extent the leader actually has total responsibility for the operation under his/her command can be questioned. There are observations that would indicate weak control. In several hospitals, the bed sections have been separated into independent departments with a nurse as head of the department and old job titles such as as head nurse and chief physician still exist. In this way, the hospital has implemented unity of command but has continued to allow separation of nurse–management and physician–management (Gjerberg and Sorensen 2006). Another example is that paper-based patient records still exist despite the introduction of electronic records. Similarly, printouts of digital radiographs have been used in the same way as old pictures in traditional meetings (although this was rare in 2008). These examples indicate that an health care organization at any given point in time has several parallel systems and structures that are waiting for a 'geriatric consultation'.

In all the Nordic countries, there is increased focus on accountability, decentralized economical responsibility with unit-based budget responsibility and improved institutional accounting practices. There is, however, an ongoing debate about how profound these changes have been. Have the formal organizational changes actually had an impact on how the core activities are being organized in the health care services? One argument has been that the changes are only superficial and the result is an even stronger decoupling between the administrative layer of the organization and the core activities of the clinics. Several scholars have argued that, although the health care organizations are changing, the changes are mostly superficial and restricted to the top level of the organizations. The core activities of the organizations – the bottom of the organization, the clinics – are still operating as normal, relatively unaffected by the changing governing structures (Vinge and Knudsen 2003).

Healthcare organizations – as all other organizations – are exposed to inconsistent demands from their surroundings. The surroundings expect the organizations to fulfil different set of goals that together are not necessarily compatible. The Nordic governance reforms do not necessarily reduce the amount of inconsistent demands but rather make them more explicit. One obvious example is demand for reduced deficits together with the demand for reduced waiting lists. Another example is the demand for unity of command together with the demand for professional autonomy. A third example is the demand for immediate efficiency together with the demand for education of health care personnel. One of the goals of the health care organizations is to ensure high-quality education of prospective health care personnel in order to ensure excellence in the next generation of health care personnel. This requires resources for hands-on training and practice. However, untrained individuals are less efficient than trained ones and require more supervision. A final example of inconsistent demands is the demand for large-scale production together with equal distribution and patient rights to have a certain amount of health care services in their vicinity. A solution, as Brunsson (1989) describes, has been to implement an organizational structure that is appropriate and legitimate in the surroundings but to decouple the core activities of the organizations. The formal organizational structure then loses its instrumental power and becomes merely a surface addition (Røvik 1992). An example is how health care organizations supposedly organized with unity of command but after closer examinations we still find split management. Another example is hospital mergers where the only results are a pure administrative fusion without changing the division of work.

All these conditions, contextual conditions as well as complexity of what would be the appropriate response, together with how structures tend to be implemented as layer upon layer of change in order to meet inconsistent demands sum up to explain the difficulties in explaining relationship 1 in the model presented in Figure 13.1. However, it does not imply that these organizational features are without effect in relationship 2 in organizing for efficiency. The problem is that we have limited knowledge about the effects of governance changes on organizational changes and performance. Much more research is needed in this area.

McKee and Healy (2002) argue that an overall perspective and focus on the overall governance and constraints of the health care organizations is enforced because of the difficulties in finding and isolating the direct relationships between internal organizational structures and efficiency. It seems easier to change the constraints of the health care organizations and then to hope that it will lead to favourable changes in the lower level of the health care organizations that will eventually increase the efficiency and quality of the organizations. The Norwegian hospital governance reform in 2002 was described as a 'tool' that would enable internal reforms and indirectly would give higher efficiency and accountability. The argument was that changing the contextual conditions of the hospitals would trigger internal changes. The overall conclusion drawn from this chapter is that the reform does seem to have accomplished this. The reforms have triggered change, although the amount of change, the type of change or the profoundness of change has been difficult to predict. We observe that the health care organizations are adapting to change in governance and that new organizational structures are being introduced. It has become a goal in it self to show ability to change.

It will be important to continue to observe how the health care organizations are developing, the types of organizational feature gaining popularity and the types being abandoned. The ideal organizational response will not be found, but the empirical basis of observation of internal structures together with observation of changes in the hospitals surroundings and external conditions could give a better foundation for steering and management and perhaps also to evaluate the effect of these changes.

Note

1. The term 'unity of command' was discussed by Luther Gulick in 'Administrative principle' as an important feature to ensure efficient administration.

References

Bentsen, E.Z. (1997) Ledelsesstrukturer og deres rationaler: en historisk forståelsesramme, in Hildebrandt, S. and Schultz, M (eds) *Fokus på sygehusledelse*. Copenhagen: Munksgaard.

Bogue, R.J., Shortell, S.M., Sohn, M.W. and Manheim, L.M. (1995) Hospital reorganisation after merger, *Medical Care* 33: 676–86.

Borum, F. and Pedersen, A.F. (2008) *Fusioner, ledelse og fortællinger: integration og polyfoni i det danske sundhedsvæsen*. Copenhagen: Handelshøjskolen.

Brunsson, N. (1989) *The Organisation of Hypocrisy: Talk, Decisions and Actions in Organisations*. Chichester: Wiley.

Calltorp, J. (2008) *Health Care Trends in Sweden*. Gothenburg: Sveriges Kommuner och Landsting.

Egeberg, M. (1989) *Institusjonspolitikk og forvaltningsutvikling: bidrag til en anvendt statsvitenskap*. Oslo: Tano.

Gjerberg, E. and Sorensen, B.A. (2006) Enhetlig ledelse: fortsatt en varm potet? *Tidsskrift for den norske lægeforening* 126: 1063–6.

Iversen, T., Østergren, K., Bryne, K. et al. (2006): *Årsrapport 2006: Beregningsutvalget for spesialisthelsetjenesten*. Oslo: Helse- og omsorgsdepartementet [Ministry of Health and Social Services].

Jakab, M., Preker, A. and Harding, A. (2002) Linking organisational structure to the external environment: experiences from hospital reform in transtition economies, in McKee, M. and Healy, J. (eds) *Hospitals in a Changing Europe*. Buckingham: Open University Press.

Järvelin, J. (2002) *Health Care Systems in Transition: Finland*. Copenhagen: WHO Regional Office for Europe on behalf of the European Observatory on Health Systems and Policies.

Kjekshus, L.E. (ed.) (2004) *Organising for Efficiency: A Study of Norwegian Somatic Hospitals*. Oslo: Unipub.

Kjekshus, L.E. (2005) Primary health care and hospital interactions: effects for hospital length of stay, *Scandinavian Journal of Public Health* 33: 114–22.

Kjekshus, L.E. and Hagen, T.P. (2005) Ring fencing of elective surgery: does it affect hospital efficiency? *Health Service and Management Research* 18: 186–97.

Kjekshus, L.E. and Hagen, T.P. (2007) Do hospital mergers increase hospital efficiency? Evidence from a national health service country, *Journal of Health Service Research and Policy* 12: 230–5.

Kjekshus, L.E. and Harsvik, T.P. (2007) Organisational change in Norwegian hospitals, *Tidsskr Nor Lægeforen* 127: 288–90.

Kjekshus, L.E. and Westlie, A. (2008) *Helseforetakenes interne organisering – INTORG 2007*. [*The Organisational Development of Norwegian Health Enteprises.*] Oslo: University of Oslo and Health Organisation Research Norway.

Levay, C. and Waks, C. (2006) *Strävan efter transparens granskning, styrning och organisering i sjukvårdens nätverk*. Stockholm: SNS.

McKee, M. and Healy, J. (2002) *Hospitals in a Changing Europe*. Buckingham: Open University Press.

Meyer, J.W. and Rowan, B. (1977) Institutionalized organizations: formal structure as myth and ceremony. *American Journal of Sociology* 83: 340–63.

Økelsrud, E.Q. (2007) *Sykehuset Innlandet*. Brumunddal: Sykehuset Innlandet http://www.sykehuset-innlandet.no/.

Powell, W.W. and DiMaggio, P.J. (1991) *The New Institutionalism in Organizational Analysis*. Chicago, IL: University of Chicago Press.

Røvik, K.A. (1992) *Den 'syke' stat: myter og moter i omstillingsarbeidet*. Oslo: Oslo University Press.

Sahlin-Andersson, K. (2003) I forandringers krydsfelt: ledelse på distance, in Borum F. (ed.) *Ledelse i sygehusvæsenet*. Copenhagen: Handelshøjskolens.

Scott, W.R., Ruef, M., Mendel, P.J. and Caronna, C.A. (2000) *Institutional Change and Healthcare Organisations: From Professional Dominance to Managed Care*. Chicago, IL: University of Chicago Press.

Selznick, P. (1957) *Leadership in Administration: A Sociological Interpretation*. Berkeley, CA: University of California Press.

SSB (2007) *Spesialisthelsetjenesten, 2006: Kostnadsveksten i spesialisthelsetjenesten fortsetter*. Oslo: Statisitics Norway. http://www.ssb.no/emner/03/02/speshelse/.

Stigen, I.M. and Opedal, S. (2005) *Helse-Norge i støpeskjeen: Søkelys på sykehusreformen*. Bergen: Fagbokforlaget.

Timm, H.U. (1997) *Patienten i centrum? Brugerundersøgelser, lægperspektiver og kvalitetsudvikling*. Copenhagen: Dsi.

Tjerbo, T. (2007) *HORN Paper* 4: *Målkonflikter og styringsdilemmaer. Utviklingen av Sykehuset Innlandet etter etableringen*. Oslo: Health Organization Research Norway.

Vinge, S. and Knudsen, M. (2003) Infrastruktur og reformer i sygehusvæsenet, in Borum, F. (ed.) *Ledelse i sygehusvæsenet*. Copenhagen: Handelshøjskolens.

Vrangbæk, K. (1999) New public management i sygehusfeltet: udforming og konsekvenser, in Bentsen, E.Z. and Borum, F. (eds) *Når Styringsambitioner møder praksis*. Copenhagen: Copenhagen Business School Press.

Vrangbæk, K. and Torjesen, D.O. (2005) Sygehuslederes opfattelse af ledelsesvilkår i Danmark og Norge, *Torjesen, Dag Olaf. I: Nordiske Organisasjonsstudier (NOS)* 7: 37–57.

fourteen

The European Union: single market pressures

Dorte S. Martinsen and Paula Blomqvist

14.1 Introduction

Although health care policies are formally the competence of the member states, and although policy reforms within health care have historically for the most been driven through domestic reforms, the internal market principles of the EU increasingly impact and challenge the national organization of health care. Particularly since the late 1990s, the principles of the internal market have reached within the formerly secluded area of national health policy. In addition, the health care systems of the Nordic member states are increasingly affected by the free movement logics of the encapsulating polity. In incremental and rather uncoordinated ways, the Nordic member states have started to adapt; meanwhile new challenges are emerging.

This chapter is structured into four main sections. Section 14.2 discusses the theoretical perspectives on EU social policy and their likely effect on national policies. Section 14.3 then analyses specific decisions of the activist European Court of Justice (ECJ) and how these have gradually formed the contours of supranational health care regulation in terms of patient mobility. Section 14.4 sets out the characteristics of the Nordic health care model in a European context in general and then Section 14.5 focuses on the implementation or adaptation carried out by the Swedish and Danish health care systems, with brief comparisons to Finland and Norway.[1]

14.2 Theoretical perspectives on European social policy

The rapid progress of European integration in the area of social policy after the 1980s surprised many. Previously, it was generally believed that the welfare states of western Europe, with their different historical trajectories, would never subject themselves to regulation from a supranational body or take to the idea of convergence towards a common 'European' model. Today, direct regulation of issues clearly within the realm of social policy are not uncommon within the EU, for instance in the areas of public health, work and safety and access to health care. In addition, far-reaching efforts have been undertaken on a voluntary basis by the member states to coordinate policies within core welfare areas such as pensions, health services provision, poverty reduction and elderly care. These developments, which were thought unlikely only a few years ago, suggest that national welfare states are not quite as 'immobile' as earlier believed (e.g. Pierson 2001). They also raise the possibility of real convergence between them, even though this might come about in a slow and uneven manner. Maurizio Ferrera (2005) argues that we see today the emergence of a new type of social politics in Europe, characterized by a diminished importance of geographical borders and nationally confined arenas of policy-making. Increasingly, European citizens can chose to which type of welfare community (i.e. a community insuring them against social risk) they want to belong, as such communities need no longer be defined by territorial borders. By the same token, policy-making processes are moving from the nation states towards the European networks and decision-making bodies.

There are, however, many questions still to be answered about the dynamics of integration in European social policy and its effects on policy-making processes within national welfare states. What are the main driving forces behind integration in this policy area and how do integration efforts affect political power balances at the domestic level? Who gains and who loses when the locus of policy-making shifts towards the supranational level? And what role do domestic political institutions play in shaping final policy outcomes as EU regulations and initiatives are implemented at the member state level?

One of the driving forces behind integration in the social policy field in recent years is undoubtedly what might be called spill-over effects from the creation of the single European market in the early 1990s. As the market came into force, observers pointed to its potential threat to the social protection systems of the member states and demanded that it be amended by measures to safeguard the systems. As a result, the project 'Social Europe' was born; a discursive platform where pro-welfare forces including politicians both to the left and right, EU civil servants, unions, lobby groups and policy experts could gather to formulate an agenda oriented towards protecting existing welfare systems in the region and to identify common goals for these. Such efforts were, however, hampered by the fact that the member states remained unwilling to delegate authority to the EU in the area of social policy. For this reason, the goals formulated under the banner of Social Europe remained vague and non-committal and few concrete measures were taken to create social regulation that could balance the pro-market orientation of the EU Treaty. Exceptions include work and safety standards in the labour market, which have been regulated through a string of binding directives during the 1980s and 1990s, and precautions taken in the wake of the bovine spongiform encephalopathy (mad cow disease) outbreak to ensure the safe transport of blood and donor organs (Blomqvist 2004).

14.2.1 *European legalism as a driving force*

In the late 1990s, social policy formation within the EU entered a new phase. The activities of the ECJ drew more political attention as the court started to deliver decisions that seemed to infringe on the autonomy of the member states in this highly sensitive political area. This was true particularly in health care, but rulings with the same orientation were also handed down in other welfare areas such as social insurance. The most controversial aspect of the rulings, which typically went further than existing regulations in ensuring the right of access to national welfare systems on the part of EU nationals from *other* member states, was that the ECJ based its decisions not on the social regulations themselves but recent articles in the EU Treaty safeguarding the four freedoms that underpinned the single market. The ECJ argued that, in order to move around freely in the region to seek work, all European citizens must have access to national social security systems on the same conditions as the inhabitants. This meant, in effect, that long-standing principles of social rights as linked to *national* citizenship and territorial borders were cast aside (Liebfried and Pierson 2000; Erhag 2004; Ferrera 2005). The recently proposed Directive on Patient Mobility from the European Commission has confirmed that the reasoning by the ECJ concerning the rights of EU nationals in the area of health will indeed be part of a common European policy in this area.

The heightened activity of the ECJ and its far-reaching implications for nation sovereignty can be seen as a sign of the increased legalism within European politics. According to scholars studying international organization, legalism became generally more important as a means to govern international relations during the 1990s. Examples include the setting-up of the North American Free Trade Agreement, the World Trade Organization, international criminal tribunes, and various quasi-legal agreements such as the United Nations' Kyoto Protocol (Goldstein et al. 1998). Among such phenomena, the ECJ stands out, however, as the extreme case of creating 'hard' (e.g. binding) legal regulations in order to govern a community of sovereign states. As observed by Garrett and co-workers (1998, p. 149), 'the accretion of power by the European Court of Justice (ECJ) is arguably the clearest manifestation of the transfer of sovereignty from nation-states to a supranational institution, not only in the European Union (EU) but also in modern international politics more generally'.

Interpretations of the increased legalism of EU integration and its implications for the member states vary. To some, the increasingly important role of the ECJ in driving the integration process forward signalled that the member states had lost control over it and that they had failed to see, in setting up the ECJ as a constitutional court and arming it with the Single European Act of 1986, what the consequences would be for their sovereignty. This so-called neo-functionalist interpretation stresses, moreover, that the activities of the ECJ have undermined the role of the nation states as political actors in the region in that its existence makes it possible for other social actors to appeal to it, thereby shifting political battles from the national political arena, with its vested power structures, to an arena outside the reach of national policy-makers (Alter 1998, 2000; Mattli and Slaughter 1998). In contrast, the intergovenmentalist perspective sees the ECJ more as an agent of the interests of the member states and argues that the member states have been basically supportive of its integration agenda. According to this view, the ECJ is not totally unrestrained by the member states but has to manoeuvre strategically in relation to them in order to preserve its political legitimacy (Garrett 1995; Garrett et al. 1998). Looking specifically at the activities of the ECJ in the area of social policy and the predominantly negative reactions of the member states to its rulings in this area so far, it seems that the neo-functionalist interpretation would have the most empirical support (e.g. Alter 2000; Liebfried and Pierson 2000; Mossialos and McKee 2002; Geer 2006). Therefore, a general implication of the strengthened role of the ECJ in health and social policy would seem to be that the sovereignty of the member states has been undermined in these areas, despite the fact that this is officially guarded by exiting EU Treaties.

14.2.2. Coordinating European health policies

Another important feature of contemporary European social policy is that a growing share is formulated on the basis of voluntary agreements between the member states, reached within the framework of the so-called 'open method of coordination' (OMC). The OMC refers to a process whereby common policy guidelines are formulated and translated into national policy objectives through agreements between the Commission and the member state in question. The subsequent process of implementing the objectives is driven forward by periodic monitoring, evaluation and peer review, based on agreed-upon indicators and benchmarks that compare the performance of the members or have been identified as 'best practice' in a given policy area (Borrás and Jacobsson 2004). The ECJ rulings in the late 1990s and early 2000s raised concerns over a legal 'spill-over effect' from the Single European Act to the area of health care; a prospect that many member states have seen as undesirable. Thus, the activities of the ECJ seem to have, to some extent, acted as a prompter for the initiation of an OMC process in health care in order to take back some political initiative in this area (Geer 2006). The process has been actively supported by the European Council and the Ministers of Health, who see a potential for deepened cooperation among the member states in the area of health. The Commission, too, has argued that the process is desirable in order to meet common health challenges among the member states, such as ageing and medical technology developments as well as the possibility of increased cross-border patient mobility. It has also identified three basic objectives for the OMC process in health care:[2]

- to insure access to health care for all within each member state, regardless of income or social status
- to promote high quality of all health services provided in all of the region
- to ensure the financial sustainability of national health care systems.

The goals were endorsed by the member states during the meeting of the European Council in Barcelona in 2002. In 2004, the OMC process in the area of health and long-term care was formally launched.[3] Since then, the Social Protection Committee (SPC) has developed a list of indicators to monitor the performance of the health care systems of the member states in relation to the common objectives. The member states have reported their performance in the form of so-called National Strategic Reports on two occasions so far, 2006 and 2008. No common policy guidelines for the area of health care have been presented yet by the Commission, however. The OMC health is still in an early phase. In addition, many member states are still sceptical about formulating common policies in this area.

Like the ECJ rulings, the OMC can be seen as a means to bypass the regular system of political decision-making within the EU, with its joint decision traps and numerous veto points (Obinger et al. 2005). The emerging research on the OMC links the adoption of this new means to coordinate interests between the member states within the EU with a more general movement towards a less hierarchical and more negotiation-based mode of governance. Therefore, the adoption of the OMC process in the area of health care could also be seen as reflecting the broader tendency to shift from traditional, hierarchical governing techniques to more network-based and informal modes of governance in European politics (Rhodes 1997).

In 2008, the creation of a common European health policy took a further decisive step, as the Commission presented a proposal for a directive on patient mobility within the EU. The proposal reflected a general desire by the members to have more clarity of the rules in this area, given the apparent risk that the rulings by the ECJ would be interpreted differently by different member states. The directive proposal is tailored closely to the ECJ rulings and thus, in effect, confirms the policies already established by the court (see below). Hence, it seems a clear case of a legal spill-over effect whereby closer political integration in the area of health care has been propelled by activism on the part of judicial bodies.

It seems safe to conclude that the EU will play a more important role as regulator and knowledge centre in the health care sector in the future; a development which implies a movement towards increased policy coordination and systems convergence in this area.

14.3 Judicial activism and health care integration

Until 1998, access to foreign health care providers in the EU was regulated solely through the system coordinating social security rights for migrant workers (i.e. Regulation 1408/71).[4] The member states, the Commission and the ECJ appeared to have found an interinstitutional consensus that European citizens were entitled to *immediate* and *necessary* health care in other member states as well as to other kinds of publicly financed health treatment, provided that they had been *authorized* beforehand by the competent national institution. The European health card regulates the right to immediate and necessary health care. Moreover, planned treatment in another member state is accessible through a form, E112, where the competent national institution prior to treatment has authorized the right to have it carried out in another member state. This institutional status quo was seriously upset from 1998 onwards when the ECJ initiated a series of case-law decisions questioning the justification for 'prior authorization' and through which the principles of the internal market have gradually been introduced into the health care policy field.[5] The ECJ first laid down that health care is a service within the meaning of the Treaty.[6] The requirement for prior authorization was, in principle, found to be a barrier to free movement. The immediate impact of the 1998 judgments was, however, modest in that they considered only *non-hospital care* (e.g. a pair of spectacles and dental treatment), and concerned the reimbursement-based Luxembourg health care system.

In subsequent rulings, the ECJ extended its interpretation across the full range of EU health care systems, including to national health systems such as the Nordic ones. The *Geraets-Smits* and *Peerbooms* judgments of 2001[7] repeated – this time with regard to the Dutch 'benefit in kind' health insurance system – that prior authorization constitutes a barrier to the free movement of services. Such a barrier could, however, be justified provided that:

- the decision on whether or not to grant treatment abroad is based on 'international medical science', and
- an equivalent treatment can be provided in the competent member state without 'undue delay' taking into consideration the medical condition of the patient, broadly defined.

The ECJ further laid restrictions upon national discretion to grant or not to grant prior authorization by emphasizing that it can only be a justified barrier to the principle of free movement if it is based on objective, non-discriminatory criteria known in advance, so national authorities cannot control the procedure arbitrarily. Requests for authorization must furthermore be dealt with within a reasonable time and refusals to grant authorization must be open to appeal (para. 90, C-157/99). In this way the ECJ initiates an emphasis on the citizens' possibility of judicial redress.

The third step towards an internal health care market took place two years later with the case of *Müller-Fauré and van Riet*.[8] In this case, the ECJ issued yet another expansive, and controversial, interpretation by introducing a distinction between hospital and non-hospital care. In the case of *hospital care*, the court restated its view that the requirement for prior authorization is justified on condition that it is exercised proportionately and that the national competent institution has no scope for acting in an arbitrary manner. The matter was, however, quite different for *non-hospital care*. The court laid down that national authorization constitutes an unjustified barrier to the free movement of services for non-hospital care. It did not further define non-hospital care. Given the increasingly blurred distinction between hospital and non-hospital care, the future implications and confusion of this judgment are rather extensive.

From the cases of *Decker* and *Kohll* onwards, it is clear that legal judgments have made a significant contribution to the integration of health care, whereas politics in the same period has been largely absent. Within a timespan of only five years, judicial activism laid down that EC law applies to a policy field which was previously taken as an 'island beyond the reach of Community law'.[9]

14.3.1 *Patient rights moving further into focus*

On May 2006, the ECJ's *Watts* case was concluded. This was the first case to specifically concern a national health system such as that in the United Kingdom, which provides health care as primarily a benefit in kind and tax financed; similar systems exist in Ireland, the Nordic countries and the southern member states.

The case concerned the topical waiting-time issue, in terms of a hip replacement needed by Mrs Yvonne Watts, a resident in the United Kingdom. Mrs Watts requested authorization to receive treatment abroad. That was refused by the competent institution on the grounds that the examining consultant stated that Mrs Watts was in no more need of a hip replacement than any of the other patients on his waiting list. Mrs Watts was told that she would have to wait approximately one year for her operation. However, upon reexamination, the consultant recommended that she be operated on within three to four months, as her situation had now become worse. Despite this reduction in waiting time, Mrs Watts went to France to have her hip replacement and, on her return, requested reimbursement of her costs of £3900. The request was again rejected, on the argument that the reduction in her waiting time would have meant that Mrs Watts would have been treated without 'undue delay'. Mrs Watts took her case to the Court of Appeal, which referred the case to the ECJ.

In its judgment, the ECJ confirmed, and indeed furthered, its previous line of health-related judgments. One of the political implications of the case seems to be that it further reduced the scope for national institutions to exercise administrative discretion. Another implication is that it brings the rights of the European patient into sharper focus – and thus strengthens the position of the patient in future cases. In so doing, it intervenes in the national sphere of governance.

Once again the ECJ stated that, regardless of the specific health care systems and different individual features, all medical services are 'services' within the meaning of the Treaty:

> It should be noted in that regard that, according to settled case-law, medical services provided for consideration fall within the scope of the provisions on the freedom to provide services . . . there being no need to distinguish between care provided in a hospital environment and care provided outside such an environment
>
> (para. 86 of the judgment)

The court thus clarified that the characteristics of the United Kingdom National Health Service do not exempt it from EC law. The internal market principles apply regardless of the way the national system is organized (para. 90 of the judgment).

It is important, however, that the ECJ did not specify in terms of time period when a waiting time for a particular treatment can be considered to be 'undue delay' or beyond 'the time normally necessary'. But it did set out a criterion for determining whether a period of waiting time is acceptable in the context of EC law and further specified that national decisions must be reviewable. The waiting time must not:

exceed the period which is acceptable on the basis of an objective medical assessment of the clinical needs of the person concerned in the light of all of the factors characterizing his medical condition at the time when the request for authorization is made or renewed, as the case may be

(para. 79 of the judgment)

Furthermore, the decision as to whether the patient faces undue delay in accessing services must be based on:

an objective medical assessment of the patient's medical condition, the history and probable course of his illness, the degree of pain he is in and/or the nature of his disability at the time when the request for authorization was made or renewed

(para. 119 of the judgment)

This may prove to be an important extension to the rights of the European patient, since it sets redress limits to the time period and even went on to specify the institutional structures that member states must provide to protect those rights. The ECJ repeated the conclusions from the previous rulings, stating that the requirement for prior authorization cannot legitimize discretionary decisions by national authorities but must be based on objective, non-discriminatory criteria and allow for decisions on authorization to be challenged in judicial or quasi-judicial proceedings (paras. 115 and 116). But the court goes beyond a simple restatement of precedent and extends member states' obligation to provide transparency and legal certainty to European citizens:

To that end, refusals to grant authorization, or the advice on which such refusals may be based, must refer to the specific provisions on which they are based and be properly reasoned in accordance with them. Likewise, courts or tribunals hearing actions against such refusals must be able, if they consider it necessary for the purpose of carrying out the review which it is incumbent on them to make, to seek the advice of wholly objective and impartial independent experts

(para. 117 of the judgment)

In this way, the *Watts* case strengthens the position of the European patient. Not only has s/he been granted rights beyond the national borders, but s/he has also been provided with a structure and judicial procedures through which to bypass the national system or challenge its decisions. National systems where judicial routes to challenge administrative decisions are weak are particularly exposed to challenge on this extension.

The last bastion for resisting the general applicability of the ECJ's previous judgments has been rejected by this judgment, as the whole range of European health care systems and services must now be interpreted against the requirements of EC law.

14.3.2 *Commission initiative and the responses of member states*

One first Commission initiative to politically codify the rulings of the ECJ was through the proposal for a Directive on services in the internal market.[10] The proposal precisely replicated ECJ's decisions in its article 23, proposing (1) an internal market for non-hospital care, where the patient has a right to seek treatment in another member state without prior authorization and subsequently have the costs reimbursed by the competent national institution; (2) a right to hospitalization in another member state, provided that the member state of affiliation offers the same treatment, and that authorization has been granted beforehand. The health ministers turned the proposal down, refusing to have their policy area regulated as part of a general directive on services, placed under the responsibility of the Directorate General (DG) on internal market.

Hereafter, it appeared clear that European health care could not be regulated solely from an overall internal market perspective, but still the judicial integration needed political codification and more transparency. On September 2006, DG Health (SANCO) communicated a consultation procedure on health services.[11] The communication called for stakeholders to state their opinions on a set of questions related to the free movement of health services. Almost 300 contributions were submitted up to 31 January 2007, and a large set of stakeholders took part. Among the contributors were member states and European Economic Area states, regional authorities, national parliaments, national organizations, international organizations, citizens, universities, commercial organizations and companies.

Initially, the Commission was supposed to adopt its proposal for a Directive on 'patient rights in cross-border health care' in late 2007, but the adoption of the proposal was postponed to 2008 (*EUobserver*, 19 December 2007). Apparently, the run-up to the presentation of the proposal contained conflicts and disagreements. The main political fault lines seem to have been internal disagreements in the College of Commissioners and Members of the European Parliament acting as veto-players.

Regarding the Commission, there appears to have been considerable disagreements between the commissioners behind the scene. Some commissioners expressed concerns about the impact of the directive on national health care systems, others pointing out the factor of timing and arguing that political timing to present the proposal was badly chosen in the shadow of the Lisbon Treaty (*EUobserver*, 7 February 2008). DG SANCO, which had been in charge of formulating the proposal, seems to have been unable to unify the College of Commissioners.

Within the European Parliament, members of the Party of European Socialists (PES) voiced strong opposition, putting forward arguments that the consequences of the proposal could become considerable, dismantling national abilities to plan health care capacities and exert budget control. The PES members argued that the proposal compromised the control instrument of 'prior authorization' also regarding hospital care, and hereby went further than legal integrative steps taken by the ECJ:

The Commission moves one step further than the decisions from the European Court of Justice. It is highly problematic that prior authorization is no longer required regarding the right to hospital treatment in another member state. That deprives the member states the instrument of economic and capacity planning and implies a risk of financially draining the national health care systems, because the patients in this way can take money along outside their own member state

> (Christel Schaldemose (PES member of the European Parliament), quoted in *Dagens Medicin*, 1 February 2008; translated from Danish)

On 2 July 2008, the Commission was finally successful in proposing the directive on patient mobility.[12] The final directive proposal is not fundamentally different from the version set to be presented in December 2007. The amendments to the December version seem rather minor; however, the timing and the reactions from the Members of the European Parliament were quite different. This time the presentation of the proposal was not vetoed. Furthermore, the proposal was presented as one part of a much larger social package, which to some extent diminishes the individual importance of the directive proposal. Currently (January 2009), the proposal is being negotiated in the Council and the European Parliament – and a long-drawn negotiation process seems likely.

14.4 The Nordic health care systems in the European context

The impact of Europeanization on national health care systems depends, naturally, on their specific organizational features. The Nordic health care systems have several features that make them distinct in a European context. First, they are financed predominantly by different sources of taxation. This means that they have public authorities as the 'third-party' financers of care rather than independent sickness funds, as is common in continental European countries. The publicly controlled financing of care also implies that access to care is open to all Nordic citizens on equal terms, rather than regulated on the basis of individual or occupation-based health insurance. The direct public control over health care systems in the Nordic countries is extended also to the provision side. In the case of primary care, provision is typically mixed, consisting of both public health centres and privately practising GPs. In Norway and Denmark, a majority of primary care physicians are privately employed, whereas in Sweden and Finland the opposite is true. In all Nordic countries, however, primary care is publicly financed. The relatively high degree of public ownership and operation of health services provision can be said to be a typical Nordic feature, even if the same applies also to other tax-based systems, like the United Kingdom and Ireland. In the case of secondary care, public provision dominates completely, as hospitals and other care institutions are normally owned and operated by public authorities. The fact that health services are both financed and provided by the same public body, typically a local government agency, means that the Nordic systems could be described as *integrated*.

Another distinct feature of Nordic health care is the crucial role of decentralized political governance. The operation of the health care systems has typically been delegated from national authorities to local, self-governing bodies, at the municipal, provincial or, more recently, regional level. In all but Norway (after its regionalization reform of 2002), the local bodies responsible for health care provisions are directly elected by the population, a feature which gives the Nordic health care systems a democratic character in international comparison. The relative independence of the municipal or provincial (or regional) health authorities in the Nordic countries means that the organization of health care provision can vary substantially from one location to another.

The exact implications of Europeanization for the Nordic health care systems remains hard to pinpoint, as much is still unknown about exactly what such a process will entail. It is clear, however, that the Nordic systems are quite distinct from the kind of insurance-based system, with independent sickness funds acting in the role of payers, that the ECJ seems to have had in mind in most of its rulings in health care so far. This is noticeable, not least when the court discusses how caregivers should be reimbursed by sickness funds, and argues that it should not matter so much for the financer whether the caregiver in question is located in the same country or not, or when it talks about the value of free competition and the creation of a non-discriminatory European 'market' also for health services.

It can be argued that three different questions, at least, can be raised when it comes to possible effects of Europeanization for the Nordic model of health organization, each with distinct policy implications. The first concerns the role of care providers and the need to develop further systems for their reimbursement in the Nordic countries. If patients in all European countries are free to move more across borders to seek care, there will be a need to standardize systems for billing and care financing and to determine the 'prices' for various treatments. Such a development has more radical implications for caregivers in the Nordic countries where, as noted above, resources have traditionally been allocated through public budgets. In effect, an open market for health services in Europe is likely to create an organizational logic where caregivers operate more independently, both financially and administratively, also in the Nordic countries. Such a development has already been initiated in some countries (particularly Sweden and Norway) through so-called purchaser–provider separation, but it is far from established everywhere.

The second question has to do with the status of patient rights in the Nordic countries and possible implication of the ECJ rulings and the proposal for a Patient Rights Directive in this respect. Generally, formal patient rights in the Nordic countries have tended to be quite weak, as health care has been provided by public authorities as part of a more general public service, open to all, rather than a service to which access is provided on basis of a specific insurance. The public provision of care and absence of individual insurance has created less need to legally specify obligations for insurers and health providers (Chapter 6). This implies that the Nordic health care systems have, in some respects, had a less 'legal' culture than some other systems in Europe, and that courts have not had an important role within them. This may be changing, as several Nordic countries, Denmark and Norway in particular, have recently sought to strengthen patient rights by formal legislation. It seems obvious that this tendency will be reinforced by a new Patient Rights Directive that stipulates – just as previous ECJ rulings – that patients in all member states should be well informed about their rights to seek care abroad and that, if prior authorization is required to do so, they must have the right to legal appeal.

The third question raised by the ongoing Europeanization of the health care sector concerns the implications for decision-making and governance within this area in the Nordic countries. As noted above, health care in the Nordic countries is largely governed by local/regional bodies, with a high degree of independence. However, implementation of European rules, court rulings or recommendations in this area calls for *national* policy adjustments, which imply that all actors within the system should adjust their working routines in a similar way, including local and regional governments. This could result in an implicit streamlining of local policies and an enhanced role for national governing bodies. Moreover, implementation of EU policy at the national level is an often complicated process, where new EU initiatives need to be interpreted, their effects investigated and the relevant actors consulted before new national regulation can be enacted or old amended. So for this reason too, EU initiatives in the area of health may have the effect of centralizing policy-making powers. It is also still predominantly as *nations* that member countries are represented within decision-making processes within the EU and can influence future policies in this area. Therefore, Europeanization in this area raises questions about how the current division of policy-making authority in health - care in the Nordic countries will be affected and how a possible shift towards a more prominent role for national policy actors will affect central–local relations in the Nordic health care systems.

14.5 The effects of European Union policies in single Nordic countries

In this section, the Europeanization effects until 2008 are analysed, primarily for the Swedish and Danish health care organizations. The responses of Finland and Norway are touched upon briefly.

14.5.1 *The Swedish system*

Prior to the early 2000s, there was virtually no recognition in Sweden that EU policies in the area of health had any direct bearing on national health policy. Since then, this has changed and national authorities, particularly the Ministry of Social Affairs (Socialdepartementet), now follow EU developments in this area closely. A series of initiatives have been taken to adjust Swedish policies in the health care sector to new EU regulations, particularly in the area of patient mobility. The fact that these initiatives have been taken up by the Ministry of Social Affairs and a national court reveals a dynamic whereby the national governing bodies appear to have strengthened their powers within the heavily decentralized system. This development has manifested itself also in the tendency to propose legislation as a means to adjust domestic policies to European precedents, which constitutes a break with previous modes of 'soft governance' and voluntary agreements between the central state and county counties as a way to coordinate policies in the area of health care.

When they were handed down, the *Kohll* and *Decker* rulings received virtually no attention in Sweden, and, if they did, their importance was played down. It was generally believed that rulings did not concern an integrated health system like the Swedish. In the early 2000s, treatment abroad was hardly a known phenomenon in Sweden, and the country was among the most reluctant in the EU to authorize such requests. Palm and co-workers (2000) reported that about 20 requests a year for health care abroad were approved in Sweden, compared with about 7000 in Luxembourg.

Soon thereafter, however, European health policies started to receive more recognition. In 2002, the Swedish Ministry of Social Affairs became part of the so-called High-Level Reflection Process concerning health matters within the EU. In the same year, the ministry appointed an expert group to investigate the organization of highly specialized health care in the country, which, like all hospital care in Sweden, is the responsibility of the county councils. In its 2003 report, the group proposed that this part of the system should be subject to special control on the part of the national government, and be led by a new national board (Ds 2003:56).[13] According to the then Minister of Health, Lars Engqvist (2004), a prime motive behind the proposal was the need for more central coordination of the provision of highly specialized care in the country, so as to be able to cooperate more effectively with other European member states in this area.

In 2004, the fact that the EU does indeed have a direct impact on health care provision in Sweden became obvious to all actors within this system. In January, the Supreme Administrative Court of Sweden (Regeringsrätten) delivered a ruling based directly on previous ECJ rulings on patient mobility, in which it overruled the refusal by a local Swedish authority to reimburse a patient for the cost of medical treatment in Germany. The patient had appealed for authorization according to the 1408/71 procedure but had been denied this on grounds that the treatment in question was not given in Sweden as it was considered medically dubious. The court noted that the Swedish health care system did not have a satisfactory procedure for applying for health care abroad on the part of individual patients and, technically, no legal demand to seek prior authorization for care abroad, although there was a well-established administrative procedure. The court also noted that the treatment given to the patient by the German care provider was effective in curing her disease. As a result, the court ordered the local health authority in question to reimburse the patient for the full cost of the treatment (about 60,000 euro), thereby setting a legal precedent that opened the possibility for Swedish patients to seek both primary and secondary care abroad without prior authorization.

The ruling was first met with confusion among local health authorities, as it was in opposition to the previously established procedure for receiving health treatment abroad, which had been based on the 1408/71 system. The court not only overthrew this procedure, it also went against the medical advice given in the case in question, which had typically been of great importance in decisions when patients demanded treatment abroad. In the year following the ruling, applications for reimbursement for care abroad rose dramatically in Sweden, and an overwhelming majority (945 out of 1101) were approved (Swedish Social Insurance Agency 2006).

The Ministry of Social Affairs reacted swiftly to these developments by setting up an investigatory expert committee to propose a new, formally regulated, system for authorizing medical treatment abroad. In February 2006, the committee delivered its report, in which it proposed a new law that would regulate the processing of such applications. The content of the law was closely tailored to the legal precedent set by the ECJ and, therefore, made a distinction between hospital care, which would require prior authorization, and outpatient care, which could be sought freely abroad on the basis of the EC Treaty articles 49 and 50. The report also noted that authorization could not be denied by local health authorities if the medical condition in question was treated within the Swedish health care system but adequate and effective treatment could not be given in the system within 'normal' time (Ministry of Social Affairs 2006). The process of legally formalizing the proposal was later paused by the new centre-of-right government that came into office in 2006. When the patient mobility directive proposal was presented by the European Commission in 2008, reactions from the Swedish Government were generally positive. It noted that new legislation will 'most likely' be necessary to adjust Swedish health care policies to the contents of the directive in order to ensure that patient rights to mobility are formalized and subject to judicial appeal. If such legislation was enacted, it would imply, in effect, that Swedish patients enjoy legal rights to medical treatment abroad but lack corresponding rights to such treatments at home, as these are not legally formalized at present (Vahlne Westerhäll 2004). Whether Sweden will introduce a legal requirement for prior authorization in order for patients to be reimbursed for hospital care abroad is still uncertain.

It can be argued that EU initiatives in the area of health have served to highlight a weak spot of the Swedish system, namely swift access to care for patients. This was acknowledged by the then Minister of Health in 2004, when he stated that Sweden meets two of the common EU health policy goals without any difficulty, namely high quality and financial sustainability, but has more problems with the third, access to care, and that this must be a priority issue in Swedish health care in the future (Engqvist 2004). Access to health services has been a controversial issue in Sweden for years because of the occasional long waiting times for treatment. The legal precedent set by the ECJ in the *Watts* case, which indicated that waiting time might indeed be a basis for patients to be entitled to treatment abroad, could, therefore, be seen as a potential threat to the Swedish system, just as to that in the United Kingdom. This problem was addressed in 2005, when the Ministry of Social Affairs negotiated an agreement with the county councils that a national waiting-time guarantee should be established within the system, ensuring that no patient in Sweden should have to wait longer than a maximum of 90 days for treatment. The new guarantee went into force in November 2005 and has led to renewed efforts by the county councils to increase the supply of care and to be ready to purchase additional services from other county councils or private caregivers should the guarantee not be met. The recent ECJ ruling in *Watts*, where the court seemed to ask for a specified maximum waiting time but also held that four months cannot be considered 'undue', indicates that the Swedish waiting-time guarantee would satisfy European demands for care delivered in reasonable time and that waiting periods for up to three months would, in most cases,[14] not constitute a basis for receiving care abroad. Therefore, even though the Swedish waiting-time guarantee resulted primarily from domestic political pressures, it appears well in line with EU policies in this area. It seems, moreover, that the implicit threat from the ECJ concerning the rights of patients to seek treatment abroad if the waiting time at home was too long may have aided the Ministry in persuading the reluctant county councils to agree to the waiting-time guarantee.

Given the adjustments within Swedish health care to meet new European policies in this area, as described above, a few final observations can be made about the possible impact of the EU on the system. First, the open endorsement of the ECJ rulings on patient mobility by the Swedish Administrative Supreme Court and Ministry of Social Affairs can be said to have strengthened the role of judicial review and formal regulation within the Swedish health care system, even though this runs against its previous tradition of more informal modes of governance. If new legislation is enacted to implement the Commission's directive on patient mobility, this tendency will be further reinforced. It can also be noted that the ECJ rulings and the Patient Rights Directive have served to highlight the fact that access to care has previously not been legally regulated in Sweden.

A second observation is that the deepened European integration in the health care area may have an important effect within the Swedish system if it creates, as it seems that it does, legitimacy for an enhanced role for national governing bodies in this area. The desire on part of the Swedish Government to strengthen its control over the system and improve the coordination of local health policies has been apparent in recent years and is reflected in a number of political initiatives, such as the waiting-time guarantee, agreements with the county councils concerning patient mobility within the country and proposals to formalize patient rights. This indicates that the Europeanization of health - care can have an important impact not only with respect to policy content but also when it comes to the distribution of power and relations between local and central actors in Swedish health care.

14.5.2 The Danish system

The impact of the judicial interpretations of the principles of the internal market on Danish health policy, while clearly visible, can be described as diffuse and restrained.

The Danish Government was one of the first governments to react to the *Decker* and *Kohll* rulings. Before the rulings, the Danish member state had held the view that internal market rules had no impact on the health care system whatsoever. The government, therefore, found it necessary to set up an interministerial working group to analyse the implications of the judgments for Danish health policy. The working group reported that these rulings contained general premises that took the scope of the judgments beyond the lawsuits themselves. Therefore, Denmark acknowledged that the cases had implications for health care systems other than that of Luxembourg and were not limited to glasses and dental treatment. The Danish report, however, contained a narrow definition of what constitutes a 'service' – and this national service definition has been maintained since. To be a service according to the meaning of Treaty Article 50, the Danish executive argued that there needs to be an element of private pay involved:

> It is the view of the working group that if, on the other hand, the treatment had been taken care of by the *public hospital sector, the Treaty's Article 49 would not have applied*. The reason is that Article 50 defines services as *services normally carried out in return for remuneration . . . Characteristic for a service is thus that a service provider offers a service in return for remuneration.*
> (Danish Report on the *Decker/Kohll* rulings 1999, p. 23; emphasis added)

The Danish way of narrowing down the definition of 'service' could keep the large majority of Danish health care services outside the definition, since they are provided as benefits in kind, free of charge and therefore with no direct remuneration.

However, in acknowledging that the principles of the internal market – under certain conditions – apply equally to health care services, the interpretation of the working group marked a decisive break with the then current Danish view. The conclusions of the report resulted in a reform of Danish health policy as from July 2000.[15] This reform allowed general and specialist medical treatment for persons insured under Group 2, as well as dental assistance, physiotherapy and chiropractic treatments for all insured persons, to be purchased abroad with subsequent fixed-price reimbursement from the relevant Danish institutions.

When the ECJ went further with its interpretations, Denmark decided to take an active position and deliver opinion in the case of *Geraets-Smits and Peerbooms*. It is interesting to see that the conclusions of the Decker/Kohll report was used as a platform for the Danish Government and largely replicated (Interview, Danish Ministry of Health, 3 April 2001). The Danish Government stated that, due to the absence of remuneration, hospital treatment did not constitute a service within the meaning of Treaty Article 50 (Report for the Hearing, pp. 76–77). Beyond making this point, Denmark argued that another precondition for a service to be Treaty-related was that it must be provided with a view to making a profit (Report for the Hearing, p. 78).

The Court, however, overruled these observations and included in the understanding of 'remuneration' in Treaty Article 50 indirect payments such as those transferred by social security funds to cover health care costs.

Through domestic policy reforms, Denmark introduced 'extended free choice' from July 2002, meaning that patients received a right to treatment outside contracted public hospitals in the event that these hospitals could not provide the necessary treatment within two months. Since October 2007, the waiting-time limit has been further reduced to one month. Denmark has hereby defined what it finds to be 'undue delay' within the health sector. This reform institutionalized the obligation to refer patients to non-contracted health care providers in the event that care cannot be provided by the public sector within the specified waiting-time guarantee. However, in making it possible to opt for treatment by non-contracted health care providers, the Danish reform had to consider the EC principle of non-discrimination. The principle obliges member states not to favour a nationally established, non-contracted (i.e. private) provider over a provider in another member state. The Danish proposal for reform directly referred to, and thus took account of the reasoning in the *Smits and Peerbooms* judgment (Legislative proposal L64, proposed 29 January 2002; adopted 19 March 2002.). The ECJ ruling thus impacted on Danish health care by granting a different exit opportunity other than private supply (i.e. health - care supply outside the national border).

It is nevertheless notable that the patient has not been granted the right to *freely* choose a foreign hospital whenever 'undue delay' of a publicly provided treatment occurs. The 'free choice' is restricted to those private and foreign hospitals with which the competent Danish authority has entered an agreement (Indenrigs- og Sundhedsministeriet: 'Frit Valg af Sygehus'). The Association for Danish Regions lists the private and foreign hospitals to which 'free choice' has been extended and with which an agreement has been concluded (http://www.sygehusvalg.dk/geoomraade.aspx). While 166 private hospitals or clinics in Denmark were listed in April 2007, only seven foreign hospitals or clinics were included, of which three were hospitals in Germany, two in Sweden, one in Spain and one is a German hospital established in Denmark. In practice, the condition that an agreement has to be concluded beforehand means that foreign hospitals are not treated on an equal footing with Danish private ones, and free movement of services has not been institutionalized when contracted hospitals in Denmark cannot provide treatment without undue delay. The central argument for restricting treatment to contracted foreign providers only is that this allows the Danish authorities to exercise control over the quality of provision through prior assessment of overseas facilities. Assuring standards and quality is still a national competence.

In several answers to parliamentary questions, the Danish Government restated that its interpretation of the concept of 'service' within the meaning of the Treaty is one that is carried out in return for remuneration and qualifies only when the insured person pays more than half of the health care costs.[16] The Danish Government thus maintained the definition of service that it formulated in the wake of the *Decker and Kohll* judgment and which exempted most Danish health care services from the impact of the principles of the internal market. As late as May 2006 the Danish Parliament was notified by the executive that this was the governing interpretation.

Meanwhile the official definition of health care *services* remained restrictive; its correctness was discussed internally in the Danish Ministry of Health. Behind the official executive stage, discussions started in the wake of the *Müller Fauré* and *van Riet* ruling – possibly earlier. Access gained to internal documents[17] shows that civil servants in the Ministry of Health raised doubt that the Danish definition was in line with the European concept of services as early as June 2003 and notified the minister thereof in an internal note. Later, in March 2004, another internal note further examined whether the Danish reinterpretation was in line with the ECJ interpretation of the concept – and explicitly stated that it was not.

Nevertheless, the official policy remained restrictive, based on the original definition. During the same period, citizens increasingly raised the question about exactly which health care treatments they were entitled to access without a prior authorization from the Danish authorities. One such question came from a Danish pensioner who had received outpatient treatment at a hospital in Germany.[18] He subsequently requested his costs reimbursed by the Danish authorities, but the competent municipality refused on the grounds that the treatment had not been authorized beforehand. The pensioner complained to the Danish Social Appeals Board. In October 2003, the National Social Appeals Board turned down the complaint, reasoning its decision on the restrictive Danish definition, consolidated by law in 2000. In the refusal, the definition, as quoted above, was explicitly referred to. Only health care for which the patient paid more than 50 per cent of the costs qualified as services within the meaning of the Treaty.

The case did not end here. The pensioner went to the Danish Ombudsman, who began to examine the case and requested the Social Appeals Board to further qualify its decision, taking the ECJ decisions further into account. An exchange of questions and answers between the Ombudsman, the National Social Appeals Board and the Ministry subsequently took place. As a result of this dialogue, addressing national interpretations and the rule of law as laid down by the ECJ, the Social Appeals Board in March 2005 decided to reconsider the case. The reexamination of the case took about 1.5 year – and in September 2006 the Board came out with its second decision on the case.[19] It stated that the European Court seemed to interpret the concept of service in a broader way than the one stated by Danish law. However, although the outpatient treatment did fall within the extended understanding of a health care service, the Board still found that the pensioner was not entitled to have his costs reimbursed, given that he had not been referred to the treatment by a GP as the Danish law requires.

Over a year later the Danish Minister of Health came out with a law proposal, admitting to the new understanding of health care service. In the meantime, the Danish Ombudsman reminded the Ministry that the Social Appeals Board is the highest authoritative level for interpreting such uncertainty.[20] The law was amended on 1 December 2008.[21] As a result, specialist treatments outside the hospital sector can now be accessed in another EU state and the costs are to be reimbursed by Danish health insurance, irrespective of whether the patient pays a part of the treatment or not. The law amendment does not, however, mean that the whole spectrum of outpatient care can be received in another EU member state, only those sets of treatments where an agreement has been established between the health insurance and the specialist doctors in Denmark.

Meanwhile Denmark has taken another step towards implementing the ECJ decisions, and Danish health care has been Europeanized a little further: the Danish Government has initiated the negotiation process on the proposal for a directive on patient rights. The Danish position is that clarification is needed, and the government, therefore, declares itself positive towards European regulation, meaning clarification, but it has some reservations regarding whether the proposal is in line with the subsidiarity principle. Forthcoming negotiations will indicate how the more specific Danish position turns out, and how a compromise will be established.

14.5.3 Finnish and Norwegian responses

Finland responded to the *Decker* and *Kohll* rulings by new guidelines given by the Social Insurance Institution, opening up patient mobility based on Article 49 of the Treaty. An amendment of the Health Insurance Act, which entered into force March 2005, legislated that an insured person can have costs refunded when treatment is given in another member state – but under a set of conditions. Although this allowed for some patient mobility, Finland has received a reasoned opinion from the Commission finding that Finland, in practice, restricts patient mobility by setting up a set of conditions for receiving treatment abroad (Sakslin 2006).

Norway is a member of the European Economic Area and has also delivered a contribution to the Commission's open consultation procedure. Norway noted that patient mobility to and from the Norwegian health system today is limited, but it expects it to increase in the future. Norway welcomed the Commission's intensions to establish further legal clarity and transparency within the area. It, however, appears to be more reluctant when it comes to how to ensure an accessible health sector for the national population, writing that it 'is a challenge to make sure that developments in the area of patient mobility and health services do not lead to greater social inequality with respect to accessibility to health services. A Commission proposal must make sure to prevent a situation where only the most resourceful patients are able to enjoy rights relating to patient mobility.' Norway furthermore finds that it should be justifiable to give higher priority to patients from the home social security system than from other member states – in order to ensure that treatment can be provided efficiently. This is a position it shares foremost with the newer member states and the United Kingdom, but a position which clearly goes against the fundamental principle of equal treatment within Community law.

14.6 Concluding remarks

The institutionalization of EU rules on patient mobility has been considerably furthered by European legalism since the mid-1990s. Although there are many factors making the integration process difficult, the impacts and challenges on health care policies in member states are increasingly identifiable. This is also true for the Nordic health care system, although its characteristics as tax financed, publicly controlled and organized, and with a decentralized structure, at first sight appear to shelter it from the market-correlating impacts of the internal market. The exact effects are still difficult to pinpoint and will become clearer with further time and developments. But the outline is there.

It seems safe to conclude that the EU will come to play a more prominent role as regulator and knowledge centre in the health care sector in the future, a development that implies a movement – albeit slow – towards increased policy coordination and some kind of system convergence.

The analytical comparison between Sweden and Denmark demonstrates that health care integration does not impact in a similar way. Instead impact, as it has unfolded in the two Nordic countries so far, depends on the national administrative, political and legal responses to the supranational events.

Nevertheless, we argue that at least three converging responses and future unavoidable challenges are identifiable. First, one natural consequence will be a need to standardize systems for billing and care financing for European patients and to determine the 'prices' for various treatments. Public health care budgets will have to be made market transparent. Second, European legalism implies an increased focus on patient rights. This goes against the Nordic tradition, in which formal patient rights have tended to be relatively weak as health care has been provided by public authorities as part of a more general public service, open to all, rather than a service to which access is provided on the basis of a specific insurance and hence a set of specific rights. Rights will become more individualized and individually enforceable. This may further cause the Nordic state–society relation to turn more 'legal', opening up more health-related court cases and more prominent roles for courts. On this aspect, it is interesting to see how the Swedish court case paved the way for further reimbursement demands for the costs of treatment in other member states. Third, regions and local authorities within the health sector are not policy-makers in the integration process as it has unfolded so far. Therefore, Europeanization seems to be tantamount to centralization. There will be an increased need to balance the interplay between the different levels of health care governance. Governing authority has taken an unexpectedly centralized turn in Sweden. In Denmark, the regions note that, as supranational competence expands into their traditional sphere of control, they will need to demand new decision-making competences similar to those of the German Länders in order to maintain their traditional domain of governance. This suggests that the Europeanization of health care could have a significant impact not only for health policy content but also for the distribution of power and relations between local, regional and central actors in Nordic health care.

Much of the future scope and direction of Europeanized health care will depend on which collective political steps will be taken as the Commission's recent proposal is negotiated and compromises are established. It will also depend on the specific wording of the final legislative text. It is far from certain that member governments will manage to establish a coherent political agreement. If this is the outcome of the current attempt at policy formulation, the ECJ will continue to be the motor of integration in the field of health care. Then the scope and direction of future developments will continue to bypass the political level and be decided by the interplay between citizens claiming their rights, private interests seeking markets, national courts interpreting European legalism and the ECJ as authoritative decision-maker.

Notes

1. In the preparation of this chapter, the authors found very little published information on the impacts of EU integration on the health care systems of Norway and Finland.
2. COM (2001) 723, 5 December 2001. Communication from the Commission on the

Future of Health Care and Care for the Elderly: Guaranteeing Accessibility, Quality and Financial Viability, p. 13.
3. COM (2004) 204 final, 20 April 2004. Communication from the Commission on Modernizing Social Protection for the Development of High-Quality, Accessible and Sustainable Healthcare and Long-term Care. Support for the national strategies using the open method of coordination.
4. A new regulation, 883/2004, was adopted on 29 April 2004 but does not enter into force before the implementation regulation is adopted by the Council. The proposal on the implementing regulation was adopted by the Commission on 31 January 2006, COM (2006) 16, and is currently negotiated in the Council Working Group on Social Affairs.
5. For a more detailed description of the series of judgments, see Martinsen (2005).
6. In the cases C-120/95, *Decker*, 28 April 1998 and C-158/96, *Kohll*, 28 April 1998.
7. Case C-157/99, *Geraets-Smits and Peerbooms*, 12 July 2001.
8. Case C-385/99, 13 May 2003. *Müller-Fauré* v *Onderlinge Waarborgmaatschappij OZ Zorgverzekeringen and Van Riet* v *Onderlinge Waarborgmaatschappij ZAO Zorgverzekeringen*. ECR 2003, p. I-04509.
9. As formulated by the Advocate General Tesauro in the 1998 cases of *Decker* and *Kohll*, which will be further examined below
10. COM (2004) 2, 5 March 2004. Proposal for a Directive of the European Parliament and of the Council on Services in the Internal Market.
11. The Communication is SEC (2006) 1195/4, 26 September 2006.
12. COM (2008) 414. Proposal for a Directive of the European Parliament and of the Council on the Application of Patients' Rights in Cross-border Healthcare.
13. The recommendations were later turned into a legal proposal (Ministry of Social Affairs 2005) but have not yet been enacted.
14. This depends, as stated by the court and later in the Commission's directive, on the nature of the disease and the degree of medical urgency in receiving treatment.
15. The policy reform entered into force by law no. 467 of 31 May 2000 and BEK no. 536 of 15 June 2000.
16. Answer to Parliamentary question no. 89, 28 June 2005; answers to parliamentary questions no. 4965, 4967 and 4969, 17 May 2006)
17. The present analysis in part builds on achieved access to internal documents, covering documents from the Ministry of Health, the National Social Appeals Board and the Danish Ombudsman.
18. This part of the analysis also builds on the achieved access to internal documents.
19. Decision S-2-06.
20. Letter from the Danish Ombudsman to the Ministry of Health, May 2007.
21. As of BEK no. 1098 and Vej. No. 70 of 19th November 2008.

References

Alter, K. (1998) Who are the 'Masters of the Treaty'? European Governments and the European Court of Justice, *International Organization* 52: 121–47.
Alter, K. (2000) The European Union's legal system and domestic policy: spillover or backlash? *International Organization* 54: 489–518.
Blomqvist, P. (ed.) (2004) *Den gränslösa välfärdsstaten*. Stockholm: Agora.
Borrás, S. and Jacobsson, K. (2004) The open method of co-ordination and the new governance patterns in the EU, *European Journal of Public Policy* 11: 185–208.
Engqvist, L. (2004) Mer statligt styre i vården. *Dagens Nyheter*, 11 May.

Erhag, T. (2004) EU-lagstiftningens påverkan på svensk socialförsäkringsrätt, in Blomqvist, P. (ed.) *Den gränslösa välfärdsstaten*. Stockholm: Agora.

Ferrera, M. (2005) *The Boundaries of Welfare*. Oxford: Oxford University Press.

Garrett, G. (1995) The politics of legal integration. *International Organisation* 49: 171–81.

Garrett, G., Kelemen, D. and Schultz, H. (1998) The European Court of Justice, national governments, and legal integration in the European Union, *International Organization* 52: 149–76.

Geer, S. (2006) Uninvited europeanization: neocfunctionalism and the EU in health policy, *Journal of European Public Policy* 13: 134–52.

Goldstein, J., Kahler, M., Keohane, R. and Slaughter, A.-M. (1998) Introduction: Legalization and world politics, *International Organization* 54: 385–99.

Liebfried, S. and Pierson, P. (2000) Social Policy. Left to courts and markets? In Wallace, H. and Wallace, W. (eds) *Policy-making in the European Union*, 4th edn. Oxford: Oxford University Press.

Martinsen, D.S. (2005) Towards an internal health market with the European Court, *West European Politics* 28: 1035–56.

Mattli, W. and Slaughter, A.-M. (1998) Revisiting the European Court of Justice, *International Organization* 52: 177–209.

Ministry of Social Affairs (2005) *Proposition (Legal proposal) 2005/06: 73. Nationell samordning av rikssjukvården*. Stockholm: Swedish Ministry of Social Affairs.

Ministry of Social Affairs (2006) *Ds 2006:4. Rätten till ersättning för kostnader för vård i annat EES-land – En översyn*. Stockholm: Swedish Ministry of Social Affairs.

Mossialos, E. and McKee, M. (eds) (2002) *EU Law and the Social Character of Health Care*. Brussels: P.I.E. Peter Lang.

Obinger, H., Liebfred, S. and Castles, F. (2005) Bypasses to a social Europe? Lessons from federal experience, *Journal of European Public Policy* 23: 545–71.

Palm, W., Nicless, N., Lewalle, H. and Coheur, C. (2000) *Implications of Recent Jurispudence on the Co-ordination of Health Care Protection Systems*. [Report produced for the European Commission Directorates – General for Employment and Social Affairs.] Brussels: Association Internationale de la Mutualité (AIM).

Pierson, P. (ed.) (2001) *The New Politics of the Welfare State*. Oxford: Oxford University Press.

Rhodes, R.A.W. (1997) *Understanding Governance: Policy Networks, Governance, Reflexivity and Accountability*. Buckingham: Open University Press.

Sakslin, M. (2006) *Training and Reporting on European Social Security. Finland: National Report*. Ghent: Ghent University Project for the EU Commission DG Employment and Social Affairs.

Swedish Social Insurance Agency [Försäkringskassan] (2006) *Slutrapport. Kartläggning av gränsöverskridande planerad vår inom EU/EES finansierad av Försäkringskassan 2004–2005*. Stockholm: Försäkringskassan.

Vahlne Westerhäll, L. (2004) EU och den svenska sjukvården: om patienters rättigheter, in Blomqvist, P. (ed.) *Den gränslösa välfärdsstaten*. Stockholm: Agora.

fifteen

The Icelandic health care system

Tinna L. Ásgeirsdóttir

15.1 Introduction

Iceland is a mountainous country in the middle of the North Atlantic Ocean, with a population of 320,000 and a total area of 103,000 km^2 (Statistics Iceland 2009). Iceland is a representative democracy and a parliamentary republic. The President of Iceland is in practice a ceremonial head of state, although granted some formal power by the constitution. The capital of Iceland is Reykjavik, the only city in the country. However, the greater capital area includes other nearby towns and urban areas located in the southwest of the country. The city of Reykjavik and the nearby towns collectively form one urban entity. In total, more than half of the population lives in this region. The rural population is located in the countryside and villages along the coastline of the country. Akureyri, the largest town outside of the capital area, has around 17,000 inhabitants. This translates into a meagre population on a relatively far-flung area of land. This fact sets its mark on health care in many ways, as will be apparent throughout this analysis of the structure, motivation, financing, provision, current reforms and challenges of the Icelandic health care system.

   The current analysis is written in the midst of a severe economic crisis in Iceland. This is a financial, currency and business crisis as well as a political crisis and has greatly affected the future prospects of the country. Before the onset of the crisis, Iceland was ranked as one of the most developed countries in the world by the United Nations Human Development Index (UNDP 2007, 2008). The economic downturn will undoubtedly lead to significant changes in the economic well-being of the Icelandic people and the availability of government funds. It is clear that the health care system will have to change along with other areas in the face of the pressing realities confronting the nation. Whereas some changes have been proposed, few have been realized and more transformations are sure to come.

This chapter will deal with the Icelandic health care system and highlight some of the challenges that are present within it. Other chapters of this book have given prominence to specific features of Nordic health care systems. This chapter will focus on how the Icelandic system compares with the other Nordic countries. Section 15.2 considers the general motivation behind the Icelandic health care system. This is followed in Section 15.3 by a description of the structure and values of the system. Section 15.4 examines financing of health care and Section 15.5 its provision. Finally, Section 15.6 will present some of the challenges facing the Icelandic health care system.

15.2 Motivation

The Icelandic health care system is deeply rooted in the Nordic model of the welfare state. A common concern in Iceland is how social arrangements meet each individual's 'right' to a certain level of sustenance. While this view of entitlement is not adhered to as firmly for all goods, health care seems to be one of the primary accepted rights. It is not simply the idea of decreasing variation in health that is envisaged but rather the decrease in variation in health by socioeconomic status. Thus, in Iceland as in the other Nordic countries, it is widely accepted that one of the principal objectives of the health care system is to improve health irrespective of the patient's financial means. Health equality, irrespective of income, refers to a lack of systematic differences in health by income. Complete income-related health equality does not, however, mean that everyone shares the same level of health, only that systematic differences in health by income do not exist.

Countries go to different lengths to attain health equality. Iceland is very committed to providing good access to health care for all citizens and thereby mitigating the health–income relationship. This has been the focus of substantial government expenditure in Iceland. While several policies aim to reduce income-related inequalities in health, near-totally subsidized medical care is by far the largest policy action.

With the decreasing impact of communicable diseases and the increase in health problems related to lifestyle, greater emphasis has been placed on the role of the individual's own behaviour in their health status. This has, however, not led to any drastic policy changes in Iceland regarding publicly provided health care. It remains the expressed goal of the Icelandic political parties to ensure all citizens have easy and equal access to good health care services. Furthermore, the Icelandic law on health care starts by stating that 'all citizens should have available to them, the greatest quality health care services that is possible to provide them with at any given time, to protect their psychological, physical and social health' (Proceedings of the Alþingi 2009a).

One may or may not subscribe to the political views in which those policies are rooted. Some argue that each individual has to be responsible for his/her own health, and that good health is a normal part of society's reward system. After all, there are many things, besides health, that those of lower financial status have less access to. However, others feel that increasing responsibility for health production is problematic. After all, poverty itself is widely accepted as one of the most significant risk factors for illness and premature death in countries where individuals bear greater responsibility. The United States is a case in point (Syme 1996). Hence, the relationship between health and income works both ways. Not only does financial abundance increase health, health itself is also important for productivity and the attainment of economic means (Grossman 1972).

15.3 Values and structure

The Icelandic health care system is founded on values similar to those generally emphasized in the other Nordic countries. These have been the major force not only behind the existence and scope of the system but also behind its general structure and financing. The Icelandic health care system can be classified as an integrated single-payer health care system financed by general taxation. The Icelandic health care system, however, differs from those of the other Nordic countries in some fundamental structural aspects. The most important ones will be highlighted here.

Probably most apparent is that the Icelandic health care system is more centralized in its governance structure, management, regulation, implementation and financing than the other Nordic countries. The Minister of Health oversees practically all health affairs. While Iceland is divided into regions, counties and municipalities, the role of local authorities in health care is almost non-existent. Funding by local taxes is not used to any extent and the involvement of local authorities in financing is limited to exceptional instances, for instance some contribution to the building costs of local nursing homes. Similarly, local authorities have played a very limited role in the management and implementation of health care services. This makes the Icelandic system distinctly different from its Nordic counterparts and it might be considered to have similarities to the National Health Service (NHS) in the United Kingdom. Basically, decision-making, enforcement and management are all concentrated at the level of the central government (Proceedings of the Alþingi 2009a).

Still, in line with other Nordic countries, Iceland has recently implemented what on the outset seems to be a decentralization, by dividing the country into seven health care regions. The purpose has not necessarily been to devolve power to the regions as much as to induce institutional mergers and increased cooperation *within* the areas. There are obvious challenges regarding the size of the population and in a rapidly specializing world of medicine, economies of scale can be difficult to realize within sparsely populated areas. The legislation that introduces health care regions states:

> Health-care institutions that provide general health care in each of the health-care regions shall cooperate in conformation of services in the region. The Minister of Health can, in cooperation with municipalities and the Association of Local Authorities in Iceland, decide to merge health-care institutions within a health-care region with regulations. Despite the separation of the country into health-care regions, patients should have equal

access to health centers or other health-care institutions where most con-
venient at each time.

(Proceedings of the Alþingi, 2009a)

In fact, the creation of health care regions was largely motivated by the need to
increase mergers and cooperation between institutions. Such mergers of institutions have systematically been taking place since the mid-1990s. This has been a
continuing development with instances of pronounced jumps along the way.
The most apparent one would probably be the 1999 merger of 10 institutions in
the east of Iceland. These included health centres, hospitals and nursing homes.
The main purpose of those mergers was to increase capabilities in the provision
of quality of care. This institutional condensation was, however, in some ways
decentralizing the system as a whole, as the larger institutions are now able to
control more of their daily decision-making than their forerunners did. They are
also more capable of managing multiple practical issues such as personnel. As
such, this has transferred to the institutions themselves a substantial amount of
the trivial decision-making that has little to do with government policy and
more to do with management.

These changes, therefore, both increase and decrease centralization. They
increase centralization as they encourage and actuate institutional mergers
within regions. They decrease centralization as they shift many local managerial
decisions to the institutions themselves. Nevertheless, the change does not
shift financing or responsibility away from the central government to other
levels of governance, such as municipalities. In fact, recent health care reforms
in Iceland have in many ways increased centralization, where the government
has taken over practically all responsibilities that local authorities previously
had. One notable example is primary health care. Systematic decentralization
from the government level to municipalities with regard to financing, as well
as management and enforcement of practical issues, has been scarce.

Other examples of increased centralization can be found in the organizational
centralization of primary health care in the capital area and the merger of the
two hospitals in Reykjavik. The new primary care institution runs almost all
primary health care in and around Reykjavik. Previous to the change, primary
care was generally provided by independent practitioners and from health care
centres. The merger of the only two hospitals in Reykjavík resulted in the creation of Landspítali University Hospital. Additionally, there is still one small
hospital in the adjacent town of Hafnafjörður.

A second structural feature in Iceland is the lack of gatekeeping by GPs. In this
respect, Iceland is similar to Sweden but differs from Norway, Denmark and
Finland. Although all Nordic countries have generally expanded patient choice
in recent years, the freedom to seek services directly from a specialist has been
and continues to be a pronounced feature of the Icelandic system. This does not
necessarily reflect deliberate ideas about how patients should move through the
health care system or a careful evaluation of the costs and benefits of possible
limits on this freedom. Limits on patient choices have also been met with strong
opposition by interest groups (Halldórsson 2003).

Yet another difference is the lower importance placed on public health policy
in Iceland as opposed to curative measures. A heavy emphasis on prevention and

communal health is something common to the other Nordic systems. Iceland does not share this emphasis. In a similar way, Iceland has not developed low-intensity care to the same extent as the other Nordic countries; rather it still relies, for example, more on inpatient care than on ambulatory care and day surgery. In terms of expenditure, Iceland directs its health care budget quite conspicuously to higher levels of care than do the Nordic counterparts (OECD 2008a).

15.4 Raising funds and financing services

The Icelandic health care system is mainly financed through taxes, even though the patient pays some minor fees at the time of service. It should be noted, however, that dental care is only subsidized for children, the elderly or when caused by birth defects, diseases or accidents. Consequently, as in other Nordic countries, dental care forms a large portion of private expenditure on health, as described by Vilhjálmsson and Sigurðardóttir (2003).

Despite fees not being directly related to earnings, some groups with limited ability to generate income, such as the disabled or retired people, pay a lower fee for health care services. Co-payments do, however, not generally take into account the patient's earnings. Around 82.5 per cent of total expenditure on health care in Iceland is publically financed. The remaining 17.5 per cent is almost exclusively financed by out-of-pocket payments (OECD 2008a). This is, with the exception of Finland, similar to the rates in the other Nordic countries.

Because of the extensive public medical services, private or employer-provided health insurance hardly exists in Iceland, although neither is prohibited by law. This is not surprising as the incentive for such insurances is negligible when the Health Services Act and the Act on the Rights of Patients state that 'every citizen has the right to the best health services available at all times, for the restoration and protection of their mental, physical, and social health' (Proceedings of the Alþingi 2009a).

The rise in health care expenditure per capita has been exceptionally rapid in Iceland over the last few decades, resulting in Iceland having one of the most expensive health care systems in the world around the start of the twenty-first century, and with health expenditure exceeding 10 per cent of gross domestic product (GDP) in 2002 and 2003. The rapid growth was curbed considerably in subsequent years and this has reduced the expenditure gap between Iceland and the other Nordic countries. Recent figures from the OECD show Iceland to have spent 9.2 per cent of GDP on health care in 2007, in line with Norway, Sweden and Denmark. In per capita spending, however, only Norway spends more than Iceland on health care, while the other Nordic countries all spend considerably less (OECD 2008a).

Iceland is a small and sparsely populated country and this may be one of the reasons for the country's high expenditure on health. It is harder to achieve economies of scale and scope in a population of 320,000 people than in larger populations. Furthermore, the geography is challenging, and ensuring access to health care, especially during the winter months, does require more outlets for health care services. What may further exacerbate hospital spending is the fact that only a few countries within the OECD have a higher share of spending on long-term care than Iceland. This is surprising in light of the very favourable demographics in Iceland. Even if the number of long-term care beds within hospitals has decreased, the capacity and utilization of nursing homes relative to the size of the elderly population is quite high. This highlights an emphasis on institutional long-term care relative to home care that is not in accordance with the current reality in the Nordic countries (OECD 2008a).

Iceland has, however, some attractive features in its health care costs. Fertility has remained high in Iceland and the problem of an ageing population is, therefore, less severe than in many countries. In fact the dependency ratio in Iceland is quite advantageous and, despite the high life expectancy, the proportion of people under the age of 65 years is very favourable. However, fertility is predicted to decline in Iceland, which will result in the same type of demographic challenges as other countries are currently facing (Statistics Iceland 2008).

Both Icelandic geography and the dependency ratio are external and have only minimal bearing on public policy. Out of the two, one would be expected to promote health expenditure and the other would be expected to decrease it. Consequently, it is not clear if the actual situation in Iceland overall would be an explanation for the nation allocating a different amount of resources to health care than neighbouring countries do.

Turning now to how resources are distributed to different segments of the system, we find that the majority of public expenditure is spent on fixed (global) budget items. This is how most institutions, be it hospitals, health centres, administrative units and the like, are financed. Similarly, most Icelandic health - care professionals are salaried employees. In that sense, authorities prioritize finances and determine the relevant importance and capabilities of each institution. However, this is countered by the fact that Icelandic patients can choose where they seek services as Iceland does not employ a gatekeeping system.

Most specialists working on ambulatory care are, however, financed on a fee-for-service basis by the government and with out-of-pocket co-payments. The government currently negotiates rates for those services with the Medical Association. Inpatient hospital care has been funded without any co-payment by patients in recent years, even though the previous Minister of Health introduced a co-payment near the end of his term that was abolished when he left office. Ambulatory hospital care has, however, involved a co-payment.

Results from Erlandsen (2008) indicate that there is a considerable potential for cost reductions in Iceland when comparing unit costs for a few standard clinical procedures. Potential savings are quite high in comparisons with the Nordic countries apart from Sweden. In spite of this, the Nordic countries themselves appear to be doing well compared with other industrialized countries. So this facet may be of less concern when examined in a larger context. The greatest pressure on total hospital spending may be the use of hospital care, particularly inpatient care, when other forms of treatment could be more cost-effective.

Evaluation of the pharmaceutical financing and expenditure in Iceland reveals that total costs are relatively high. The rapid growth in pharmaceutical expenditure was previously a concern but has now been curbed substantially (OECD 2008a). However, the expenditure is still a considerable challenge, especially considering the favourable demographics and the relatively low use of prescription drugs. This high outlay partly reflects the high prices of pharmaceuticals in Iceland and the frequent use of expensive drug choices in treatments.

Progress has been made in curbing the high prices of pharmaceuticals in recent years, especially the prices of branded drugs, but less progress has been made in lowering the prices of generic drugs. Similarly, limited progress has been made in directing use towards less costly options. The cost-sharing structure on prescription drugs has involved incentives towards the use of expensive drugs, although some changes have been proposed and revisions are being prepared. Action has been taken to stop pharmacies continuing their practice of offering rebates to patients on their co-payments of brand-name drugs, as that allowed pharmacies to direct use towards more expensive products, solely through the patients' co-payments.

The small size of the Icelandic market is partly to blame for the high prices. There is a continuous discussion about practical solutions that would allow for a Nordic pharmaceutical market (Friðriksdóttir et al. 2008).

The Icelandic Health Insurance is a recently founded public institution that is intended to administer and transact purchases of health care services on behalf of the government. The main goal of the institution is to strengthen the government's role as a purchaser of health services, leaving this institution as the only purchaser. At the same time, the creation of this institution was meant to introduce a purchaser–provider split. The institution is meant to conduct cost-analysis and this will be the first time that such analysis will be systematically carried out in Iceland, even though such analyses have been suggested, for example in the OECD *Economic Survey: Iceland* (OECD 2008b). The Icelandic Health Insurance is intended to execute its role by taking into consideration economic efficiency and equal access (Proceedings of the Alþingi 2009b).

When founding the Icelandic Health Insurance, policy-makers were inspired by the Swedish purchaser–provider split of the early 1990s. However, the implementation in Sweden also provided a cautionary tale. Total expenditure rose quite sharply with large-scale introduction of activity-based financing (ABF). Therefore, the Icelandic Health Insurance will introduce negotiations and contracting slowly. The effects that this new system will have on fixed costs and ABF remain to be seen.

As discussed in earlier chapters, ABF has been tried in a limited number of cases. Furthermore, extensive efforts have been undertaken to structure diagnosis-related group (DRG) costs in Iceland and prepare the hospitals for allocation of resources based on diagnostic groups. Several issues have, however, not been resolved as they pertain to the situation in Iceland. For example, the country has only one major hospital. How DRG pricing should be defined is, therefore, a challenge, and using hospitals in different countries with different currencies, labour-market regulations and so forth is easier said than done. The transition that DRG offers away from historical costs may be more limited in Iceland than in other countries, or at least more complex.

15.5 Provision

While there is a general consensus in Iceland about the public financing of the health care system, there has been extensive discussion on what is the best way to provide health care. This debate has to some extent been a response to developments within health care systems in neighbouring countries, such as the Nordic ones and the United Kingdom. As in the other Nordic countries, the question of private or public health care has revolved around the private or public provision and production within a system that would still be publicly financed and controlled.

A recent comparison presented in a report by the OECD (2008b) reveals that private provision has not been used to the same extent in Iceland as in the other Nordic countries, currently accounting for approximately one quarter of publicly financed health services. In a small country such as Iceland, numbers such as these can, however, be greatly influenced by the provision of a few large institutions. For example, the fact that the Landspítali University Hospital takes up one-third of the Icelandic health care budget and is a state-run hospital is important in this context. Therefore, it needs to be kept in mind that there are areas of Icelandic health care that are quite extensively privatized already. This is most notable with regard to specialist care, which is provided by independently run private practices when not serviced directly in hospitals.

Icelanders have followed closely the developments in other Nordic health care systems that have increased emphasis on incentives in the provision of health - care. However, Iceland has been slower itself in terms of implementation in general, although there are exceptions, for example specialist care, which is financed on a fee-for-service basis.

Health centres providing primary care are located throughout the country and are sometimes run jointly with small hospitals or health institutions. The centres outside the capital area are all publicly run, based on fixed budgets. Even if the locations of the primary care units have been chosen with geographic access in mind, there have been some concerns about access rationing through waiting times. Such problems have, however, been most apparent in Reykjavik.

In the capital area, most GPs provide services at health care centres, most of which are under public provision and financed through one institution, Primary Health Care of the Capital Area (PHCCA). This institution operates 15 health clinics, of which one is fairly independent in its affairs even though it is under the administration of the board of the PHCCA. The health care clinics offer various medical and nursing services, general medical services, general nursing care, infant or maternity services, school nursing, vaccinations for adults, health care for the elderly and so on. The activities of the health clinics are directed towards neighbourhood services and they are expected to serve inhabitants of particular parts of the capital city area. A few GPs still see patients privately, as remnants of an old system, even if government policy of recent years has been that all primary care should preferably be provided within health centres.

In the capital area, one health care centre is privately run, without any direct administrative affiliation with PHCCA. It is, however, financed publicly according to a contract with the Ministry of Health. In the tender process for this project, it was specified that the goals were to increase access and efficiency while guaranteeing the public conformable and comprehensive services. The contract involves an incentive scheme where some of the payments are based on services given. The outcome of this experiment has been examined and reported. The results were favourable on the three activities examined: costs, performance and the satisfaction of the users (Ministry of Health, 2008).

The debate on the appropriateness of private or public provision in industrialized countries seems to generally raise greater political debate regarding specialist care than primary care. It is, therefore, interesting that Icelanders have chosen to use private provision for specialist care but public provision for primary care. Obstacles for GPs are formidable, and those interested in practising have limited opportunities besides applying for positions at the public health centres described above, when such positions come available. In this way, the number of individuals in general practice is publicly determined and, consequently, also the amount of services delivered. By comparison, specialists can start practising with little impediment. They can open private clinics and start servicing patients under the public insurance on a fee-for-service basis. This does not require the specialist in question to wait for a position to become available or to negotiate the amount of services he or she would like the state to purchase. There is, however, an upper limit on services provided by specialties as a whole. The entrance of a new provider can thus limit the potential for other providers within the same field. Specialist practices have thus grown rapidly and, because of the somewhat limited access to GPs and extensive patient choice, it might be assumed that specialists provide considerable services that in other countries are provided by GPs. The distribution of specialist services seem quite random, with some areas apparently over-serviced while others are lacking same type of specialist care. There is nothing that really indicates, on the part of the government purchasing those services, what type of services should be provided, by whom, where and in what amounts. It is not known if this has led to service provision rooted in supplier-induced demand.

Pharmacies in Iceland are privately run, but their service provision has to be handled by a licensed pharmacist who can be held professionally accountable. Ownership, however, is not restricted to pharmacists and anyone can run a pharmacy. There are currently no restrictions on the number of pharmaceutical outlets in a particular area.

The size of the Icelandic market clearly leads to little competition. This has sparked discussion on whether provision should be limited to Icelandic pharmacies or not. Specifically, the idea of a Nordic market through which Icelanders could order their medicine by mail has been suggested, although not realized.

15.6 Challenges

Industrialized societies spend increasing proportions of their GDP on health - care. Although expenditure growth has been curbed somewhat recently, the sustainability of health care systems is under pressure. Demographic changes have so far had a limited effect on expenditure in Iceland, as the ageing of the population has not been as pronounced as in the other Nordic countries. Demographic changes are, however, predicted to happen in Iceland as elsewhere.

This development of increased expenditure holds true for both tax- and insurance-based systems. The Icelandic health care system is financed through general taxes and is very centralized at the government level. Taxes are not collected specifically for health care and so expenditure comes out of the general fiscal budget. In such a system, the opportunities for political bargaining are substantial. This is further emphasized by the fact that Icelandic Health Ministers, as other Ministers, are professional politicians relying on democratic elections and have, because of the centralized system, many decisions concerning local expenditure directly in their hands. This decreases the sense of trade-offs by the managers of health care services.

As Iceland does not employ a gatekeeping system, incentives within the system are all the more important. Unfortunately, incentives to use relatively expensive health care products and services rather than less-costly and often equally effective care are numerous. This is apparent in many respects, but one particular area, primary versus other health services, will be discussed below.

In Iceland, the mainly salaried GPs have few economic incentives to attract patients. This working environment has been shown to decrease the productivity within primary care in Iceland substantially (Ministry of Health 2008). What further decreases the availability of GP services is that they face substantial barriers in setting up practice. This differs substantially from the situation in specialist care, where opening a private practice is based on very minimal requirements. In theory, GPs and primary health services are supposed to be patients' first point of contact within the system. In reality, specialists and emergency care units are involved in a substantial amount of what could be classified as primary care. What is the most effective or cost-effective way for patients to move through a health care system will not be considered here. It can, however, be clearly stated that the declared aim of primary care being the patient's first point of contact with the health services has not been attained in Iceland.

The fact that this goal has not been achieved can hardly be surprising given the structure of the system and the incentives within it. The interplay between a highly regulated primary care system with less than optimal productivity and the less-regulated services of specialist ambulatory care, financed on a fee-for-service basis, is likely to lead to outcomes that are not consistent with the idea of primary care being the first point of contact within the system. Consequently, secondary and tertiary care may be accessed in instances where primary care would suffice. Supplier-induced demand within systems employing a fee-for-service financial mechanism in Iceland has not been estimated, but the potential for such a problem certainly exists. However, regardless of whether such a demand exists, simply the existing interplay between primary care and specialist care warrants attention.

There are other examples of how incentives within the system increase the use of relatively expensive services. Outpatient hospital care and home care could surely be used to a greater extent where currently inpatient services are employed. It has often been suggested that out-of-pocket payment for inpatient hospital care should be considered for a number of reasons, including to decrease incentives for using very expensive resources when not needed (OECD 2008b). Consistency and egalitarian views are another reason as co-payments within the system are quite different and based on treatments needed by patients. The focus on institutional long-term care rather than less-costly measures such as home care is also a feature that sets the Icelandic health care system apart from its Nordic counterparts.

A further example involves the high cost of pharmaceuticals in Iceland (OECD 2008a). One of the main reasons for this appears to choices of drugs by Icelandic doctors and patients, where more expensive drugs are used in Iceland than in the other Nordic countries. In short, estimates of technical efficiency suggest that the good health outcomes of Iceland could be attained at a lesser cost (OECD 2008b). How best way to facilitate the substitution of generic drugs, where available and appropriate, is currently debated.

Cost-effectiveness has been relied on to a significantly lesser extent in Iceland than generally in the industrialized world and information regarding the cost-effectiveness of different possibilities has not been gathered. This was expressed in a report by the OECD on Iceland (OECD 2008b, p. 16): 'What is clearly needed is a prioritization of public health care spending based on cost–benefit analysis of different kinds of services'. The report continue by saying that it is 'important to improve the cost-effectiveness of health care in Iceland, which seems to be lacking, in order to be better prepared for the unavoidable long-term pressures due to population ageing' (OECD 2008b, p. 86). This is surely true, but is undoubtedly related to another problem. Because there is little population research in Iceland, there are few results on which policy can be based. Because of their scarcity, studies conducted in the context of Iceland are of particular value to Icelandic policy-makers, who are otherwise left to rely on intuition and results from people, places and times that may be very different from the current Icelandic reality. However, cost analysis may be a coming trend in Iceland with the foundation of this newly established institution and the evaluation of the cost-efficiency of different kinds of treatments and provision.

Within a system where patients have extensive choices in where they seek treatment, incentives need to be carefully reviewed. The structure of the cost-sharing scheme could be used more effectively to direct patients to the most appropriate level of care. Currently co-payments are not structured according to the cost of the services being provided. It is sometimes the case within the Icelandic health system that when a patient uses a more expensive measure in terms of total costs the patient's co-payment can frequently be lower than if a less costly measure was used. Examples of this can be found in the cost-sharing structure of some drug treatments, as well as inpatient versus outpatient care.

A great deal of scarce resources is utilized in centralized health production in Iceland. It is, therefore, important to ask if their allocation alleviates income-related health inequalities, as laid out in the introduction to this chapter. Importantly, the relative equality in health care delivery and financing may not be the same as income-related equality in health. For one thing, there may be income-related differences in the use of the health care system. Furthermore, medical care is not the only input in the production of health. There are still opportunities for differences based on finances, even in societies such as Iceland where a strong social-welfare system should keep people out of desperate poverty and where medical services are largely provided through government funding. For example, financial means can help people to invest in their health through elements such as fitness centres, nutritional counselling and better living conditions. Therefore, the efforts of the Icelandic Government may or may not have dramatic effects regarding variations in health.

A study on income-related health inequality in Iceland revealed a statistically significant relationship between health and income (Ásgeirsdóttir 2007a). But this relationship was smaller than that reported for other countries using the same methodology. Because of methodological differences, it is only possible to compare the outcome in Iceland with that in Sweden and Finland of the Nordic countries. Iceland has a similar income-related inequality as Sweden. Finland appears to suffer a greater level of income-related health inequality. Comparison with the international results suggests that health inequality, though it exists, is relatively limited in Iceland compared with other countries and is similar or marginally more favourable than that of the other Nordic countries (van Doorslaer et al. 1997). It can be concluded that the goal of income-related health equality has been attained to a greater extent in Iceland than in many other countries. The same can be said for the other Nordic countries, albeit to differing extents. This is important as it relates to the founding principles on which these systems are based and ideologies in which they are to a large extent rooted.

As indicated above, health-related inequality based on socioeconomic inequality is not pronounced despite certainly occurring in Iceland and it may be quite similar to that in other Nordic countries. This would not be changed by a changing cost-sharing scheme as the total share of private to public expenditure would not have to be affected. Similarly, gender differences in health have been decreasing over the years, for example with respect to longevity. However, there is one area in which equity has been lacking and that is between diagnostic groups. What seems to determine the extent of individual co-payments is not the severity of the illness or the individual's financial deprivation, it is rather the form of treatment needed, for example drugs, ambulatory care or inpatient hospital care, that determines the amount of co-payment. This could also be adjusted by a change in the cost-sharing structure within the Icelandic health - care system.

15.7 Concluding remarks

The Icelandic people enjoy good access to health care services that are of a very high quality. Health outcomes are generally favourable, with life expectancy among the very highest in the world. Other markers are also encouraging, such as infant mortality, which is among the lowest in the world. As in any other health care system, there are several challenges, some of which will be highlighted here.

The good health of the Icelandic population has fiscal importance as the government takes financial responsibility for the medical care demands of its citizens, to the point where nongovernmental funding of such consumption has been negligible for several decades. The same holds true for disability-related income replacements, both long and short term. This means that the Icelandic Government has a considerable stake in the health of its populace, both directly through health care expenditure and through the impact that an individual's bad health can have on the labour market. As the Icelandic Government is responsible for a wide variety of income replacements, it is sensitive to the effects of its policies on health and the effect of health on the labour market. Risky lifestyle choices in Iceland, as in the industrialized world in general, have attracted the attention of policy-makers. There is a large difference between what is currently acknowledged as a healthy lifestyle and what most individuals practise. This difference seems difficult to alter and is projected to be the source of leading health issues facing Icelanders in the coming decades.

Substantial progress has been made on many fronts in terms of lifestyle choices. Smoking, for example, has declined substantially and some progress has been made with regard to other substances, legal and illegal. There are, however, still areas of concern. Despite the fact that the average per capita consumption of alcohol in Iceland is lower than in most other European countries, drinking habits of Icelanders have traditionally differed from those in neighbouring countries and are characterized by lower frequency of consumption. However, when many people do use alcoholic beverages, they consume them to the point of intoxication and binge drinking of hard liquor is quite common. These patterns are slowly changing and Icelanders are starting to spread their consumption over more occasions (Ólafsdóttir 1998).

The most pressing public health concern is obesity. Currently, the Icelandic people are among the heaviest in Europe. The increase in weight has been quite rapid in Iceland, with 7.5 per cent of the population being obese in 1990, but over 20 per cent in 2007 (Steingrímsdóttir et al. 2002; Ásgeirsdóttir 2007b; Gísladóttir et al. 2009). Currently, the Icelandic people are heavier than their Scandinavian counterparts (OECD 2008a).

In recent decades many parts of the industrialized world, including the Nordic countries, have implemented substantial changes in their health systems. Many of these changes have been summarized under the term 'new public management' (NPM). Many Icelandic policy-makers have looked with interest toward these changes in the Nordic countries, for example, changes allowing a greater role for market forces and the use of economic incentives for providers of health care. The organizational structure of the Icelandic system has undergone some changes so that it can improve its handling of a more market-oriented system. For example, the Icelandic Health Insurance has been set up to achieve an increased purchaser–provider split by acting as a purchaser of health care services for the government. The relative role of the private sector is, however, substantially smaller in Iceland than in the other Nordic countries.

The Icelandic health care system is, for all general purposes, providing the citizens of Iceland with quality services. The average lifespan of an Icelander is long and his or her health is generally good during this long life. However, this is accomplished at a relatively high cost. There are several reasons for this. First, Icelanders are paying a price for very minimal restrictions to their choices of where to seek services. Second, specific segments of the system have limited incentives to optimize as future budgets will be based to a large extent on historical costs. Third, cost-effectiveness has received limited attention in Iceland until fairly recently, although there is now growing attention to health economics at the university level. Fourth, the cost-sharing structure frequently directs individuals to very expensive health care options even where less-costly measures could be utilized. The current Icelandic health care system provides good services, but it can be argued that the enviable health status of the Icelandic people could be attained with less resource use.

Acknowledgments

The author would like to thank Sveinn Magnússon at the Ministry of Health, Sigurður Gylfi Magnússon, historian at the Reykjavík Academy, and Ásgeir Haraldsson Professor of Medicine at the University of Iceland, for information provided and helpful comments.

References

Ásgeirsdóttir, T.L. (2007a) *Lifestyle Economics: A Health and Labor-market Analysis of Iceland.* Saarbrücken: VDM Verlag Dr. Müller.
Ásgeirsdóttir, T.L. (2007b) Holdafar: hagfræðileg greining. [*Physique: An Economic Analysis.*] Reykjavík: Public Health Institute of Iceland [Lýðheilsustöð]
Erlandsen, E. (2008) *OECD Economic Studies No. 44: Improving the Efficiency of Health-Care Spending: What Can be Learnt from Partial and Selected Analysis of Hospital Performance.* OECD, Paris: OECD.
Friðriksdóttir, Á., Ingimundardóttir, B.M. and Ásgeirsdóttir, T.L. (2008) *Contractual Report C08:06: Rekstrarumhverfi á lyfjamarkaði. [The Business Environment of the Icelandic Pharmaceutical Market.]* Reykjavík: Institute of Economic Studies [Hagfræðistofnun Háskóla Íslands].
Gísladóttir, E., Þorgeirsdóttir, H., Guðlaugsson, J.Ó., Valdimarsdóttir, M., Jónsson, S.H. and Þórlindsson, Þ. (2009) *Tíðni ofþyngdar og offitu fullorðinna Íslendinga frá 1990 til 2007. [Prevalence of Overweight and Obesity in the Adult Population of Iceland 1990–1007.*]) Reykjavík: Public Health Institute of Iceland [Lýðheilsustöð].
Grossman, M. (1972) On the concept of health capital and the demand for health, *Journal of Political Economy* 80: 223–55.
Halldórsson, M. (2003) *Health Care Systems in Transition: Iceland* (Bankauskaite, V. (ed.)). Copenhagen: WHO Regional Office for Europe on behalf of the European Observatory of Health Systems and Policies.
Ministry of Health (2008) *Samanburður á rekstri heilsugæslunnar á höfuðborgarsvæðinu við samning um rekstur heilsugæslustöðvarinnar í Salahverfi. [A Comparison of Primary Health Care within the Capital Area.]* Reykjavík:Government of Iceland.
OECD (2008a) *Health Data 2008.* Paris: OECD.
OECD (2008b) *Economic Surveys: Iceland 2008.* Paris: OECD.
Ólafsdóttir, H. (1998) The dynamics of shifts in alcoholic beverage preference: effects of the legalization of beer in Iceland, *Journal of Studies on Alcohol* 59:107–17.
Proceedings of the Alþingi [Vefútgáfa Alþingistíðinda] (2009a) *Lög um heilbrigðisþjónustu 40/2007. [Health Service Act 40/2007.*]. Reykjavík: Government of Iceland; http://www.althingi.is.
Proceedings of the Alþingi [Vefútgáfa Alþingistíðinda] (2009b) *Lög um sjúkratryggingar 112/2008. [Health Insurance Act 112/2008.]* Reykjavík:Government of Iceland; http://www.althingi.is.

Statistics Iceland [Hagstofa Íslands] (2008) *Statistical Series, 2008–03: Mannfjöldaspá. [Population Forecast.]* Reykjavik: Statistics Iceland; www.hagstofa.is

Statistics Iceland [Hagstofa Íslands] (2009) *Geography and Environment.* Reykjavik: Statistics Iceland; www.hagstofa.is

Steingrímsdóttir, L., Þorgeirsdóttir, H. and Ólafsdóttir, A.S. (2002) *Research Report No. 5: Hvað borða Íslendingar? Könnun á mataræði Íslendinga 2002. [What do Icelanders Eat? A Dietary Survey 2002.]* Reykjavík: Icelandic Nutritional Council [Manneldisráð].

Syme, S.L. (1996) Rethinking disease: where do we go from here? *Annals of Epidemiology,* 24: 559–68.

UNDP (2007) *Human Development Report 2007.* New York: United Nations Development Programme.

UNDP (2008) *Human Development Report 2008.* New York: United Nations Development Programme.

van Doorslaer, E., Wagstaff, A., Bleichrodt, H. et al. (1997) Income-related inequalitites in health: some international comparisons, *Journal of Health Economics* 16: 93–112.

Vilhjálmsson, R. and Sigurðardóttir, G.V. (2003) Bein útgjöld íslenskra heimila vegna heilbrigðisþjónustu. [Out-of-pocket health care costs among population groups in Iceland.] *Læknablaðið [Icelandic Medical Journal]* 89: 25–30.

Index

The index entries appear in word-by-word alphabetical order.
Entries in italics indicate information contained in tables and figures.

Absenteeism, 90, 186, 261
Accountability, professional, 153–4,
    165
Activity-based funding (ABF) schemes,
    15, 16–17
  Denmark, 35, 46–7, *61*, 112, 114
  effects of, 45–6, 47, 116, 118, 121
  Finland, 46
  Iceland, 322
  institutional response to, 279
  Norway, 45–6, *61*, 111, 114, 116,
    118, 185
  Sweden, 44–5, 110
ADEL Reform, 16, 78, 91–2, 245
Ageing, 58, 85, 91, 195, 321, 325
Alma Ata Declaration, 233, 234
Aspirations, 7, *8*, 10–11, 78, 83–4, 99
Association of Finnish Local
    Authorities (AFLA), 71
Autonomy
  and efficiency, *156*, 199
  see also Fiscal autonomy;
    Professional autonomy

Behaviour *see* Lifestyle/behaviour
    issues

Case managers, 243, 252
Centralization/decentralization,
    10–11, 31–5, 63–4, 74–5, 123,
    186
  blame avoidance, 48, 60, *67*, 68,
    118
  in Denmark, 34–5
  European context, 23, 303–4, 313
  in Finland, 33–4, 169
  and fiscal sustainability, 180, 181–3,
    186
  future policy issues, 93–5, 99–100
  in Iceland, 318–19
  institutional response to, 278–9
  mix/balance of, *8*, 11–12, 80–1
  Nordic policy overview, 14–15
  in Norway, 32–3, 60, *61*, 68, 112
  policy veto, 75–6
  primary health care reforms, *248*,
    249

Centralization/decentralization –
 Contd.
 in Sweden, 31–2, 59–60
 see also Governance/management
 structures
Collegiality, 170–1
Committee on Public Sector
 Responsibilites (Sweden), 31, *66*,
 70, 111, 115, 201–2
Complaint procedures, 136–9
 as individual influence mechanism,
 128, 136, 145
 usage trends, 139
Confidentiality, 136
Continuity of care, 91, 204, 234–5,
 242, 245–6, 250–2
 see also Coordination issues;
 Integration
Coordination issues, 35, 60, *61*, 74
 and future policy, 91–2
 governance structure, 108–9, 114,
 115–16, 280, 287
 open method of coordination
 (OMC), 297–8
 primary health care reform, 236,
 237, 240–1, 242–3, 246, 250–2
 vertical integration, 199, 202–4
 see also Continuity of care;
 Integration
Coronary heart disease, service equity
 case study, 223–4
Cost-containment strategies, 192–5
 demand side measures, 193
 investment decisions, 195
 resource utilization improvements,
 194–5
 supply side measures, 194
Cost-efficiency, 92, 120–1, 326,
 328–9
Coverage, extent of, 180, 196
Cultural changes, 58

Dagmar Reform, 16, 165, 244
Decentralization *see* Centralization/
 decentralization
Demand inconsistencies, 290–1
Demographic issues, 195, 324–5
 ageing, 58, 85, 91, 195, 321, 325
 organizational demography, 275–6,
 278, *282*, 283–4
 population size/density, 57, 243–4,
 250, 317–18, 320–1

Dental services, 224–5, 226
Diagnosis-related grouping (DRG)
 systems, 15, 17, 23, 44–7, 114
 Denmark, 46–7, 112
 effects of, 45, 116, 121, 194
 Finland, 46, 113
 Iceland, 322
 Norway, 17, 45, 111
 Sweden, 44, 45, 110
Digitalization, 276, *282*, 285, 287, 290
 see also Information technology
 developments
Diversity (of provision), 198–211
 payment structures, 207–8
 public–private mix, 204–6, 209–10
 scale and scope, 200–2
 vertical integration, 199, 202–4

Economic context, 58, 59–60, 316
 future policy issues, 82–3, 86, 101–2
Efficiency, *61*
 autonomy and, *156*, 199
 centralization/decentralization
 issues, 33–4, 59–60, 80–1, 95,
 117–18
 country-specific hospital
 comparisons, 210
 and hospital choice, 116–17
 market orientation, 23–4, 247
 pharmaceutical developments, 5
 prospective payment system, 15, 45,
 47, 116, 121, 194
 resource utilization, 194–5
 scale effects on, 115–16
 technological developments, 5
 see also Cost-efficiency;
 Performance
Employment issues, 82–3, 90, 186,
 261, 264
Empowerment *see* Patient rights and
 empowerment
Epidemiological issues, 58, 85
Equity, 10–11, 59–60, *62*, 74–5, 135,
 214–30
 conceptual definitions, 7, *8*, 9,
 214–16, 258
 coronary heart disease case study,
 223–4
 dental service utilization, 224–5,
 226
 governance structures and, 117–18,
 120, 249

hospitalization rates, 219–23
and knowledge-informed
    management, 227–8
mechanisms for, 228
new perspectives, 226–7
and occupational health care, 90,
    203, 226
primary health care access, 219–23,
    250
priority setting, 217–19, 228–9
resource distribution, 216–17
service utilization, 219–26, 229–30
see also Health inequalities
European Court of Justice (ECJ),
    296–302
European Union, 57–8, 59, 76, 93,
    294–314
    Danish system and, 308–11
    Finnish system and, 312
    future policy issues, 18–19, 96–7,
        102
    judicial activism and health care
        integration, 298–303
    Nordic health care systems' context
        in, 303–5, 312–13
    Norwegian system and, 312
    open method of coordination
        (OMC), 297–8
    social policy perspectives, 294–8
    Swedish system and, 305–8
Exclusion, 268

Family Doctor Act (Sweden), 27, 36,
    245
Financing and payment, 8, 23, 44–7,
    114
    budget overruns, 56, 61
    centralization/decentralization of,
        31–5, 109, 181–3, 186, 195–6
    co-payments, 225–6, 247, 320, 321,
        322, 325
    cost-containment strategies, 192–5
    Europeanization issues, 304, 313
    fiscal autonomy, 183–7, 184, 185,
        186
    fiscal federalism, 181–3
    future policy issues, 92–3
    Icelandic system, 320–2
    institutional response to changes,
        279
    intergovernmental transfers/grants,
        109, 181–6, 184, 196, 216–17, 244

payment structures, 207–8
primary health care summary, 248
see also Activity-based funding (ABF)
    schemes; Fiscal sustainability;
    Health care spending; Taxation
Fiscal autonomy, 183–7, 184, 185,
    186
Fiscal sustainability, 5–6, 74, 180–96
    cost-containment strategies, 192–5
    and fiscal autonomy, 183–7, 184,
        185, 186
    fiscal federalism and
        decentralization, 181–3
    future challenges, 195–6
Formalization policies, 48
    see also specific policies
Freedom to Establish Private Practice
    Act (Sweden), 27, 245
Funding see Financing and payment
Future policy issues, 78–103
    common challenges, 78–81
    contextual shifts, 81–6, 101–2
    coordination, 91–2
    European Union's impact, 96–7,
        102
    financing and payment, 92–3
    fiscal sustainability, 195–6
    local government reconfiguration,
        93–5, 99–100
    pragmatism, 97–8
    provider choice, 89–91
    provider diversification, 87–9

Gatekeeping, 193, 246, 247, 248, 251,
    317
General Practitioners (GPs)
    and care coordination, 92, 237
    continuity of care, 91
    Danish reforms, 30, 235–8, 248
    Finnish reforms, 29, 241–4, 248
    gatekeeping role, 193, 246, 247,
        248, 251, 317
    governance structures, 111, 112–13
    Icelandic system, 323–4, 325
    list patient reform, 29, 111, 238–9,
        245–6, 250, 251
    Norwegian reforms, 29, 238–41, 248
    payment structures, 207–8
    recruitment problems, 100, 206,
        207–8, 211, 238, 250
    Regular General Practitioner (RGP)
        scheme, 141, 207, 211

General Practitioners (GPs) – *Contd.*
  Swedish reforms, 27–8, 244–7, *248*
  visit distribution, 220–3
  see also Patient choice; Primary
    health care
Globalization pressures, 17, 56–9, 76,
    82–3
  future funding issues, 93
Goals, 6–7, *8*, 10–13, 78
  future policy, 99
Governance/management structures,
    8, 9–10
  in Denmark, 156–60, 172–3
  and equity, 227–8
  in Finland, 167–71, 172–3
  Nordic, 287–9
  in Norway, 160–4, 172–3
  and professional autonomy
    classifications, 155–6, *156*
  in Sweden, 164–7, 172–3
  unitary management, 158–64,
    172–3
  see also Centralization/
    decentralization; Institutional
    management; New public
    management (NPM); Political
    governance structures

Health 2015 programme, 42–3
Health and Medical Services Act
    (Sweden), 132–3, 134, 140, 165,
    244
Health Care Act (Finland), 38, 203
Health centres
  choice of, 90, 100
  coordination issues, 236–7, 252
  development of, 79
  Finnish, 242, 244
  Icelandic, 323–4
  merger of, 170, 203, 206
  prevention and rehabilitation role,
    236–7
  private provision, 88
  Swedish, 245–6
  waiting times, 135
  see also Primary health care
Health improvement, 255–70
  health problem prioritization,
    260–2
  mechanisms for, 266–8
  policy development, 258–60
  responsibility for, 256–7, 264–8

stable/changing agendas, 268–9
see also Public health
Health inequalities, 43, 255–70
  causes of, 266
  comparisons of, 263, *263*
  definitions of, 262–3
  in Iceland, 317–18, 326–7
  policy development, 258–9
  problematization of, 260–2, 268,
    269–70
  reduction methods, 268
  service utilization statistics, 219–26,
    229–30
  stable/changing agendas, 268–9
  see also Equity
Health insurance, *8*, 11, 96, 123
  in Denmark, 29–30, 91, 100, 311
  in Finland, 29, 91, 101, 168, 312
  health care expenditure and,
    187–92, *187*, *188*, *189*, *190*
  in Norway, 28
  primary health care reform, 235
  in Sweden, 27, 91
Health Insurance Act (Finland), 312
Health professionals
  policy development role, 64
  see also Professional autonomy
Health promotion, 43–4
  see also Public health
Health/state enterprises, 25, 32–3, 84,
    99, 204–5
Health technology assessment (HTA),
    226–7, 229
Healthcare Act (Denmark), 135–6,
    138
Health care spending, 58, *59*, 187–92,
    320–2, 324–5
  future prediction of, 195–6
  per capita, 188–9, *1892*
  private health insurance's role,
    191–2
  public financing share, *190*, 190–1
  share of gross domestic product,
    187–91, *187*, *188*, 320
Healthy Throughout Life 2002–2010,
    44
Home-care services, 88, 239, 240, 249
Hospital Act (Norway), 32–3
Hospitals
  analytical framework, 275–6
  conceptual changes, 287–8, *288*
  hospitalization rates, 220–3

organizational demography, 275–6,
278, *282*, 283–4
organizational structure, 275, 276,
278, *285*, 285–92, *288*
physical arrangements, 275, *278*,
284–5
and primary health care
relationship, 240–1, 280
public/private mix, 13, 28, 30, 88–9,
204–5, 209–10
response to governance changes,
276–80, *278*, 281, *282–3*, 283–7
see also Institutional management;
Norwegian hospital reform
(2002); Patient choice

Icelandic health care system, 316–29
challenges, 324–7
financing, 320–2
motivation, 317–18
provision, 323–4
structure of, 318–20
values, 318
Implementation (policy), 65
Incentive schemes
efficiency, 15, *61*, 84, 123, 194,
325–6
municipal co-ordination/
amalgamation, 60, *67*, 69, 71–2,
114
Industry
and future policy issues, 82–3
policy development role, 64–5
see also Pharmaceuticals/
pharmaceutical industry
Information access/provision, 5, 57,
134, 136, 266
Information technology
developments
continuity of care, 243
digitalization, 276, *282*, 285, 287,
290
patient information, 5
research and development role,
244
supervisory role, 94
Injury, patient, 137–9
Institutional management, 274–92
analytical framework, 275–6
response to governance changes,
276–80, *278*, 281, *282–3*, 283–7
Insurance *see* Health insurance

Integration (service), 25, 113, 115–16,
199, 202–4
European judicial activism, 298–303
primary health care, 240–1, 246, *248*
see also Continuity of care;
Coordination issues
Interest groups, *8*, 54–5, 64, 65, 127–8
see also Patient organizations
Investment decisions, 195

Knowledge base
internationalization of, 57
Knowledge management, 229, 230

Legitimacy, public health system,
122–3
Life expectancy, 43–4, 261–2, *262*,
327
Lifestyle/behaviour issues, 5, 41, 85,
264–7, 317–18, 328
List patient reform, 29, 111, 238–9,
245–6, 250, 251
Lønning Committee, 217–18

Management structures *see*
Governance/management
structures
Market orientation, *8*, 23–30, 79–80,
110, 194–5, 200
institutional response to changes,
280
Nordic policy overview, 14
see also Private provision;
Purchaser–provider models
Mental health problems, 261
Mental health services, 240, 243
Municipalities/counties/regions
amalgamation of, 60, *61–2*, *67*,
69–72, 110–11, 114–16
quality differences, *61*, 80–1, 112,
115–16, 201–2
and state relations, *62*
Municipalities Health Service Act
(Norway), 141

New public management (NPM), 4,
21, 60, 151, 172–4, 200
in Denmark, 158, 159, 160
in Finland, 172
in Iceland, 328
in Norway, 60, *61*, 161
in Sweden, 165

Non-clinical services, 205, 209–10
Nordic health policy, existence of,
13–15
Nordic health care model
concept of, 6–10, *8*
and equity, 228
existence of, 17–19, 79, 247, 252,
269–70
summary of characteristics, 13
Norwegian hospital reform (2002), 25,
32–3, 84, 111–12, 114, 118–19
effects of, 120, 121–2, 185, 210–11,
291
Nursing homes, 239, 240–1, 249

Obesity, 5, 328
Occupational health services, 29, 39,
101
equity issues, 90, 203, 226
Open method of coordination (OMC),
297–8

Participation (public), 4, 7, *8*, 9, 11
future policy, 78, 99
and health improvement, 264, 266
see also Patient organizations
Patient choice, 5, *8*, 10, 14, 36–8,
89–91
in Denmark, 38, 112, 142–3, 237,
248, 309–10
and equity, 226, 230
European context, 300–2, 304–5,
309–10, 313
in Finland, 38, 142, 168, 243–4,
248
fiscal implications, 114, 193
health improvement, 264–7
as individual influence mechanism,
128, *128*, 139–43, 145–6, 147
in Norway, 37, 111, 141, *248*
performance and, 116–17
primary health care reform, 237,
243–4, 246, *248*, 250–2
in Sweden, 36–7, 140–1, 205–6, 246,
248
see also Patient rights and
empowerment
Patient empowerment *see* Patient
rights and empowerment
Patient fees, 193
Patient Injuries Act (Finland), 138
Patient Injury Act (Norway), 137–8

Patient injury legislation/
compensation schemes, 137–9
Patient involvement mechanisms,
126–47
collective influence, 127–31, 143–4,
146
future implications, 147
individual influence, 128, *128*, 129,
131–43, 144–7
see also Patient organizations
Patient ombudsman schemes, 137–9,
145
Patient organizations, 5, *65*, 127–31,
128, 143–4
efficiency of, 131, 144, 146
numbers and size of, 129–30, 143–4
politicization of, 130–1, 144
Patient Rights Act (Finland), 138, 142,
144
Patient Rights Act (Norway), 37, 111,
134–5, 137, 139, 141
Patient rights and empowerment, 5,
23, 36–8
in Denmark, 38, 135–6, 310
European context, 300–2, 304–5,
310, 313
in Finland, 37–8, 135, 138, 142,
144
fiscal implications of, 193
as individual influence mechanism,
128, 129, 144, 146–7
legislation development reasons,
132
in Norway, 37, 111, 134–5, 137,
139, 141
in Sweden, 36–7, 132–4, 205–6
see also Patient choice; Patient
organizations
Performance
and governance reform, 291
problems, 55–7, *61*
standards and monitoring, 117–18,
237, 239, 249–50, 286, 310
see also Efficiency; Quality
Personnel/organizational
demography, 275–6, *278*, *282*,
283–4
Pharmaceuticals/pharmaceutical
industry
developments and efficiency, 5
Europeanization, 57–8, 96
in Iceland, 321–2, 324, 326

pharmacy systems, 28–9, 30
provision restrictions, 6, 85, 192
Pharmacy Act (Norway), 28–9
Physiotherapy, 238
Planning, service, 108–9, 114, 169
Policy application, 7, *8*, 10, 13–15, 79
Political context, 83–6, 102
Political governance structures, 9, 16,
    107–23, 275
  administrative cost reduction, *61*,
    75
  effects of reform, 120–3, 210
  Europeanization effects, 305
  as existing around 1990, 108–10
  explanation of reforms, 115–20
  reforms implemented during 1990s
    and early 2000s, 110–14, 280–1
  see also Centralization/
    decentralization; Political
    processes
Political processes, 9–10, 53–76, 127
  country specifics, 65, *66–7*, 68–73
  implementation arena, 65, *67*
  management of, 69, 72–3, 75
  multi-level governance arena, 63–5,
    67, 93–5, 99–100, 107, 109
  parliamentary arena, 63, *66*, 127
  performance problems and process
    initiation, 55–7
  problem formulation and policy
    options, 59–60, *61–2*, 63, 255–6
  see also Centralization/
    decentralization
Population
  ageing, 5, 58, 85, 91, 195, 321, 325
  changes in, 5, 85
  size/density, *3*, 57, 243–4, 250,
    317–18, 320–1
Pragmatism, 97–8
Preventive health services, 41, 236–7,
    252
  see also Public health
Primary Care Act (Sweden), 79
Primary Health Care Act (Finland), 38,
    79, 168, 241–2
Primary health care
  concept of, 234
  country-specific summary, *248*
  Danish reforms, 30, 235–8, *248*
  equity issues, 220–3, 226, 250
  Finnish reforms, *29*, 241–4, *248*
  governance structures, 111, 112–13

historical perspective, 233–4
Icelandic provision, 323–4, 325
list patient reform, 29, 111, 238–9,
    245–6, 250, 251
Norwegian reforms, 29, 238–41, *248*
payment structures, 207–8
public/private mix, 27–30, 205–6,
    237–8, 247–9, *248*, 303
recruitment problems, 100, 206,
    207–8, 211, 238, 250
Swedish reforms, 27–8, 244–7, *248*
see also General Practitioners (GPs);
    Health centres; Patient choice
Priority setting, 217–19, 228–9,
    230
Private health insurance *see* Health
    insurance
Private provision, 13, 22–3, 27–30
  in Denmark, 29–30, *248*
  in Finland, 29, 168, 169, 206, *248*
  future policy, 18–19, 88–9, 100–1
  home-care services, 88, 239, 249
  hospital, 13, 28, 30, 88–9, 204–5,
    209–10
  in Iceland, 323–4
  in Norway, 28–9, *248*
  nursing home, 239, 249
  patient choice and, 198
  primary health care, 27–30, 205–6,
    237–8, 247–9, *248*, 303
  in Sweden, 27–8, 205–6, *248*
Professional autonomy, 151–74
  changing pattern of, 171–4
  conceptual framework of, 155–6,
    156
  in Denmark, 156–60
  in Finland, 167–71
  in Norway, 160–4
  in sociology of professions, 152–5
  in Sweden, 164–7
Prospective payment systems (PPS), 17
  and efficiency, 116, 194
  see also Activity-based funding (ABF)
    schemes; DRG systems
Provider choice *see* Patient choice
Provider diversification, 84, 87–9
Public Authorities Collaboration in
    Rehabilitation Act (Finland), 243
Public health, *8*, 10, 23, 39–44
  Danish strategies, 43–4
  factors affecting, 264
  Finnish strategies, 41–3

Public health – *Contd.*
  health improvement and inequality
    reduction, 255–70
  in Iceland, 319–20, 328
  Norwegian strategies, 40–1
  programmes as policy source, 257–8
  responsibility for, 256–7, 264–8,
    269, 317–18
  Swedish strategies, 39–40
  system legitimacy, 122–3
Public relations, *283*, 284
Purchaser–provider models, 14, 23–6,
    87
  Denmark, 26
  Finland, 25–6
  Iceland, 322, 328
  Norway, 25, *61*
  Sweden, 23–4, 85–6, 110, 120–1

Quality
  emphasis on, 56, 59, 83, 84–5
  and hospital choice, 116–17, 172
  market-based mechanisms and, 24,
    79–80
  national standards and monitoring,
    117–18, 237, 239, 249–50, 286,
    310
  regional differences in, *61*, 80–1,
    112, 115–16, 201–2
  scale effects on, 115–16
  see also Performance
Quality of life, 44

Rationing, service, 85, 96–7, 192, 193
Referral procedures
  gatekeeping, 193, 246, 247, *248*,
    251, 317
  socioeconomic differences, 222,
    223, 226
Reform
  approaches to, 15–17
  definition of, 22
  study framework, 22–3
  timing of, 15–17
Regionalization *see* Municipalities/
    counties/regions
Regular General Practitioner (RGP)
    scheme, 141, 207, 211
Rehabilitation services, 191–2, 203,
    236–7, 243, 252
Resource distribution, equity of,
    216–17

Resource utilization, efficiency
    improvements, 194–5
Responsibility
  governance structure reforms, 108,
    114
  for health, 256–7, 264–8, 269,
    317–18
  population responsibility, 242
Ring fencing, surgical, 276, 279, 281,
    286, 287

Scale effects, 5, 59, 75, 115–16, 121,
    123
  in Denmark, 60, *61*, 69, 119, 122
  diversity and, 199, 200–2
  in Finland, *61*
  in Iceland, 317–18, 320–1
  in Norway, 32–3, *61*
  in Sweden, *61*
Service, concept of, 309, 310–11
Single European Act, 296–7
Socioeconomic differences *see* Health
    inequalities
Specialised Medical Care Act
    (Finland), 38
Specialization issues, *61*, 80–1,
    115–16, 324
  Europeanization, 306
  gatekeeping, 193, 246, 247, *248*,
    251, 317
  public–private partnership, 206
  ring fencing, 276, 279, 281, 286,
    287
State–region–municipality relations,
    62
Status and Rights of Patients Act
    (Finland), 37–8
Sustainability *see* Fiscal sustainability
Sweden's New Public Health Policy,
    39–40

Taxation, *8*, 9, 11–13
  in Denmark, 35, 60, *62*
  earmarked, *8*, 9, 35, 185–6, 188
  and employment issues, 82–3
  in European context, 303
  in Finland, 34
  and fiscal sustainability, 180–7
  Icelandic, 318, 320
  insurance premiums and, 27, 28,
    30
  limitations to, 58, 82, 93

in Norway, 33
public support for, 93, 123, 188
regional level elimination, 19, 60,
    62, 114
and service equity, 216–17
share of autonomous local taxes to
    total tax revenue, 184, *184*
in Sweden, 31–2
Technological advances, 5–6, 57, 85,
    195
    health technology assessment
        (HTA), 226–7, 229
    knowledge management, 229, 230
*The Danish Government Programme on
    Public Health and Health Promotion
    1999–2008*, 43–4
The Patient is Right, 133

Unions, policy development role,
    64–5
Unitary management, 158–64,
    172–3
Unity of command, 276, 278, *283*,
    290, 292
Universality, 4–5, 9, 10, 256, 102
Urbanization, *62*, 71
Utilization, service, 219–26

Value tensions, 59
Vertical integration, 25, 199, 202–4

Waiting-time guarantees, 45, 90,
    194
    in Denmark, 136
    in Finland, 117, 135
    in Norway, 45
    in Sweden, 133–4, 307–8
Waiting lists/times, 85
    in Denmark, 136, 309–10
    and European Union, 96–7,
        300–2
    in Finland, 135
    fiscal issues, 193, 194
    and hospital choice, 117
    in Norway, 45, 116, 134
    patient's rights legislation, 134–6
    standards and monitoring, 117–18
    in Sweden, 307–8
    see also Waiting-time guarantees
Wealth, societal, 83
Welfare state
    European Union and, 294–5
    Nordic model, 4–6, 18
    policy models, 256, 269–70
    social democratic regime, 127